AF552691

ATLAS OF MICROSCOPY

To the memory of

Dr. T. E. Wallis

Pharmacognosist *par excellence*,
whose meticulous microscopy
has served as our inspiration

ATLAS OF MICROSCOPY OF MEDICINAL PLANTS, CULINARY HERBS AND SPICES

By

BETTY P. JACKSON

Ph.D., B.Pharm., B.Sc. (Lond), F.R.Pharm.S., F.L.S.

and

DEREK W. SNOWDON

B.Pharm. (Lond), F.R.Pharm.S.

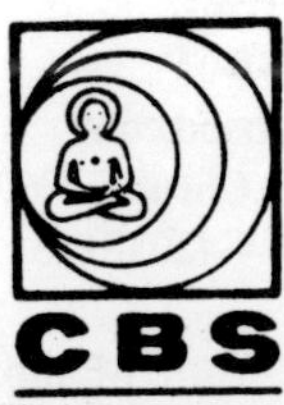

CBS PUBLISHERS & DISTRIBUTORS PVT. LTD.

NEW DELHI • BENGALURU • CHENNAI • KOCHI • MUMBAI • PUNE

ISBN : 81-239-0025-2 (CBS Pubs.)
ISBN : 1-85293-081-0 (Belhaven Press)

First Indian Reprint : 1992
Reprint : 2000, 2005

This edition has been reprinted in India by arrangement with Belhaven Press (A Division of Pinter Publishers), UK

Published by Satish Kumar Jain and produced by V.K. Jain for
CBS Publishers & Distributors Pvt. Ltd.,
CBS Plaza, 4819/XI Prahlad Street, 24 Ansari Road, Daryaganj,
New Delhi - 110002, India. • Website: www.cbspd.com
e-mail: delhi@cbspd.com, cbspubs@airtelmail.in
Ph.: 23289259, 23266861, 23266867 • Fax: 011-23243014

Branches:

- ***Bengaluru:*** Seema House, 2975, 17th Cross, K.R. Road, Bansankari 2nd Stage, Bengaluru - 560070
  • Ph.: +91-80-26771678/79 • Fax: +91-80-26771680
  • E-mail: cbsbng@gmail.com, bangalore@cbspd.com
- ***Pune:*** Bhuruk Prestige, Sr. No. 52/12/2+1+3/2, Narhe, Haveli (Near Katraj-Dehu Road By-pass), Pune - 411041
  • Ph.: +91-20-64704058/59, 020-32392277 • E-mail: pune@cbspd.com
- ***Kochi:*** 36/14, Kalluvilakam, Lissie Hospital Road, Kochi - 682018, Kerala • Ph.: +91-484-4059061-65
  • Fax: +91-484-4059065 • E-mail: cochin@cbspd.com
- ***Chennai:*** 20, West Park Road, Shenoy Nagar, Chennai - 600030
  Ph.: +91-44-26260666, 26208620 • Fax: +91-44-42032115
  • E-mail: chennai@cbspd.com
- ***Mumbai:*** 83-C, Ist Floor, Dr. E. Moses Road, Worli, Mumbai-400 018, Maharashtra Ph.: +91-9833017933, 022-24902340/24902341
  • E-mail: mumbai@cbspd.com

Printed at :
J.S. Offset Printers, Delhi

CONTENTS

PREFACE

Some twenty years ago our book Powdered Vegetable Drugs was published, which provided an Atlas for use by analysts and others in the identification and authentication of medicinal plant materials. It is now out of print, and with the opportunity to produce a new work we have been able to consider the possibility of extending its usefulness to include other areas of analysis where microscopical criteria are of established or potential value. One particular field which is inadequately covered in the currently available literature is the microscopy of culinary herbs and spices, and as certain medicinal products such as Ginger and Clove, described in the earlier book, also have culinary uses, a logical expansion seemed to be to include some of the more important herbs and spices commonly used in food products. By widening the scope in this way it is hoped that this present work will provide a more useful reference not only for forensic scientists and others engaged in the evaluation of powdered drugs, but also for analysts in the food and allied industries who are concerned with the authentication of raw materials.

Accordingly, we have prepared drawings and descriptions for some twenty culinary herbs and spices for inclusion in this volume. We have also added to the coverage of powdered drugs with monographs on Ajowan, Hemlock, Opium, Rhatany, Senna Fruit and Visnaga, which were not in our earlier book. In addition, we have incorporated monographs on Grass and Lucerne as these, in powdered form, may be used to standardise Prepared Digitalis.

Although chemical methods of analysis, especially chromatography, are now accepted as standard techniques for the identification of many vegetable materials, microscopical structure is long established as providing a most useful and reliable criterion. Microscopy is particularly applicable to the examination of mixtures when individual components can readily be recognised whereas no satisfactory chromatographic identification would be possible. Microscopy also has the advantages of requiring only small quantities of the material and, once the technique has been acquired, a conclusion as to whether or not a sample is genuine can be reached very rapidly.

As this book is intended primarily for use in the verification of materials, for ease of location we have arranged the contents in alphabetical order according to their commonly accepted names. We have also provided separate indices of Synonyms and Botanical Sources.

All the drawings in this book have been made solely by ourselves from previously authenticated samples. For the drugs and spices, which usually occur commercially in the powdered form, number 60 grade powders were prepared for examination, but for the culinary herbs, which are more usually available in the whole or broken condition, fragments of a suitable size were examined. The drawings were made at a magnification of 500, using a camera lucida, from fresh mounts prepared as described in the section on Practical Methods. In preparing the drawings our aim has been to illustrate the diagnostic characters for each material and we have excluded cell contents which are common to a morphological group but are not otherwise diagnostic, for example, aleurone grains and fixed oil globules in seeds. The descriptions, similarly, are intended to give a detailed account of the actual characters seen in the fragments rather than the full histology of the plant organ from which the materials are derived. We have quoted dimensions of cells and other particles only when they are of value in distinguishing between closely similar materials.

One of us (D.W.S.) wishes to express thanks to the School of Pharmaceutical Sciences, Sunderland Polytechnic, for kindly according laboratory facilities during the execution of some of this work.

Finally, we would like to thank Belhaven Press, and especially Dr Iain Stevenson, for undertaking to publish this work and for the care and co-operation shown throughout its production.

Betty P. Jackson
Derek W. Snowdon
1990

PRACTICAL METHODS

When using this book to authenticate a given sample it will be necessary to make microscopical preparations of the material in order to compare the structures present with those drawn and described in the relevant monograph. It is appreciated that users may not be familiar with all the mountants employed and the techniques involved in making such preparations, and the following notes are given for guidance.

Solution of Chloral Hydrate

In the microscopical examination of vegetable materials the most diagnostic features are specific cell types and calcium oxalate crystals, and they are best observed in a *Chloral Hydrate* mount. However, before the details can be discerned it is essential to 'clear' the preparation in order to allow the chloral hydrate solution to penetrate the tissues and remove entrapped air bubbles. The procedure is as follows.

Add two or three drops of the solution to the material on a microscope slide and apply a cover glass. Heat *very gently* by passing the slide to and fro over a very low flame (the use of a micro burner is recommended). As soon as bubbles start to appear stop the heating and, if necessary, run more solution under the cover glass. If the material contains considerable amounts of starch or mucilage it will probably be necessary to repeat the heating several times, and it is important to ensure that sufficient liquid is always present to prevent the preparation from drying out. When a satisfactory preparation has been made, lift the cover glass and add one or two drops of *Solution of Chloral Hydrate and Glycerol* to inhibit the formation of crystals of chloral hydrate during the subsequent examination of the slide.

The clearing process removes starch granules and all water-soluble cell inclusions.

Alcohol and Water

To examine a material (usually in the powdered form) for the presence of starch granules a mount is prepared as follows.

To the material on a slide add one or two drops of *Alcohol* and mix until thoroughly wetted. Add one or two drops of water and apply a cover glass; on examination the starch granules should readily be recognisable. If necessary, their identity can be confirmed by allowing a drop of *Solution of Iodine* to run under the cover glass and observing the blue-black staining of the granules.

N.B. If the material to be examined contains a high proportion of oil (for example, some powdered fruits and seeds), cloudiness will occur when the water is added, which will render subsequent examination unsatisfactory. It is, therefore, recommended that most of the oil be removed from such materials, using a suitable solvent (ether or chloroform), before examining for starch granules.

Phloroglucinol and Hydrochloric Acid

To establish lignification in cells and tissues the procedure is as follows.

To the material on a slide add one or two drops of *Solution of Phloroglucinol*, mix and allow the solvent to evaporate almost completely. Add one or two drops of *Hydrochloric Acid* and apply a cover glass. Examine immediately; a red colour indicates the presence of lignin. The reaction is semi-quantitative, i.e. heavy lignification gives a deep red colour and slight lignification a pale pink; the colour gradually fades.

N.B. As in the examination for starch granules, described above, when the hydrochloric acid is added after the alcoholic solution of phloroglucinol, cloudiness will occur if large amounts of oil are present in the sample. With such materials the test for lignin should ideally be carried out after removal of the oil.

Lead Acetate Solution of Ruthenium Red and *Alkaline Solution of Corallin*

These dye solutions are sometimes used to confirm the presence of certain types of mucilage. The solution should be added directly to the material on a slide and a cover glass applied. Examine, and if some particles appear to have *absorbed* the colour allow a drop of distilled water to run under the cover glass and re-examine. A *permanent* colouration of the particles is positive.

Solution of Potassium Hydroxide

Flavonoid glycosides such as diosmin and hesperidin sometimes occur in cells in the crystalline form and their identity can be confirmed by the use of this reagent. The solution is added to the material on a slide and the preparation examined immediately; the crystals slowly dissolve giving a yellow colouration.

REAGENTS

Alcohol, Ethyl Alcohol 95%

For most purposes this can be replaced by Industrial Methylated Spirit (66 O.P.).

Chloral Hydrate, Solution of

Chloral Hydrate	50 g
Distilled Water	20 ml

Dissolve, using gentle heat if necessary.

Chloral Hydrate and Glycerol, Solution of

Solution of Chloral Hydrate	90 ml
Glycerol	10 ml

Mix.

Corallin, Alkaline, Solution of

Corallin	0.125 g
Anhydrous Sodium Carbonate	7.4 g

Mix the dry materials. Divide into ten portions each of 0.75 g and transfer to bottles of about 15 ml capacity. Seal. For use, add 10 ml Distilled Water to the contents of a bottle and shake to dissolve. The solution deteriorates on standing, but in a closed container is usable for 10 to 14 days.

Hexanol, n-Hexanol.

Hydrochloric Acid, Hydrochloric Acid of the British Pharmacopoeia. (Wt/ml about 1.8; Content of HC1 35 to 39% w/v).

Iodine, Solution of

Iodine	2 g
Potassium Iodine	3 g
Distilled Water	to make 100 ml

Mix the two solids in a measure and add about 5 ml of the Water. Agitate until dissolved. Slowly dilute to volume with further Water.

Store in a closed, well-filled container.

Phloroglucinol, Solution of

Phloroglucinol	1 g
Alcohol (95%)	to make 100 ml

Dissolve.

Store in a closed container.

Potassium Hydroxide, Solution of

Potassium Hydroxide	5 g
Distilled Water	to make 100 ml

Dissolve.

Store in a closed, well-filled container.

Ruthenium Red, Solution of

Ruthenium Red	8 mg
Lead Acetate	1 g
Distilled Water, recently boiled and cooled	10 ml

Dissolve.

This reagent deteriorates rapidly on storage, particularly if exposed to the atmosphere. Its useful life is only two or three days.

Atlas of Microscopy of Medicinal Plants, Culinary Herbs and Spices

ACONITE

Aconitum napellus L. (agg.) Ranunculaceae

Aconite Root, Wolfsbane Root

A greyish-brown powder with a faint odour and a taste which is sweetish at first, then gives a persistent sensation of numbness.

The diagnostic characters are:

(*a*) The abundant *starch granules*, which are simple and spherical or compound with two, three, four or occasionally up to six components; some of the larger granules show a radiate or slit-shaped hilum.

(*b*) The fairly numerous *sclereids*, which occur singly with associated thin-walled parenchyma or, occasionally, in small groups; they are large, vary from oval to square to subrectangular in outline and have moderately thickened, pitted walls and a large lumen. Occasional *fibrous sclereids* occur, derived from the stem bases; these are considerably elongated, rectangular cells, blunt ended with moderately thickened walls and numerous pits.

(*c*) The abundant *parenchyma of the cortex and stele*. The cells are fairly large and vary from rounded to elongated rectangular in outline; the walls are sometimes quite markedly thickened and are frequently somewhat uneven; they have few, indistinct pits. The cells are filled with starch granules.

(*d*) The fragments of the *outer layer*, dark brown to almost black in colour; in surface view the cells appear subrectangular with moderately thickened walls; they are rather unevenly pigmented

(*e*) The *vessels*, which are fairly large and are found singly or in small groups; the walls are lignified and have numerous slit-shaped pits with indistinct borders. A few vessels also occur with reticulate, spiral or annular thickening.

(*f*) The occasional *fibres* from the stem bases; they are lignified, rather thin-walled, and have numerous well-marked pits.

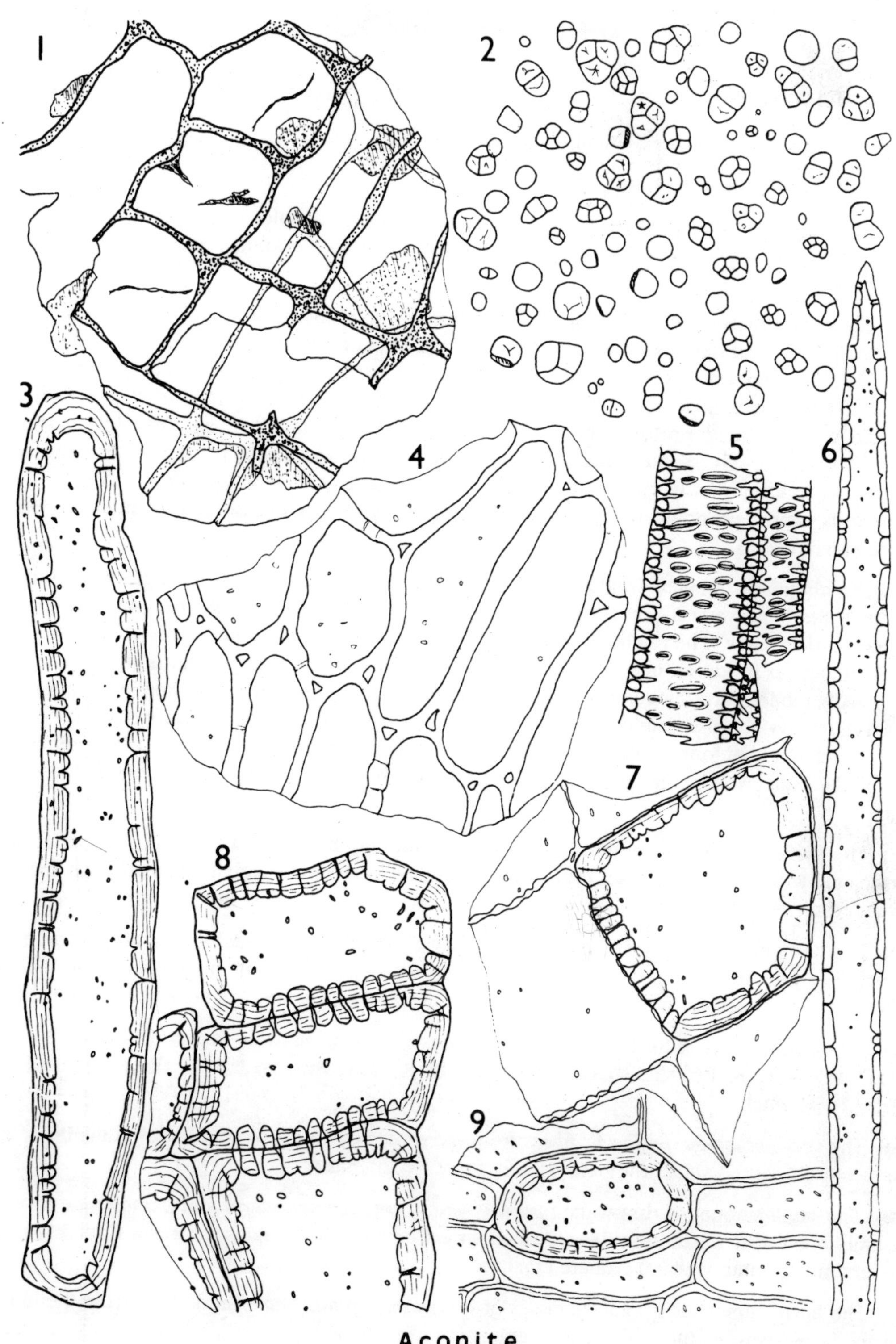

Aconite

×330

1 Outer layer in surface view showing pigment.
2 Starch granules.
3 Fibrous sclereid from the stem base.
4 Thick-walled parenchyma.
5 Fragments of bordered pitted vessels.
6 Part of a fibre from the stem base.
7 A single sclereid with associated thin-walled parenchyma.
8 Part of a group of sclereids.
9 A single sclereid with associated thicker-walled parenchyma.

AFRICAN RAUWOLFIA

Rauwolfia vomitoria Afz. Apocynaceae

A pale yellowish-brown powder with little odour and a bitter taste.

The diagnostic characters are:

(*a*) The fairly abundant *starch granules*, which are mostly simple, spherical to ovoid with a circular, slit-shaped or stellate hilum; a number of compound granules also occur with two or three components.

(*b*) The very numerous *sclereids* from the phelloderm and phloem; they occur singly or in groups of two or more and may be found attached to fragments of thin-walled parenchyma; they show considerable variation in size and are sometimes very large; the shape varies from more or less isodiametric to elongated rectangular or some of the larger sclereids may be very irregular in outline with rounded protuberances. The walls of the isodiametric and irregularly shaped sclereids are strongly striated and moderately or heavily thickened; those of the rectangular sclereids are usually only moderately thickened and have few, faint striations; all types have numerous simple or branched pits. The isodiametric sclereids occasionally contain *prisms of calcium oxalate*.

(*c*) The abundant lignified fragments of the xylem composed of *vessels, tracheids* and *xylem parenchyma*. The vessels are sometimes very large and may be broken; they have numerous small, bordered pits. The tracheids usually occur associated with the smaller vessels and they also have numerous bordered pits. The xylem parenchyma is composed of longitudinally elongated cells with moderately thickened walls and numerous pits which may be simple or bordered. *Medullary rays* are also found associated with the xylem tissue; they are composed of lignified cells which in radial longitudinal section are rectangular, moderately thick walled with numerous pits in the radial walls; in tangential longitudinal section the medullary rays are one to three cells wide.

(*d*) The *fibres*, which are frequently fragmented and may be found scattered or, more usually, associated with the xylem tissue; they are lignified and have moderately thickened walls and few, rounded pits.

(*e*) The *calcium oxalate crystals*, which are fairly abundant; they are found scattered or, more usually, in longitudinal files in parenchymatous cells associated with fragments of the phloem tissue. They are usually in the form of *single or twinned prisms* but are very irregular in shape.

(*f*) The fragments of reddish-brown *cork* composed of two or three layers of thin-walled cells which are polygonal to slightly elongated in surface view; the majority of these fragments are strongly lignified.

(*g*) The very occasional *pericyclic fibres* from the rhizome; these are very large, unlignified, with unevenly thickened walls; they are usually found fragmented.

(*h*) The small amount of thin-walled *parenchyma from the phelloderm* and *phloem*; the cells are usually filled with starch granules although an occasional cell contains a brownish secretion and others may contain calcium oxalate crystals.

(*i*) The fairly numerous irregular masses of yellow *amorphous material* derived from the lumina of the larger vessels; most of these fragments are lignified.

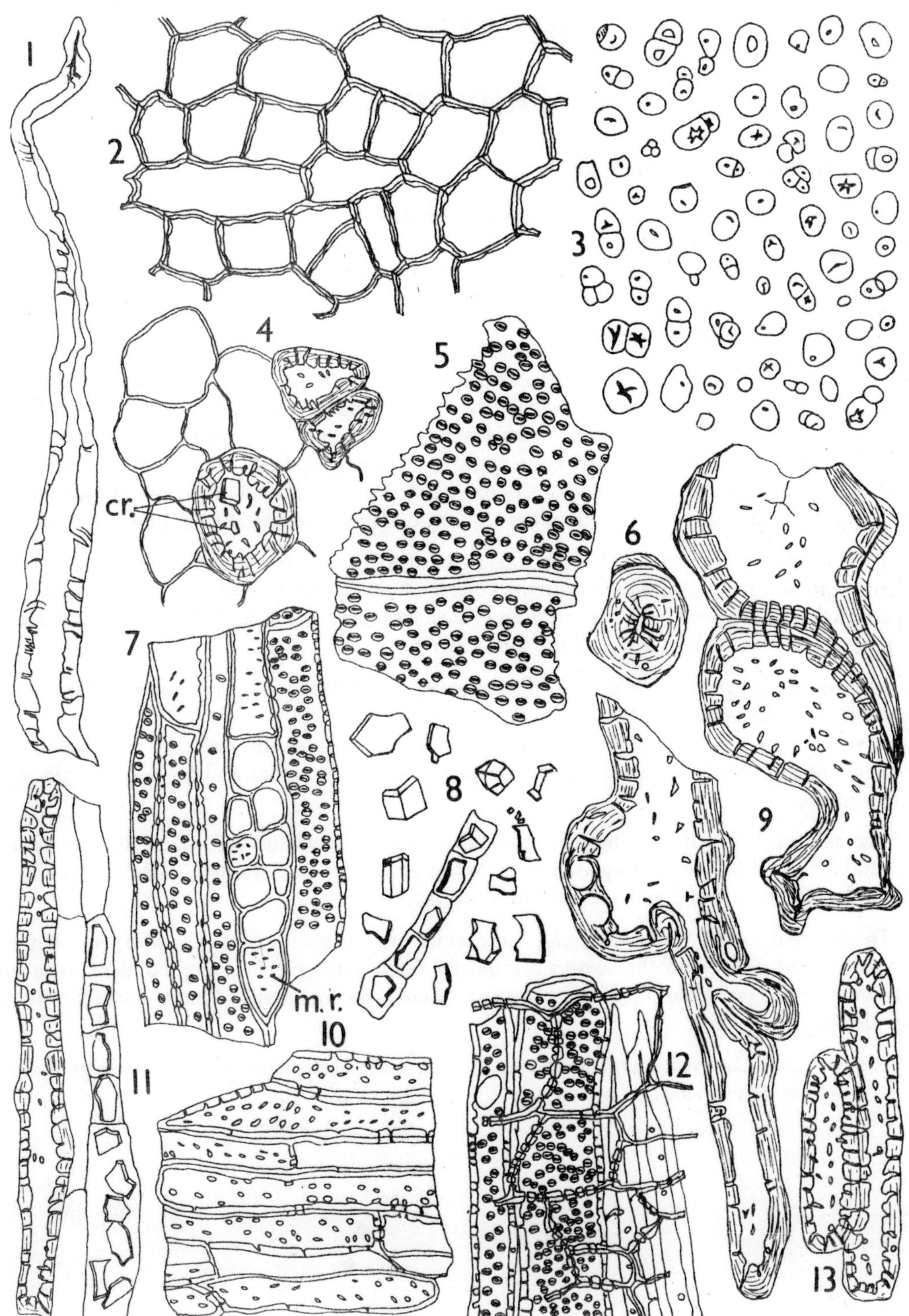

African Rauwolfia

×330

1 Part of a pericyclic fibre from the rhizome.
2 Cork in surface view.
3 Starch granules.
4 Isodiametric sclereids, one containing calcium oxalate prisms (cr.), and associated thin-walled parenchyma of the phelloderm.
5 Fragment of a large vessel with bordered pits.
6 A thick-walled isodiametric sclereid.
7 Part of a group of tracheids, vessels and xylem parenchyma with a medullary ray (m.r.) in tangential longitudinal section.
8 Crystals of calcium oxalate, some contained in parenchyma.
9 Parts of large, irregularly shaped sclereids.
10 Xylem parenchyma in longitudinal section.
11 Elongated sclereids associated with thin-walled phloem tissue and parenchyma containing calcium oxalate crystals, in longitudinal section.
12 Part of a medullary ray of the xylem in radial longitudinal section with underlying vessels and fibres.
13 Elongated sclereids.

AJOWAN

Trachyspermum copticum (L.) Link. Umbelliferae

Ajowan Fruits

A mid yellowish-brown powder with a strong odour of thymol and a numbing, unpleasant and lingering taste.

The diagnostic characters are:

(*a*) The *epicarp* composed of a layer of cells which, in surface view, are large, irregularly polygonal with unevenly thickened walls; the *cuticle* is strongly striated. The majority of the cells are extended to form *protuberances* of varying size which are very characteristic; the smaller ones are ovoid to pear-shaped and slightly constricted at the base, the large ones are more finger-like and rounded at the tip; all have a thick, very much wrinkled and reticulated *cuticle*. Fragments of these protuberances occur scattered and are a very diagnostic feature of the powder.

(*b*) The fairly numerous orange-brown fragments of the *vittae*, composed of thin-walled cells, polygonal in surface view, with slight thickening at the corners; larger fragments show the presence of septa at fairly frequent intervals. These fragments are usually found associated with the parenchyma and collenchyma of the mesocarp.

(*c*) The thin-walled *parenchyma and collenchyma of the mesocarp* which is not abundant and is usually found associated with the fragments of the vittae.

A layer of *sclereids* also occurs in the mesocarp at the apex of the mericarp, and occasional fragments of this layer may be seen; the cells are small and irregular and have thick walls with numerous pits.

(*d*) The *endocarp*, which is a single layer of fairly large, thin-walled cells, elongated in surface view and arranged with their long axes more or less parallel to one another. This layer is almost always associated with the pale, yellowish-brown *testa*.

(*e*) The lignified groups of *fibro-vascular tissue* which are fairly abundant. The *fibres* are slender, thin-walled and pitted and the *vessels* are mostly small with spiral or annular thickening but occasional larger, bordered-pitted vessels occur. Small groups of lignified *pitted parenchymatous cells* are very infrequent.

(*f*) The very abundant *endosperm* composed of thick-walled cells containing aleurone grains and *microrosette crystals of calcium oxalate*.

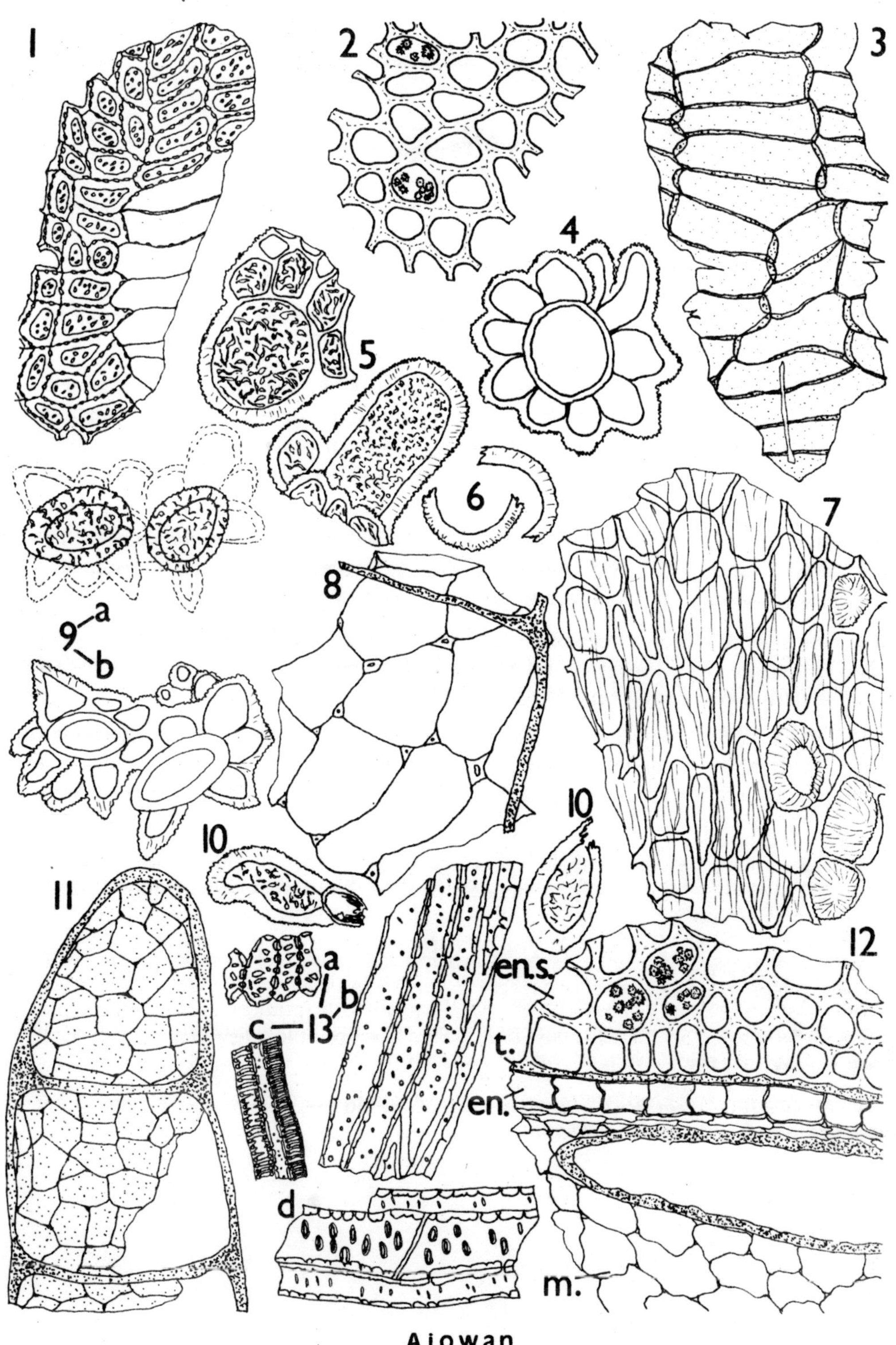

Ajowan

×330

1 Part of the sclereid layer of the mesocarp.
2 Endosperm containing microrosette crystals of calcium oxalate.
3 Endocarp in surface view.
4 The base of a large protuberance on the epicarp with surrounding cells showing smaller protuberances.
5 Large protuberances of the epicarp in side and oblique surface views.
6 Fragments of protuberances.
7 Epicarp in surface view with some smaller protuberances.
8 Collenchyma of the mesocarp with a fragment of a vitta.
9 Part of the epicarp showing protuberances (a) from the top level and (b) focused at a lower level.
10 Detached protuberances.
11 End part of a vitta showing transverse septa.
12 Part of the mericarp in transverse section showing the endosperm (en.s.) containing microrosette crystals of calcium oxalate, the testa (t.), endocarp (en.) and collenchyma of the mesocarp (m.) with part of a vitta.
13 Elements of the fibro-vascular tissue showing (a) pitted parenchymatous cells, (b) pitted fibres, (c) narrow vessels and tracheids and (d) parts of fibres and a larger, bordered-pitted vessel.

ANISE

Pimpinella anisum L. — Umbelliferae

Aniseed, Anise Fruits

A medium brown powder with a characteristic, aromatic odour and taste.

The diagnostic characters are:

(*a*) The *epicarp* composed of a layer of colourless cells with unevenly thickened and pitted walls; in surface view the cells are seen to be arranged with three or four rows of straight-walled, somewhat elongated cells alternating with wider areas of irregularly shaped cells with slightly sinuous walls; scattered *stomata* occur in the areas of sinuous-walled cells. The *cuticle* is strongly striated.

(*b*) The *covering trichomes*, which are nearly always found detached from the epicarp. They are conical, slightly curved and usually unicellular although occasionally the lumen is divided by a single transverse septum; the walls are thickened and distinctly warted.

(*c*) The very numerous brown fragments of the *vittae* composed of thin-walled cells, polygonal to elongated in surface view. The larger fragments which include the whole width of the vittae show them to be fairly narrow and frequently branched.

(*d*) The *sclereids of the mesocarp*, which are usually found in groups in a single layer, often associated with thinner-walled unlignified parenchymatous cells. Individual sclereids are square to rectangular in outline with a large lumen and uniformly thickened walls traversed by numerous pits.

(*e*) The *endocarp* composed of a single layer of very thin-walled cells, elongated in surface view and arranged with their long axes approximately parallel. This layer is usually found adherent to fragments of the vittae.

(*f*) The *testa* composed of a single layer of brown cells, polygonal in surface view, with thin, sometimes slightly beaded, walls.

(*g*) The abundant *endosperm* with numerous *aleurone grains* containing *microrosette crystals of calcium oxalate*; the cells have moderately thickened walls.

(*h*) The fragments of lignified *fibro-vascular tissue* composed of small, thin-walled fibres and vessels with spiral and annular thickening.

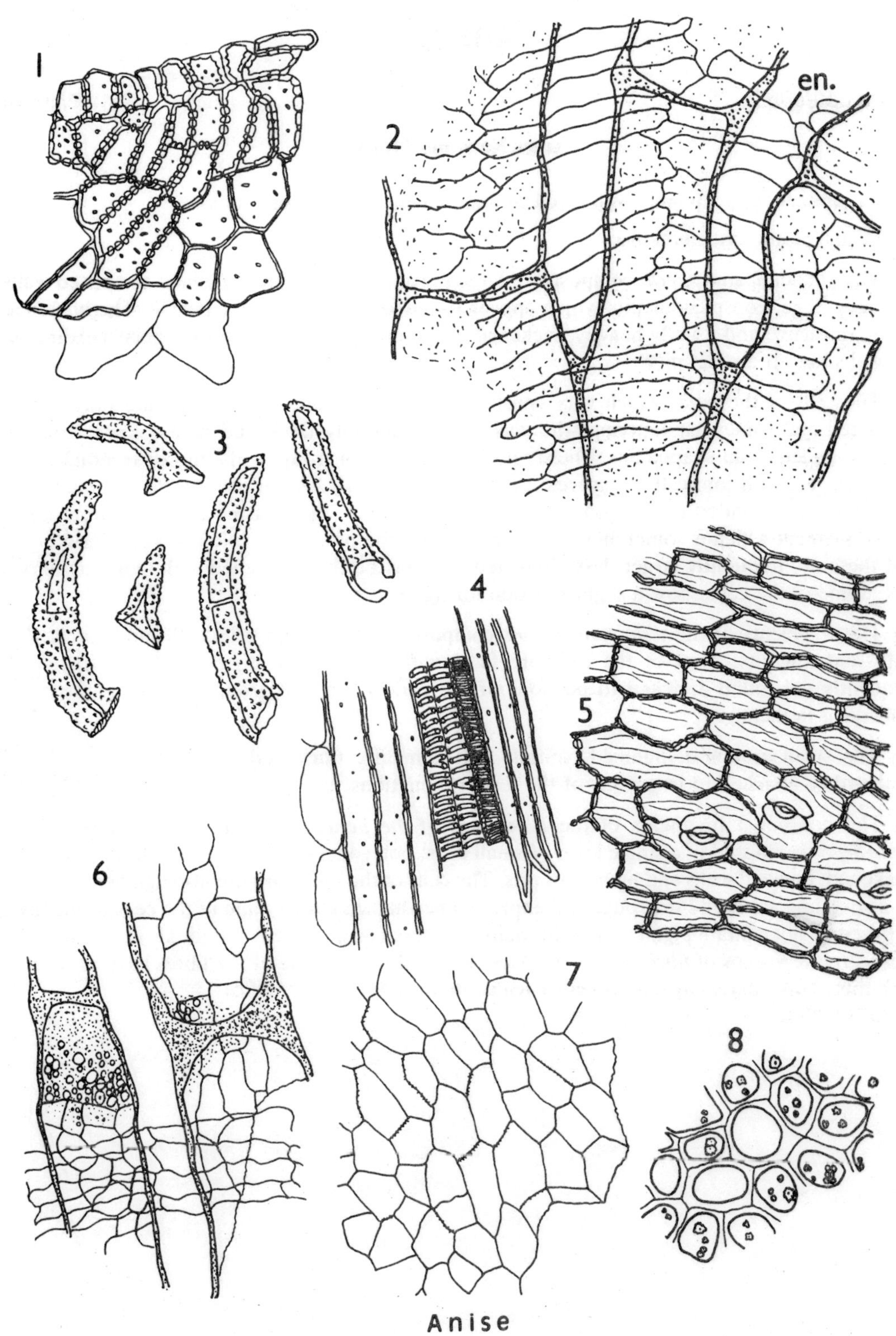

Anise

×330

1 A group of sclereids from the mesocarp with adjacent unlignified parenchyma.
2 Branching vittae (shown in outline only) and underlying endocarp (en.) in surface view.
3 Covering trichomes.
4 Part of a group of fibro-vascular tissue.
5 Epicarp in surface view showing stomata and striated cuticle.
6 Part of two vittae showing transverse septa and part of the underlying endocarp in surface view.
7 Testa in surface view.
8 Endosperm containing microrosette crystals of calcium oxalate.

ARECA

Areca catechu L. Palmae

Areca Nuts, Betel Nuts

A dark cinnamon-brown powder with no odour and a bitter, slightly astringent taste.

The diagnostic characters are:

(*a*) The abundant *endosperm* composed of large polygonal cells with irregularly thickened walls and very large, conspicuous pits which appear rounded to oval in surface view. The walls are highly refractive and usually heavily thickened; occasional fragments show irregular beading on the walls but no distinct pits.

(*b*) The cells of the *testa*, which vary considerably in shape but the majority are tangentially elongated and somewhat tapering; the walls are moderately thickened with a few scattered, small, rounded or slit-shaped pits. These cells usually occur in groups consisting of several loosely packed layers with intercellular spaces; they are occasionally seen in transverse sectional view when they are rounded to polygonal or irregular in outline. Most of the cells contain reddish-brown pigment which is sometimes concentrated near the periphery; colourless cells also occur and these are frequently larger, less elongated and may be thicker-walled with more numerous pits. Some of the cells show a slight reaction for lignin.

(*c*) The fragments of the *testa ruminations* composed of polygonal cells with moderately thin walls and few pits; most of the cells are filled with dark brown pigment. These fragments frequently are found attached to portions of the endosperm and groups of vessels are often embedded in them.

(*d*) The small groups of lignified, spirally and annularly thickened *vessels* which are found scattered or attached to fragments of the testa ruminations.

(*e*) The occasional fragments of the *inner part of the pericarp* which may be present. The *endocarp* is composed of a single layer of small cells, polygonal in surface view, with moderately thickened, lignified walls and numerous pits. The cells of the *mesocarp* are also lignified; they are elongated and are found in groups and appear somewhat similar to some of the cells of the testa but they do not contain pigment and the walls are more conspicuously pitted; also present in the mesocarp are groups of *fibres* with very thick, lignified walls; some of the fibres have associated with them small parenchymatous cells each containing a *nodule of silica*.

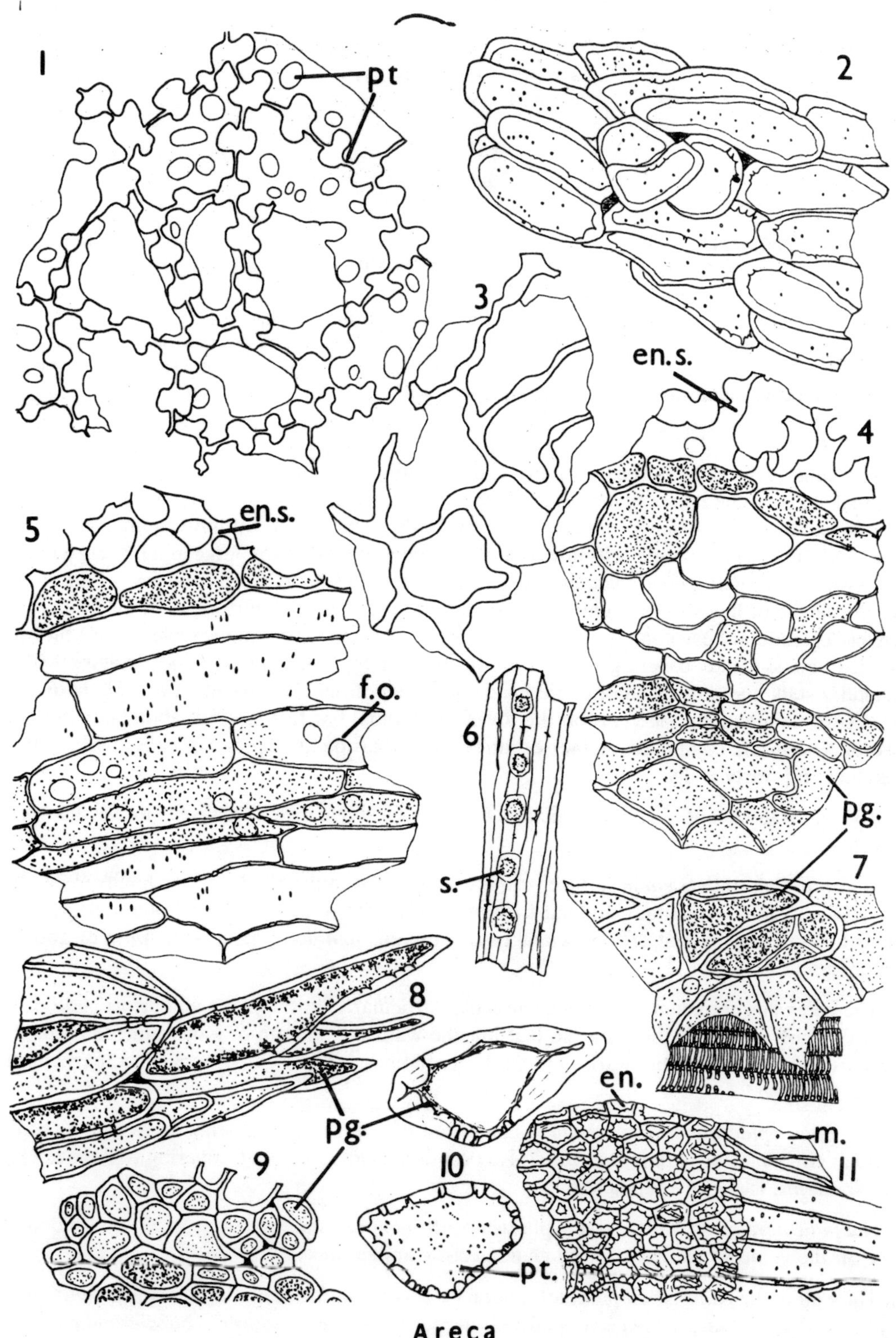

Areca

×330

1 Part of the endosperm showing pits (pt.).
2 Cells of the mesocarp.
3 Part of the endosperm without pits.
4 Part of a testa rumination in transverse sectional view showing pigment (pg.) in some of the cells and part of the adjacent endosperm (en.s.).
5 Part of a testa rumination in longitudinal view showing pigment and globules of fixed oil (f.o.) in some of the cells and part of the adjacent endosperm (en.s.).
6 Fibres of the mesocarp with associated parenchymatous cells containing silica nodules (s.).
7 Part of a testa rumination in longitudinal view showing cells containing pigment (pg.) and part of a group of annularly thickened vessels.
8 Elongated cells of the testa containing pigment (pg.).
9 Cells of the testa containing pigment (pg.), in transverse sectional view.
10 Isolated cells of the testa showing conspicuous pits (pt.) and the concentration of pigment (pg.) around the periphery of the lumen in one of the cells.
11 Fragment of the inner part of the pericarp in surface view showing endocarp (en.) and mesocarp (m.).

BASIL

Ocimum basilicum L. Labiatae

Sweet Basil

Usually occurs in commerce as the dried, much-broken leaves with scattered pieces of slender stems and a few brownish flowers; varying amounts of small brown fruits are also present. It has a strong, aromatic and characteristic odour and a characteristic, slightly bitter taste.

The diagnostic characters are:

(*a*) The cells of both epidermises of the leaf are large and thin-walled in surface view; the anticlinal walls on the *upper epidermis* are sinuous to wavy and those on the *lower epidermis* are more markedly wavy; *diacytic stomata* occur on both surfaces but are more numerous on the lower epidermis. The palisade cells underlying the upper epidermis are large and loosely packed. Yellowish-brown *glandular trichomes* occur fairly abundantly and are of two types; the larger ones are sessile or have a short, unicellular stalk and they occur in depressions in the epidermis; each has a glandular head composed of four radiating cells with a common cuticle raised to form a spherical, bladder-like covering. Those of the second type are smaller and capitate with a unicellular stalk and a rounded or ovoid head composed of one or two cells. *Covering trichomes* also occur, mainly along the veins on the lower epidermis, but they are not abundant; they are uniseriate, conical, composed of two or three and occasionally up to six cells, with slightly thickened and warty walls.

(*b*) The leaf is dorsiventral and in *sectional view* shows a single layer of palisade under the upper epidermis.

(*c*) The *epidermis of the stem* in surface view is composed of thin-walled, longitudinally elongated cells with occasional stomata; glandular trichomes and scattered covering trichomes are present, similar to those on the leaf. The vascular tissue contains *lignified vessels* with spiral or annular thickening.

(*d*) The *calyx* has abundant covering trichomes, particularly on the outer epidermis and on the lobes; they are similar to those on the leaf but the walls are smooth or have faint, longitudinal striations and are not usually warty. Glandular trichomes are also fairly numerous, particularly the capitate type.

(*e*) The *outer epidermis of the corolla* is composed of elongated cells with thin, sinuous walls; glandular trichomes of both types occur, also occasional smooth-walled covering trichomes. The *inner epidermis* is slightly papillose.

(*f*) The *pollen grains* are fairly large, spherical with six pores and furrows; rounded, raised areas occur on the exine which have a very characteristic appearance.

(*g*) The wall of the *fruits* is composed of several layers of cells including a *thin-walled epidermis*, a very dense dark brown *pigment layer* and an inner *sclerenchymatous layer*. The sclerenchymatous layer is composed of small, columnar cells with strongly thickened inner and radial walls; each cell contains a *prism crystal*; when seen in surface view the cells are polygonal with beaded thickening on the walls.

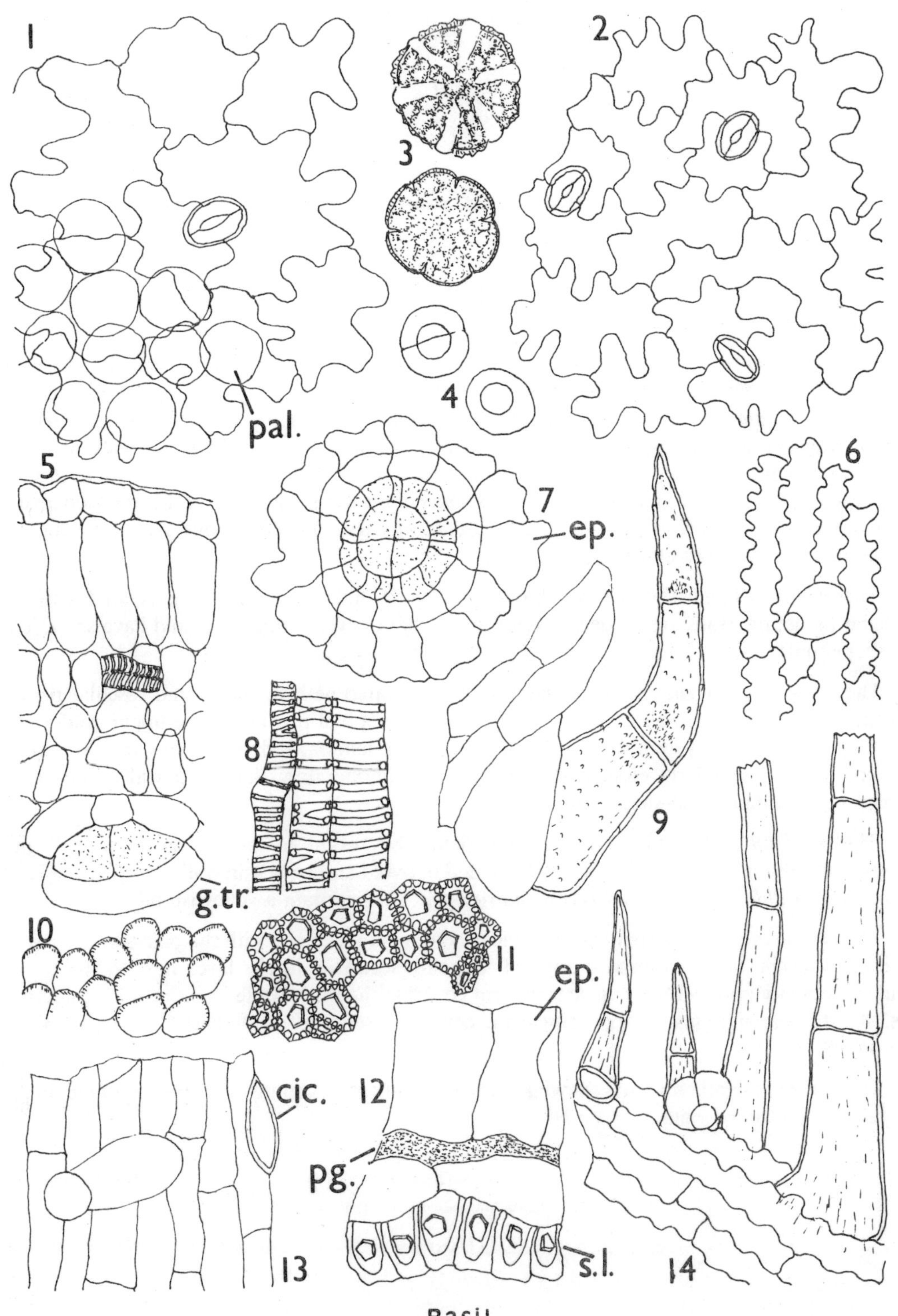

Basil

×330

1 Upper epidermis of the leaf in surface view with part of the underlying palisade (pal.).
2 Lower epidermis of the leaf in surface view showing diacytic stomata.
3 Pollen grains.
4 Capitate glands in surface view.
5 Part of the lamina in sectional view showing a multicellular gland (g.tr.) in the lower epidermis.
6 Outer epidermis of the corolla in surface view.
7 A multicellular gland on the epidermis of the leaf, in surface view, showing radiating epidermal cells (ep.).
8 Part of a group of vessels from the stem.
9 Epidermis over a vein on the lower epidermis of the leaf with a covering trichome.
10 Inner epidermis of the corolla in surface view.
11 Sclerenchymatous layer of the fruit wall in surface view, seen from above.
12 Part of the fruit wall in sectional view showing the epidermis (ep.), pigment layer (pg.) and sclerenchymatous layer (s.l.).
13 Epidermis of the stem in surface view with a capitate gland and a cicatrix (cic.).
14 Outer epidermis of the calyx in surface view showing a capitate gland and covering trichomes.

BAY

Laurus nobilis L. — Lauraceae

Bay Laurel Leaf, Sweet Bay Leaf

Usually occurs in commerce as whole or slightly broken dried leaves which are thick and coriaceous, brown or greenish-brown with a characteristic spicy odour and taste.

The diagnostic characters are:

(*a*) The *upper epidermis* which, in surface view, is composed of irregularly shaped cells with considerably thickened cellulosic walls and large, conspicuous pits giving an irregular and beaded appearance; stomata are absent; the underlying palisade cells are fairly large and loosely packed. The *lower epidermis* is composed of cells with slightly sinuous, unevenly thickened walls with few pits; the walls are less-markedly thickened than those of the upper epidermis but some show a faint reaction for lignin; numerous *paracytic stomata* are present, the guard cells of which give a positive reaction with *Phloroglucinol and Hydrochloric Acid*. In the regions over the veins the epidermal cells are more elongated.

(*b*) The abundant lignified *fibres*, which occur in groups and are frequently associated with the vascular tissue; the walls are moderately and somewhat unevenly thickened and have scattered, slit-shaped pits.

(*c*) The numerous *sclereids*; some of these occur associated with the fibres and vascular tissue, but the majority are in small groups in the palisade mesophyll just below the upper epidermis, and they are particularly abundant at the margins of the lamina. Individual cells vary in outline but are usually irregularly elongated and they have moderately thickened walls with fairly numerous, rounded or slit-shaped pits.

(*d*) The large *oil cells*, which are very abundant; they occur in the spongy mesophyll and occasionally also in the palisade; they are rounded to ovoid and have thin walls which give a faint reaction with *Phloroglucinol and Hydrochloric Acid*; they contain a yellowish oil.

(*e*) The *lamina in sectional view* shows the leaves to be dorsiventral with the palisade composed of several layers, with scattered groups of sclereids occurring in the layer next to the upper epidermis; a moderately thick *cuticle* is present covering the thick-walled cells of both epidermises. At the leaf margins a large, single oil cell is present, associated with sclereids in the mesophyll.

(*f*) The groups of lignified *vessels* showing spiral or annular thickening or, in the larger elements, reticulately thickened walls.

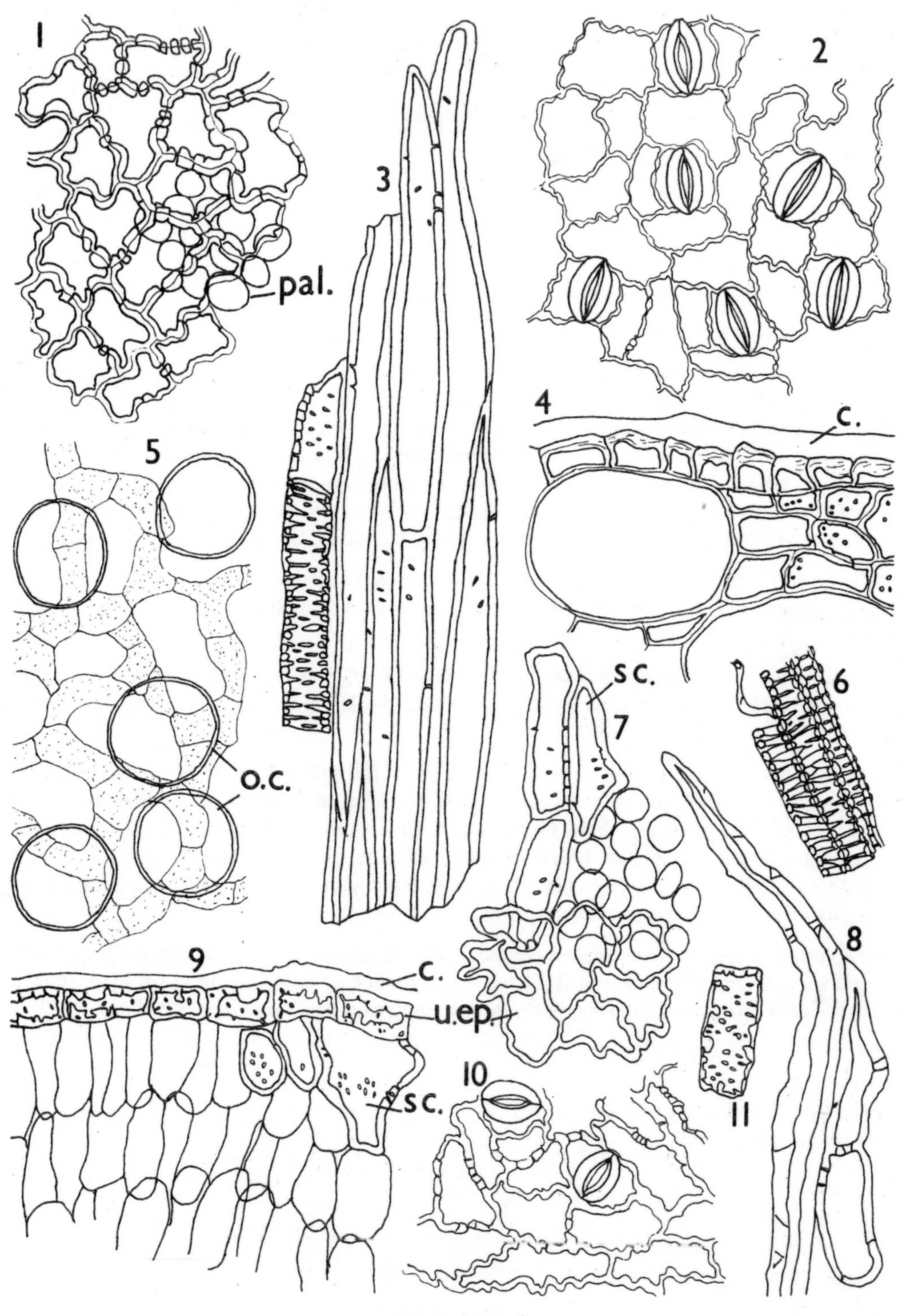

Bay Leaf

×330

1 Upper epidermis in surface view with part of the underlying palisade (pal.).

2 Lower epidermis in surface view with paracytic stomata.

3 Part of a group of fibres and sclereids with an associated reticulately thickened vessel.

4 Part of the lamina from near the margin, in sectional view, showing the thick cuticle (c.), lower epidermal cells with thickened walls, a large oil cell and sclereids in the mesophyll.

5 Oil cells (o.c.) and associated spongy mesophyll cells.

6 A group of vessels from a vein.

7 Upper epidermis (u.ep.) in surface view showing a group of sclereids (sc.) in the underlying palisade.

8 Sclereids and part of a fibre.

9 Part of the lamina in sectional view showing the cuticle (c.), upper epidermis (u.ep.) and underlying palisade with a group of sclereids (sc.).

10 Lower epidermis in surface view showing the more elongated cells over a vein.

11 An isolated sclereid.

BEARBERRY

Arctostaphylos uva-ursi (L.) Spreng. Ericaceae

Bearberry Leaves

A greenish-fawn powder with a slight odour and a very astringent taste.

The diagnostic characters are:

(*a*) The fragments of the *lamina in surface view*. The *upper epidermis* is composed of large, polygonal to rectangular cells with straight walls which are distinctly thickened and pitted, appearing irregularly beaded; stomata are absent; the underlying palisade cells are fairly large and closely packed. The cells of the *lower epidermis* are similar to those of the upper epidermis but they are usually smaller; numerous large, almost circular *anomocytic stomata* are present and where these occur the thick *cuticle*, which is present on both epidermises, is discontinuous, and on focusing up to a higher plane these breaks in the cuticle are clearly seen as circular apertures.

(*b*) The *prisms of calcium oxalate*, which are found scattered and in the cortical parenchymatous cells of the veins; the crystals are variable in size and the smaller ones often form small aggregates.

(*c*) The occasional groups of *fibres* with thick, lignified walls and few pits; they are frequently associated with parenchymatous cells containing prisms of calcium oxalate. Occasional groups of lignified *tracheids* and *vessels* are also present.

(*d*) The fragments of the *leaves in sectional view*; sections through the whole lamina rarely occur but fragments of the thick cuticle showing marked curvature and with part of the underlying epidermis attached are fairly abundant. Occasional fragments show the multiple palisade and the spongy mesophyll cells, many of which contain granular orange-brown pigmented matter. Fragments of the *midrib and larger veins* in sectional and surface views show the presence of similar pigment in the cells of the cortex.

(*e*) The very occasional *covering trichomes*, which are unicellular, conical and moderately thick-walled and may be slightly swollen at the base. Occasional fragments of the lower epidermis in surface view show the presence of *cicatrices* where the trichomes have been attached.

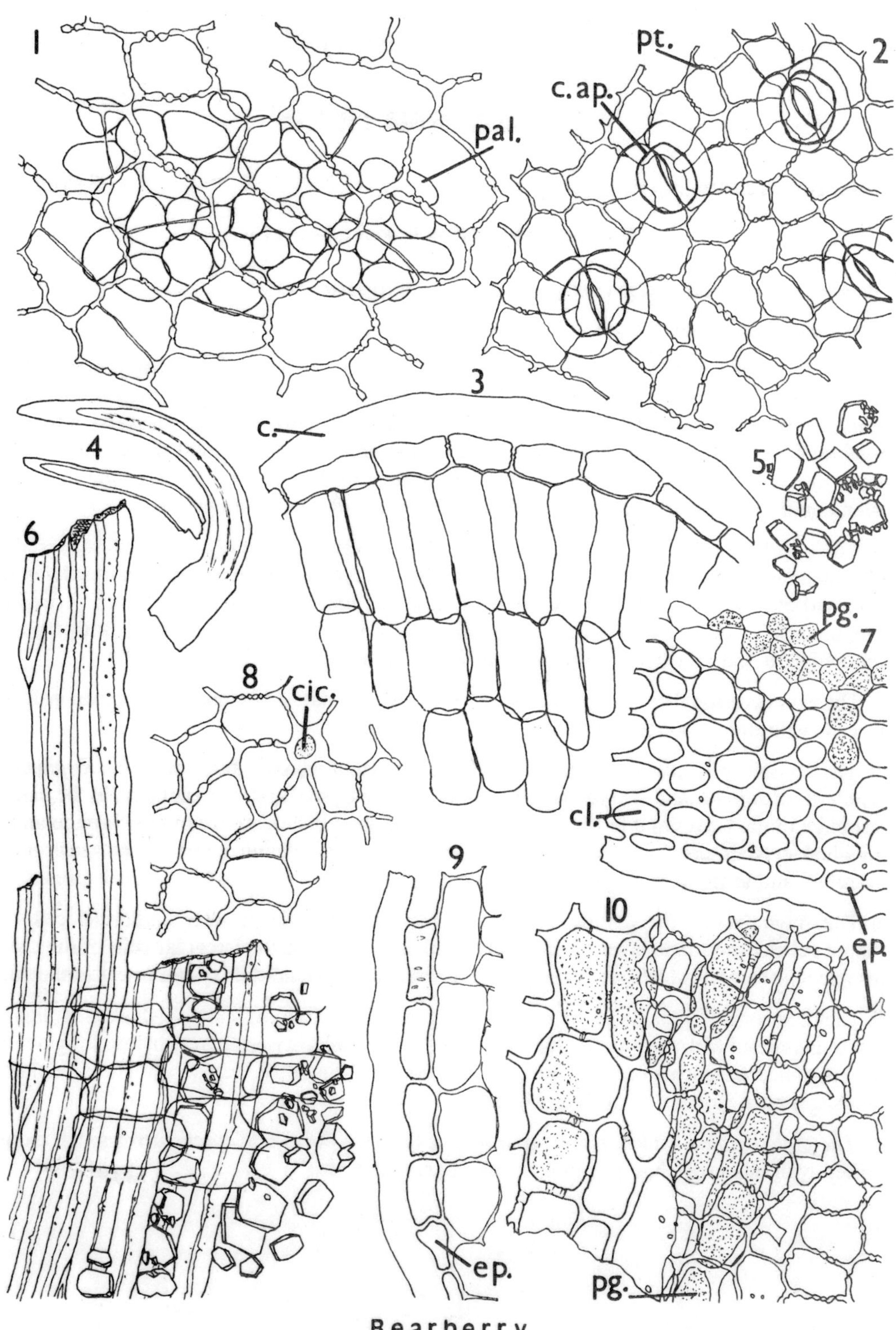

Bearberry

×330

1 Upper epidermis in surface view with part of the underlying palisade (pal.).
2 Lower epidermis in surface view showing stomata, pitted walls (pt.) and circular apertures (c.ap.) in the cuticle.
3 Part of the lamina in sectional view showing the thick cuticle (c.), upper epidermis and cells of the multiple palisade mesophyll.
4 Covering trichomes.
5 Calcium oxalate crystals.
6 Part of a group of fibres with associated parenchymatous cells and crystals of calcium oxalate.
7 Part of the midrib in sectional view showing the lower epidermis (ep.), collenchyma (cl.) and parenchymatous cells of the cortex containing pigment (pg.).
8 Lower epidermis in surface view showing a cicatrix (cic.).
9 Part of a vein in longitudinal view showing the cuticle, epidermis (ep.) and underlying parenchyma.
10 Epidermis (ep.) over a vein, in surface view, with underlying parenchyma containing pigment (pg.).

BELLADONNA HERB

Atropa belladonna L. Solanaceae

Belladonna Leaf, Deadly Nightshade Leaf

A dark green powder with a faint odour and a slightly bitter taste.

The diagnostic characters are:

(*a*) The fragments of the *lamina in surface view*. The *upper epidermis* is composed of cells with a slightly sinuous outline and a strongly striated *cuticle; anisocytic stomata* are present but are not numerous; the underlying palisade cells are fairly small and tightly packed. The cells of the *lower epidermis* have more sinuous walls than those of the upper epidermis and the striations on the cuticle are sometimes less clearly marked; numerous anisocytic stomata are present. In the regions over the veins the epidermal cells are straight-walled and elongated.

(*b*) The *glandular trichomes*, which are not very numerous; they usually are found scattered and are sometimes fragmented. They are of two types; one type has a uniseriate, multicellular stalk composed of from two to four cells and a subspherical unicellular head; the second type has a short unicellular stalk and an ovoid to pyriform head with four to seven cells. Both types are occasionally found attached to fragments of the epidermises.

(*c*) The very occasional *covering trichomes*; these are uniseriate and conical, composed of four or five cells with thin, smooth walls.

(*d*) The conspicuous *idioblasts* composed of parenchymatous cells filled with *microsphenoidal crystals* of *calcium oxalate*. These occur in the spongy mesophyll and, occasionally, in the palisade mesophyll of the leaves and in the parenchyma of the stem. They are frequently broken and the individual crystals are found scattered. A few *prisms* of calcium oxalate also occur in the mesophyll and in the parenchyma of the stem.

(*e*) The fragments of the *lamina in sectional view* showing the tabular epidermal cells with striated cuticle, the single layer of thin-walled palisade cells and the irregular cells of the spongy mesophyll, several of which are densely packed with microsphenoidal crystals of calcium oxalate.

(*f*) The occasional fragments of the *stem* showing the fairly large, reticulately thickened, lignified vessels associated with thin-walled lignified fibres and lignified xylem parenchyma. Fragments of the unlignified parenchyma from the pith and cortex frequently include idioblasts containing microsphenoidal crystals of calcium oxalate.

(*g*) *The pollen grains*, which are subspherical with three pores and three furrows; the exine is marked with numerous fine pits in a radiating arrangement.

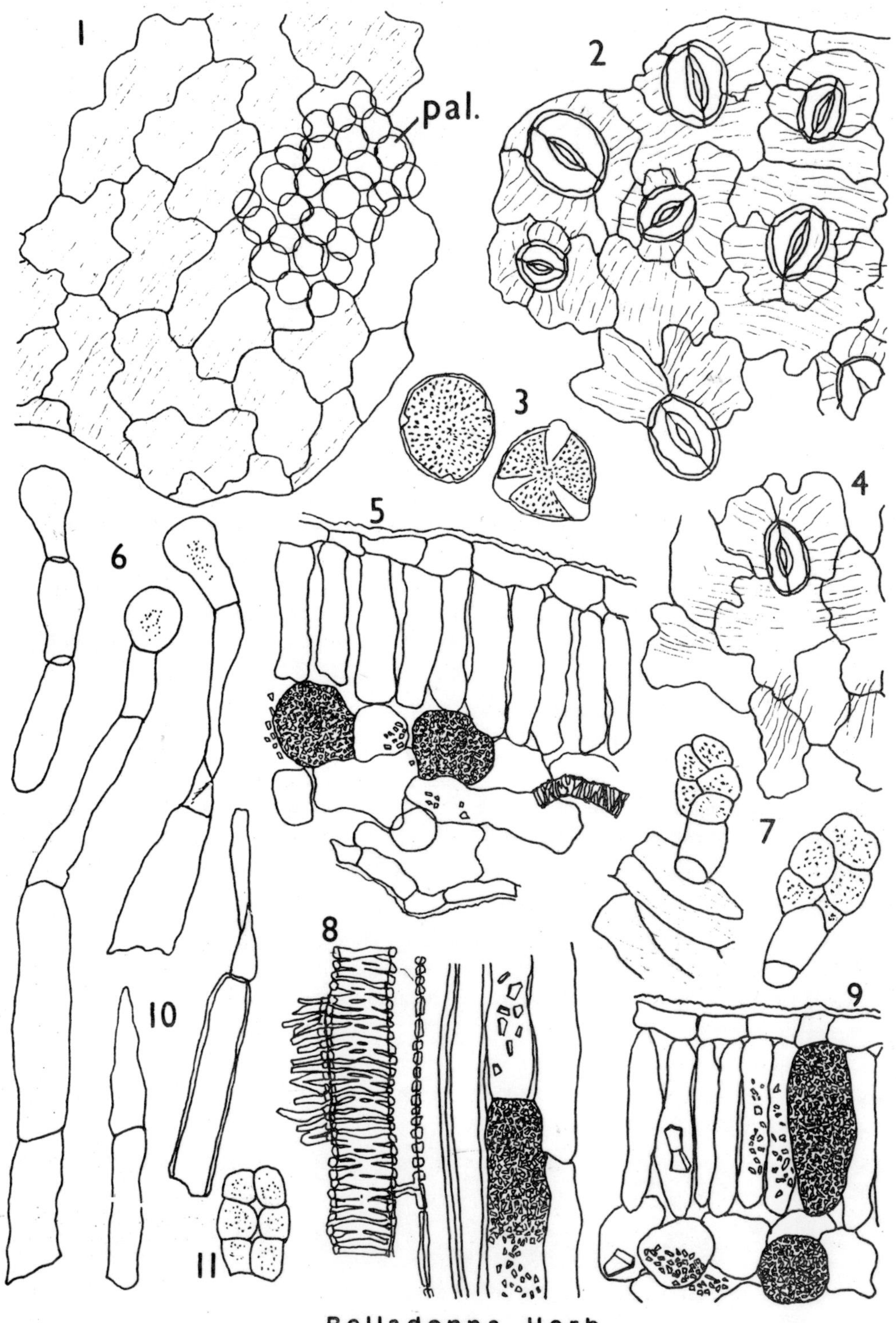

Belladonna Herb

×330

1 Upper epidermis in surface view showing cuticular striations and part of the underlying palisade (pal.).
2 Lower epidermis in surface view showing cuticular striations and numerous anisocytic stomata.
3 Pollen grains.
4 Upper epidermis in surface view showing an anisocytic stoma.
5 Part of the lamina in sectional view showing two idioblasts in the spongy mesophyll and scattered microsphenoidal crystals of calcium oxalate.
6 Glandular trichomes with uniseriate, multicellular stalks and unicellular heads.
7 Glandular trichomes with unicellular stalks and multicellular heads, one attached to a fragment of the epidermis over a vein.
8 Fragments of the inner tissues of the stem in longitudinal sectional view showing reticulately thickened vessels, xylem parenchyma, fibres and unlignified parenchymatous cells containing calcium oxalate crystals.
9 Part of the lamina in sectional view showing the upper epidermis, an idioblast in the palisade and other cells containing scattered prisms and microsphenoidal crystals of calcium oxalate.
10 Part of a covering trichome.
11 Multicellular head from a glandular trichome.

BELLADONNA ROOT

Atropa belladonna L. Solanaceae

A pale fawnish-brown powder with little odour and a faint, slightly bitter taste.

The diagnostic characters are:

(*a*) The abundant *starch granules*, which are simple and spherical or compound with two to four or more components; some of the granules show a faint, rounded or slit-shaped hilum.

(*b*) The abundant *parenchyma of the cortex, pith* and *medullary rays* composed of large, ovoid to elongated cells with thin walls. Some of the cells are densely packed with *microsphenoidal crystals of calcium oxalate* and in some others a few, scattered microsphenoidal crystals may be found; the remainder are filled with starch granules.

(*c*) The *vessels* and *fibres* of the xylem, which are lignified and occur in groups of interlocking cells. The cells have somewhat oblique end walls and numerous closely arranged bordered pits; occasional reticulately thickened vessels also occur. The fibres are thin-walled and have simple pits which may be fairly numerous; they usually occur associated with the vessels. Lignified xylem *parenchyma* is also found scattered and associated with the vessels and fibres; the cells are elongated rectangular in sectional view and have moderately thickened walls and numerous simple pits.

(*d*) The occasional fragments of tawny-brown *cork* composed of cells with slightly thickened walls which may give a slight reaction for lignin; the cells are elongated and somewhat irregular in surface view.

(*e*) The very occasional fragments of *sieve tissue* composed of small elongated elements, some showing faint sieve areas on the oblique end walls.

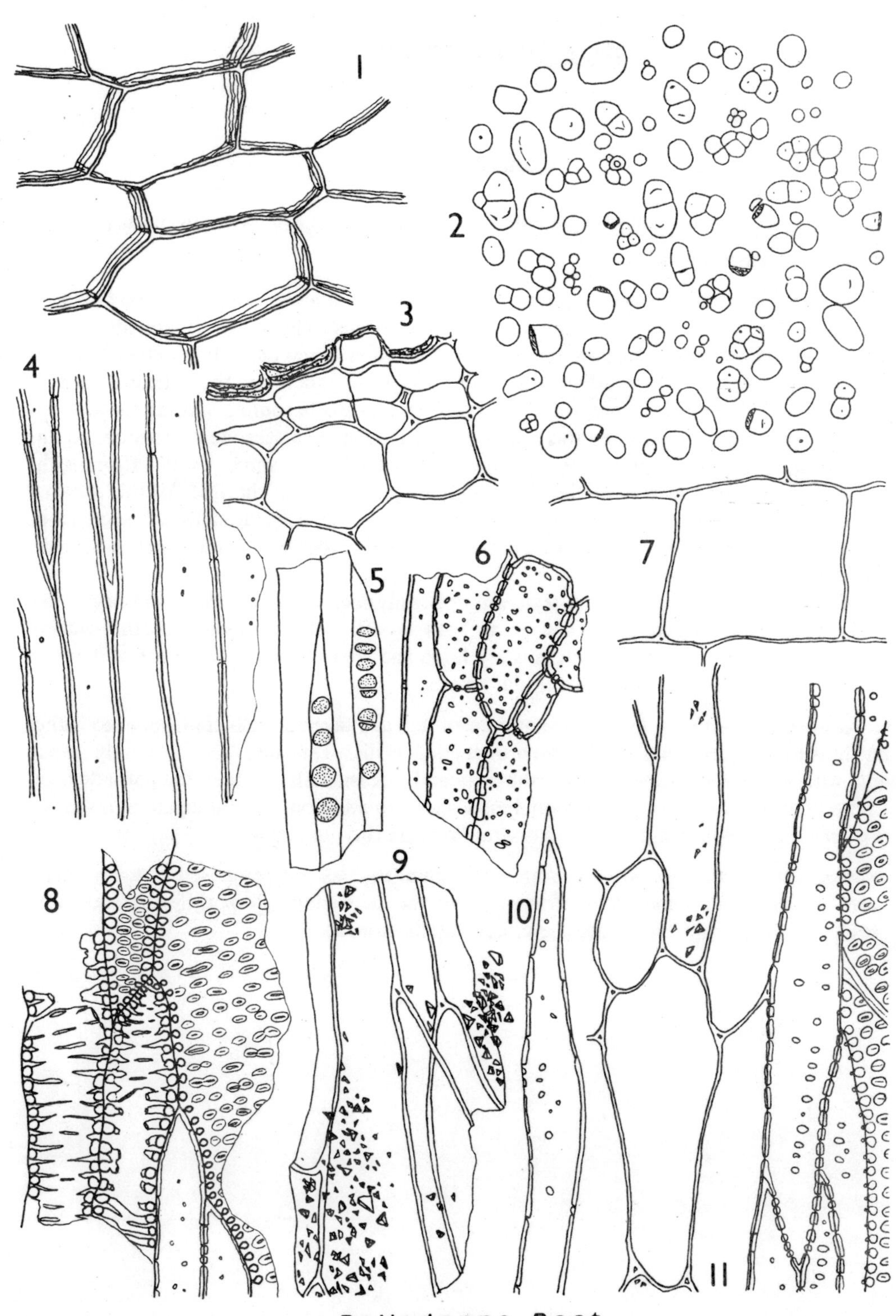

Belladonna Root

×330

1 Cork in surface view.
2 Starch granules.
3 Cork and outer tissues in sectional view.
4 Part of a group of fibres.
5 Sieve tissue.
6 Xylem parenchyma and part of a fibre.
7 Cells of a medullary ray in radial longitudinal section.
8 Reticulately thickened and bordered pitted vessels associated with fibres.
9 Parenchymatous cells containing microsphenoidal crystals of calcium oxalate.
10 Part of a fibre.
11 Part of a vessel, fibres and a medullary ray in tangential longitudinal section.

BLACK MUSTARD

Brassica nigra (L.) Koch — Cruciferae

Mustard Seeds

A light brown powder with little odour and a taste which is bitter at first and then strongly pungent.

The diagnostic characters are:

(*a*) The characteristic dark brown fragments of the *palisade layer of the testa in surface view* composed of small, polygonal cells with thick, lignified walls. The larger fragments show a distinct network duc to the fact that the individual cells vary in height according to their position in relation to the large cells of the adjacent hypodermis, those underlying the anticlinal walls of the hypodermal cells being the longest and the intervening cells becoming shorter towards the centre of each hypodermal cell; when the palisade layer is seen in surface view, from above, the narrow tips of the longer cells are arranged as lines of small cells with sinuous walls, forming the network, and on focusing to a lower level the shorter cells between the lines of the network appear as larger cells with straight walls. In *sectional view* the palisade cells are seen to be thickened on the basal and anticlinal walls, and the longer cells taper towards the apex, where the anticlinal walls are slightly sinuous.

The *epidermis* and *hypodermis* of the testa are not easily seen in surface view, but occasional fragments of the seed in sectional view show both layers to be composed of thin-walled, colourless cells, and those of the hypodermis are large and rounded with the longer cells of the palisade layer extending to fill the intercellular spaces.

(*b*) The *parenchyma of the endosperm* composed of a single layer of cells, polygonal to rather irregular in surface view with moderately thickened walls. This layer is frequently found associated with the brown *pigment layer* of the testa and, occasionally, some of the palisade layer may also be attached. Fragments in sectional view show, in addition, several layers of *collapsed parenchymatous* cells adhering to the endosperm layer on the inner side.

(*c*) The fragments of the *embryo*, which are very abundant and are composed of fairly small, thin-walled parenchyma; some of the fragments of the cotyledons show differentiation into epidermis and palisade and, in surface view, developing stomata.

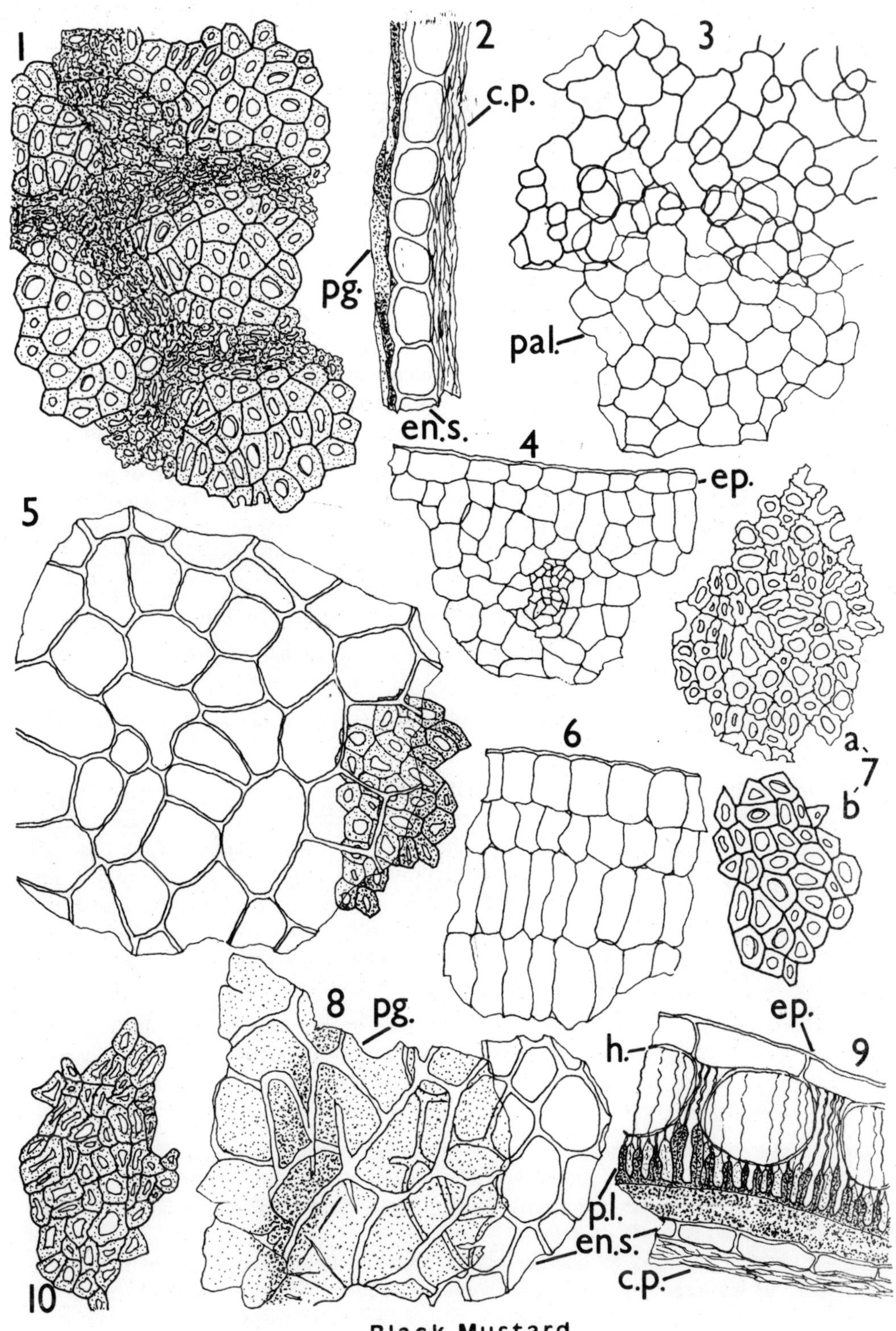

Black Mustard

×330

1 Palisade layer of the testa in surface view, seen from above, showing part of the network arrangement.
2 Endosperm layer (en.s.), in sectional view, with attached pigment layer of the testa (pg.) and underlying collapsed parenchymatous cells (c.p.).
3 Epidermis of a cotyledon in surface view showing developing stomata and part of the underlying palisade (pal.).
4 Part of a cotyledon in sectional view showing the epidermis (ep.) and underlying mesophyll.
5 Endosperm layer in surface view with part of the palisade layer of the testa, seen from below.
6 Parenchyma of the embryo.
7 Palisade layer of the testa in surface view, (a) seen from above and (b) seen from below.
8 Pigment layer of the testa (pg.) in surface view with part of the underlying endosperm (en.s.).
9 Part of the seed in sectional view showing the epidermis (ep.), hypodermis (h.), palisade layer (p.l.) and pigment layer of the testa, with underlying endosperm (en.s.) and collapsed parenchymatous layers (c.p.).
10 Palisade layer of the testa in surface view, from below, showing less uniform cells.

BLACK PEPPER

Piper nigrum L. Piperaceae

Pepper

A dark greyish-brown powder with black specks; it has a strong, characteristic, spicy odour and a burning taste; it is strongly sternutatory.

The diagnostic characters are:

(*a*) The *epicarp*, which is always adherent to the outermost sclerenchymatous layers of the mesocarp. In surface view the cells cannot readily be distinguished, but the layer is recognised by the areas of dark brown pigment in which are embedded small *prism crystals of calcium oxalate*.

(*b*) The *sclereids of the outer mesocarp* which do not form continuous layers but occur in groups separated by ill-defined parenchyma and may be two or three cells in depth. The sclereids vary considerably in size and shape but are usually polygonal to rectangular with moderately thickened walls and fairly numerous pits, although sometimes the walls are much more heavily thickened; all have dark brown contents. These cells frequently are found isolated or in small groups with adhering fragments of thin-walled tissue; they are fairly abundant.

(*c*) The *parenchyma of the mesocarp* composed of large, polygonal, thin-walled cells with associated larger, thin-walled *oil cells*.

(*d*) The very occasional groups of small, lignified, spirally or annularly thickened *vessels* from the vascular strands. Groups of large, *fibrous sclereids* from the stem also occur infrequently.

(*e*) The *endocarp* composed of a single layer of lignified cells which are more uniform in size and shape than the sclereids of the outer mesocarp. In *sectional view* the cells are seen to be strongly thickened on the inner tangential walls and the radial walls are also thickened at the base but taper towards the outer tangential walls, which are relatively thin. In *surface view* the cells are polygonal and, when seen from above, show distinct pits in the side walls; in median focus the side walls appear markedly convoluted and, when seen from below, pits are absent and the lumens are small and irregular. This layer is nearly always found adherent to the layers of the testa.

(*f*) The *testa* composed of a narrow outer area with one or more layers of collapsed cells containing *reddish-brown pigment* and an inner *hyaline layer* composed of rather indistinct, colourless, thin-walled cells, polygonal in surface view. The layers of the testa are usually found adherent to the endocarp and may also be associated with the outer layers of the perisperm.

(*g*) The numerous fragments of the *parenchyma of the perisperm* composed of thin-walled, polygonal or ovoid cells; the majority are packed with minute *starch granules* which are clumped together to form very dense masses completely filling the cells. Scattered among the starch-filled cells are smaller, rounded to ovoid *oil cells*.

A few small, single, rounded to angular starch granules (from the parenchyma of the mesocarp) also occur scattered.

WHITE PEPPER

A pale brown to cream powder with the odour of Black Pepper and a similar but slightly less pungent taste. Microscopically, it differs from Black Pepper in that the epicarp and outer sclerenchymatous layers of the mesocarp are not present; it consists mainly of perisperm with associated fragments of the testa and endocarp, and strands of vascular tissue.

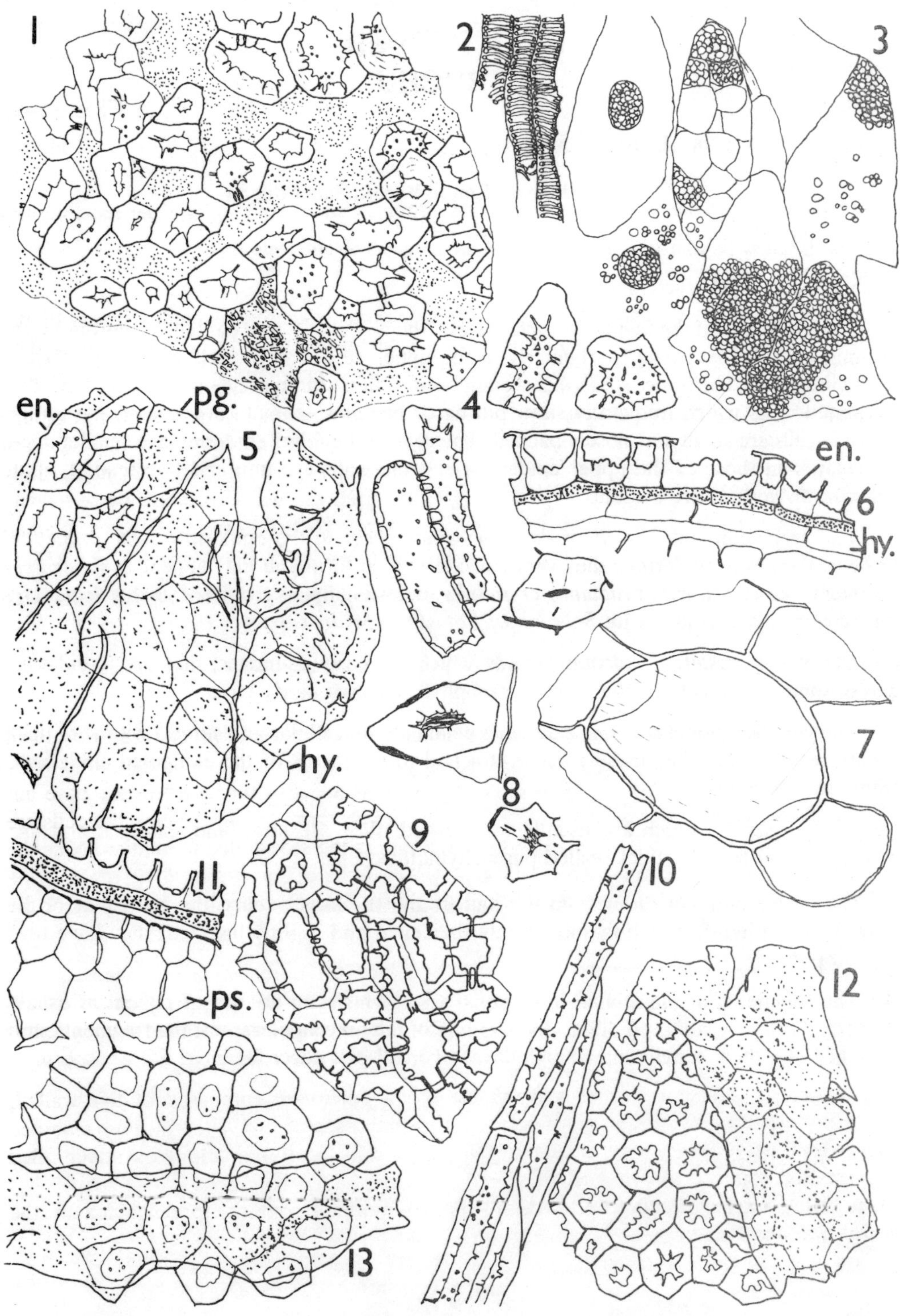

Black Pepper

×330

1 Two layers of sclereids of the outer mesocarp with adhering epicarp containing pigment and calcium oxalate crystals, in surface view.
2 Part of a group of vessels from a vascular strand.
3 Perisperm cells containing densely compacted masses of starch granules and some loose starch granules.
4 Isolated sclereids from the outer mesocarp.
5 Cells of the endocarp (en.) in surface view with underlying pigment layer (pg.) and hyaline layer (hy.) of the testa.
6 Endocarp (en.), pigment layer and hyaline layer (hy.) of the testa in sectional view.
7 Parenchyma of the mesocarp with an oil cell.
8 Sclereids with strongly thickened walls.
9 Endocarp in surface view, seen from above.
10 Fibrous sclereids from the stalk.
11 Endocarp, layers of the testa and outer parenchyma of the perisperm (ps.) in sectional view.
12 Endocarp cells in median focus with associated pigment layer of the testa in surface view.
13 Endocarp cells seen from below, with associated pigment layer of the testa, in surface view.

BUCHU

Agathosma betulina (Berg.) Pillans Rutaceae

Buchu Leaves, Round Buchu, Short Buchu

A greenish-yellow powder with a characteristic aromatic odour and taste.

The diagnostic characters are:

(*a*) The fragments of the *lamina in surface view*; the epidermal cells contain numerous crystals of diosmin and also *mucilage* (particularly in the upper epidermis) which stains with *Solution of Ruthenium Red*. The *upper epidermis* is composed of fairly large polygonal cells with moderately thickened walls which frequently show pitting or beading; stomata are absent; the underlying palisade cells are small and closely packed. The cells of the *lower epidermis* are smaller and more irregular than those of the upper epidermis and the walls are thin and not beaded; abundant *anomocytic stomata* are present.

(*b*) The very abundant *crystals of diosmin*, which occur in the epidermal cells, particularly in those of the lower epidermis; they vary considerably in form and may appear as *sphaerocrystalline masses* or as *feathery* or *radiating crystals* or, occasionally, as groups of small *acicular crystals*; they give a yellow colour with *Solution of Potassium Hydroxide*.

(*c*) The *cluster crystals of calcium oxalate*, which are fairly abundant; they are found scattered and in some of the cells of the spongy mesophyll; they are fairly large.

(*d*) The very occasional *covering trichomes* which are unicellular and conical with very thick and slightly warty walls; they usually occur attached to fragments of the elongated epidermal cells from over the veins.

(*e*) The *oil glands*, which are usually fragmented; they are large and spherical and are surrounded by moderately thick-walled parenchymatous cells.

(*f*) The fairly abundant *fibres* from the midrib and the larger veins; the walls may be heavily thickened and lignified or only moderately thickened and slightly lignified; they have few, slit-shaped pits.

(*g*) The fragments of the *lamina in sectional view*, which are not very frequent as usually the epidermal cells are ruptured due to the swelling of the mucilage present; the fragments show the presence of a thick cuticle and a single layer of small palisade cells.

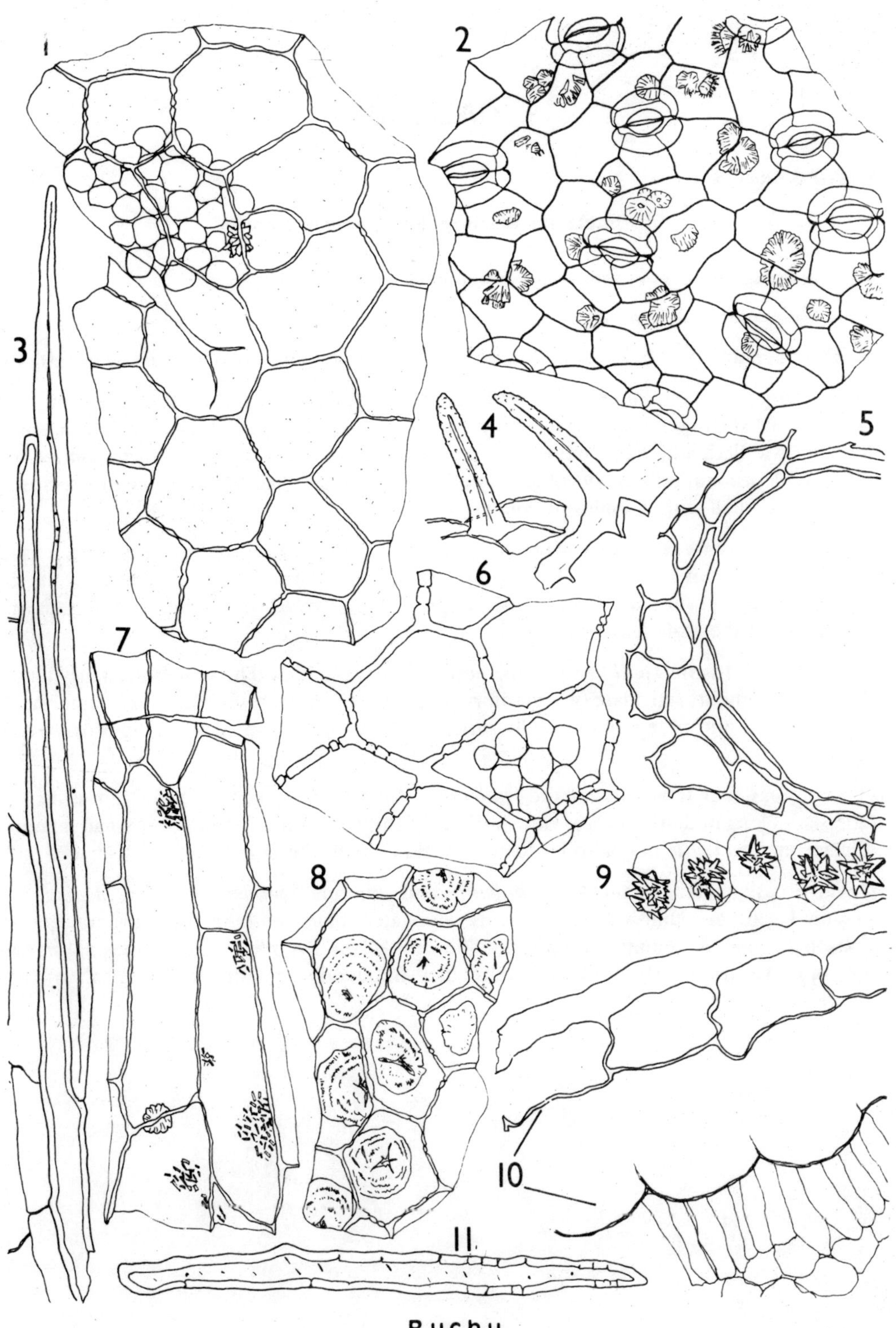

Buchu

×330

1 Upper epidermis in surface view with underlying palisade and a cluster crystal of calcium oxalate.
2 Lower epidermis in surface view showing anomocytic stomata and numerous radiating masses of diosmin.
3 Fibres and adjacent parenchyma.
4 Covering trichomes.
5 Part of an oil gland with surrounding thick-walled parenchyma.
6 Upper epidermis in surface view showing thicker-walled cells and underlying palisade.
7 Epidermis from over a vein in surface view, with groups of acicular crystals of diosmin.
8 Upper epidermis in surface view showing sphaerocrystalline masses of diosmin.
9 Cells of the spongy mesophyll containing cluster crystals of calcium oxalate.
10 Part of the lamina in sectional view showing the thick cuticle, ruptured cells of the epidermis, palisade and part of the spongy mesophyll.
11 Single fibre with moderately thickened walls

CALAMUS

Acorus calamus L. — Araceae

Calamus Rhizome, Sweet Flag Rhizome

A pale brownish-buff powder with a spicy odour and a bitter, slightly pungent taste.

The diagnostic characters are:

(*a*) The fairly abundant *starch granules*, which are small, spherical to ovoid and nearly all simple.

(*b*) The very abundant *parenchyma*, which is mainly developed as *lacunose tissue*, composed of rounded cells surrounding numerous large, irregularly shaped air spaces. The cells are moderately thick-walled and have numerous very conspicuous pitted areas; they contain starch granules. Occasional cells are developed as *oil cells*; these are slightly larger than the surrounding cells and are filled with globules of volatile oil.

(*c*) The *calcium oxalate crystals* which are occasionally found scattered but are more frequently found in parenchymatous cells. The *prisms* are small and form an incomplete crystal sheath surrounding the groups of fibres. Fairly large *cluster crystals* also occur in the cells of the hypodermis of the scale leaves.

(*d*) The lignified *vessels and fibres* of the fibro-vascular bundles. The vessels are fairly large and have spiral, annular, reticulate or scalariform thickening. The fibres are not very numerous; they are thin-walled and pitted and partially surrounded by an inconspicuous calcium oxalate prism sheath.

(*e*) The occasional fragments of the *epidermis of the rhizome* composed of thin-walled cells, somewhat elongated in surface view with a slightly irregular outline. A small amount of collenchymatous tissue may also be found associated with the epidermis.

(*f*) The occasional fragments of the *epidermis* and adhering *hypodermis of the scale leaves*. The epidermal cells are thin-walled and more elongated than those of the rhizome epidermis; occasional rounded stomata are present. The cells of the hypodermis are polygonal in surface view and have irregularly thickened walls; they frequently contain cluster crystals of calcium oxalate.

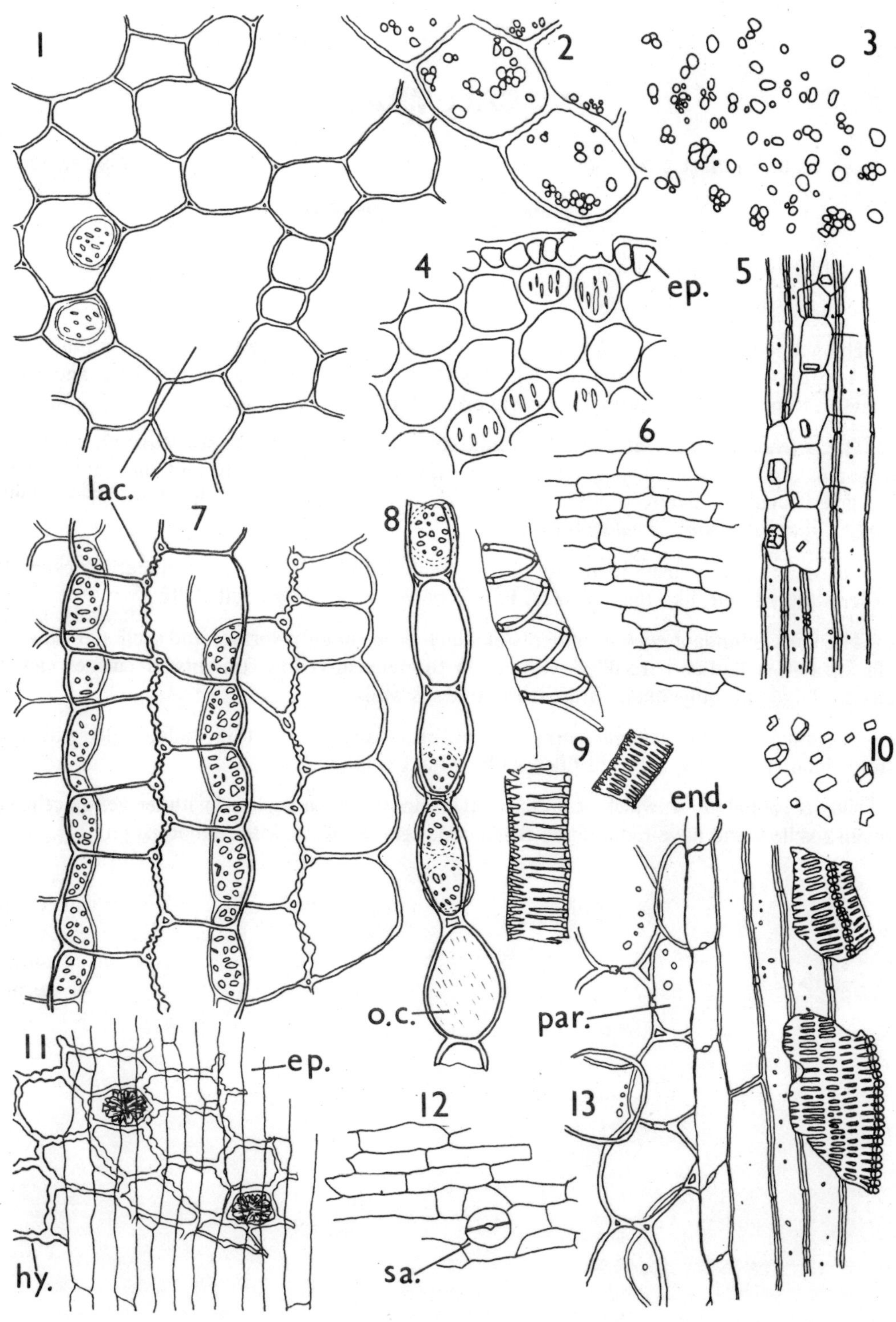

Calamus

×330

1 Parenchyma forming the lacunose tissue (lac. = lacuna) in transverse section.
2 Parenchyma containing starch granules.
3 Starch granules.
4 Epidermis (ep.) and collenchyma of the rhizome in sectional view.
5 Fibres with part of a calcium oxalate prism sheath.
6 Epidermis of the rhizome in surface view.
7 Part of the lacunose tissue (lac. = lacuna) in longitudinal section.
8 Parenchyma of the lacunose tissue with an oil cell (o.c.).
9 Fragments of spirally and reticulately thickened vessels.
10 Prisms of calcium oxalate.
11 Epidermis (ep.) and hypodermis (hy.) of the scale leaves in surface view, with calcium oxalate cluster crystals in the hypodermis.
12 Epidermis of the scale leaves in surface view showing a stoma (sa.).
13 Parenchyma (par.), endodermis (end.), fibres and fragments of a scalariformly thickened vessel, in longitudinal section.

CALUMBA

Jateorhiza palmata (Lam.) Miers — Menispermaceae

Calumba Root, Colombo Root

A yellowish-brown powder with a greenish tinge; it has little odour and the taste is bitter but not astringent.

The diagnostic characters are:

(*a*) The abundant *starch granules*, which are mostly simple but a few compound granules occur with two or three components; the hilum is distinct, cleft or irregularly stellate and usually situated eccentrically; striations are visible on only a few of the granules.

(*b*) The *sclereids*, which are usually found in groups. Individual sclereids are irregularly rectangular and are sometimes quite large; the walls are greenish-yellow and unevenly thickened and have irregularly arranged pits; striations are sometimes visible. Each cell usually contains a number of small *prisms of calcium oxalate*.

(*c*) The *vessels*, which usually are found fragmented; they are large, reticulately thickened or bordered pitted and, like the sclereids, have greenish-yellow, lignified walls.

(*d*) The fairly abundant *cork*, fragments of which occur in both surface and sectional views; the cells are thin-walled and are filled with yellow to greenish-yellow contents. In surface view the cells are large and polygonal, with slightly sinuous walls.

(*e*) The abundant *parenchyma* composed of irregularly ovoid, thin-walled cells with small intercellular spaces; the cells are filled with starch granules.

(*f*) The occasional *fibres*, which occur in small groups usually associated with the vessels; they are greenish-yellow and have moderately thickened, lignified walls with numerous pits.

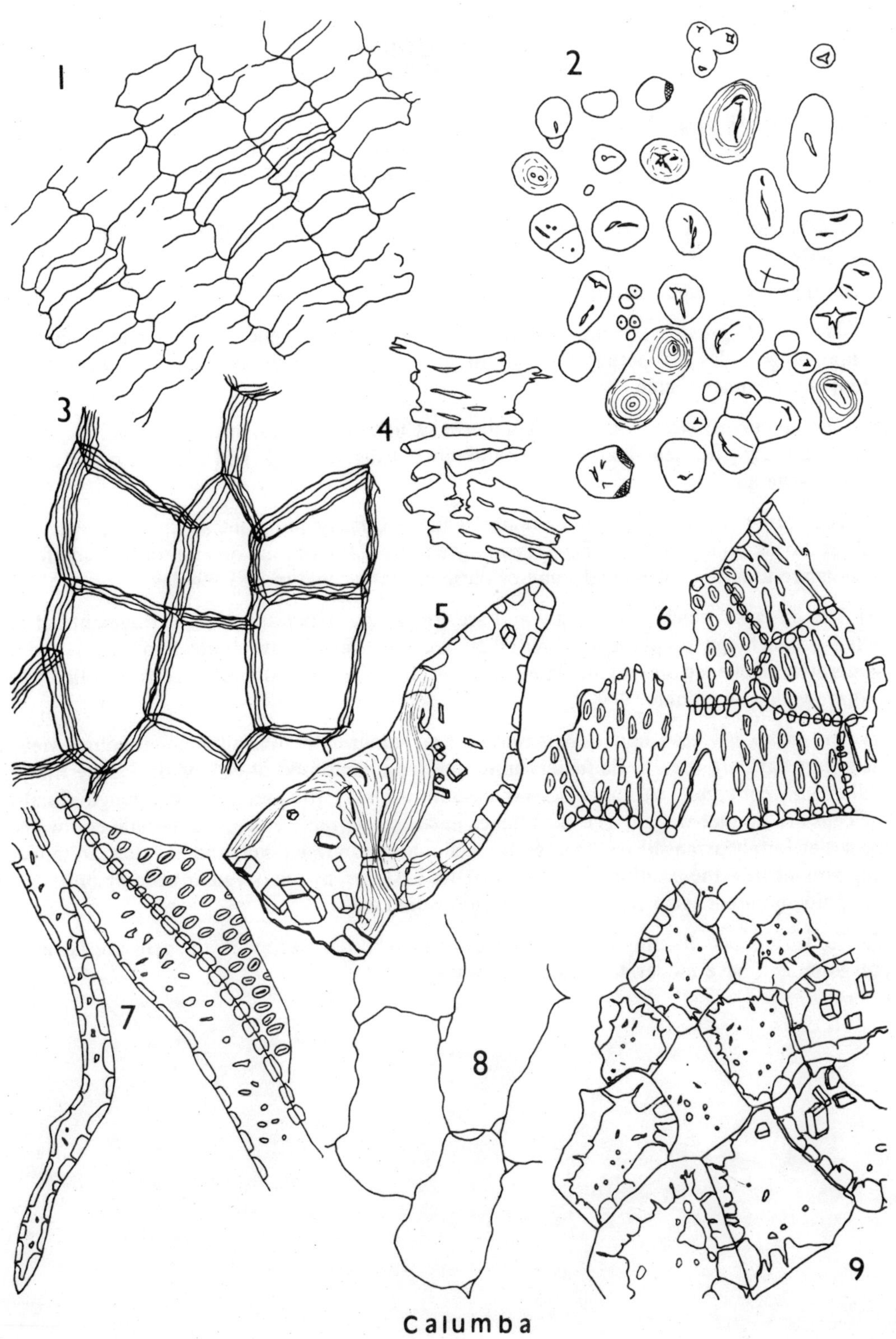

Calumba

×330

1 Cork in sectional view.
2 Starch granules.
3 Cork in surface view.
4 Fragment of a reticulately thickened vessel.
5 Large sclereids with unevenly thickened walls and containing prisms of calcium oxalate.
6 Fragments of bordered pitted vessels.
7 Fibres associated with a bordered pitted vessel.
8 Parenchyma.
9 Part of a group of sclereids.

CANELLA

Canella alba Murray — Canellaceae

Canella Bark, Wild Cinnamon Bark

A bright yellowish-fawn powder with an aromatic odour reminiscent of eucalyptus and a pungent, slightly bitter taste.

The diagnostic characters are:

(*a*) The *starch granules*, mainly simple and rather small, spherical to slightly polyhedral; compound granules also occur with two, three, four or more components; a small point or cleft hilum is sometimes visible.

(*b*) The abundant *sclereids* of the phelloderm, which occur singly or in small groups; they are large and heavily thickened on the inner and radial walls; the thickened walls are pitted and show marked striations.

(*c*) The *cluster crystals of calcium oxalate*, which are fairly abundant; many are present in the cells of the medullary rays and these crystals are fairly regular in size and uniformly radiate; other crystals are found scattered and some of these are larger and more irregular.

(*d*) The *oil cells*, which occur singly and are frequently found adherent to fragments of large-celled parenchyma or phloem tissue; they are very large, subspherical to ovoid and have moderately thickened and slightly lignified walls. In uncleared mounts the cells are filled with oil and are yellow in colour.

(*e*) The *medullary rays* and *sieve tissue* of the phloem. In tangential longitudinal view the medullary rays are seen to be mainly uniseriate and composed of cells with slightly thickened walls, many containing cluster crystals of calcium oxalate; when seen in radial longitudinal view the cells are thinner-walled. The sieve tubes have considerably elongated oblique end walls and the scalariformly arranged sieve plates are well marked in radial longitudinal view; in tangential longitudinal view the position of the sieve plates is shown by the irregular beading on the walls. The phloem parenchyma is composed of thin-walled cells.

(*f*) The very occasional fragments of pale brown *cork*; in surface view the cells are fairly large, polygonal and have moderately thickened walls.

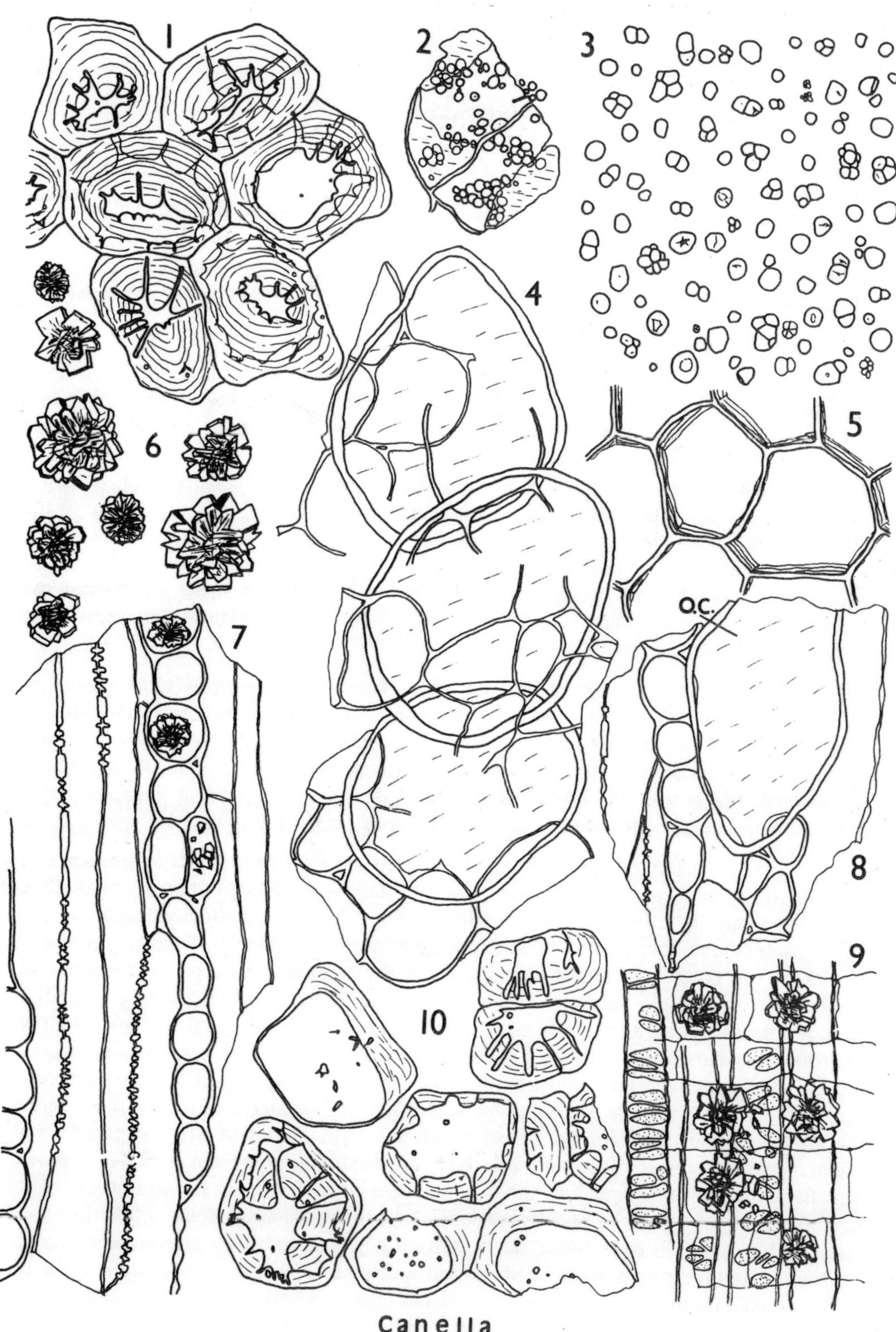

Canella

×330

1 Part of a group of sclereids in surface view showing the moderately thickened radial walls and heavily thickened inner walls.
2 Parenchymatous cells containing starch granules.
3 Starch granules.
4 Oil cells with adherent parenchyma.
5 Cork in surface view.
6 Calcium oxalate cluster crystals.
7 Part of the phloem in tangential longitudinal section showing parts of medullary rays with some of the cells containing cluster crystals of calcium oxalate, and adjacent sieve tubes with beading on the oblique end walls.
8 Part of the phloem in tangential longitudinal section showing part of an oil cell (o.c.).
9 Part of the phloem in radial longitudinal section showing the medullary ray cells, some containing cluster crystals of calcium oxalate, and the underlying sieve tubes with scalariformly arranged sieve plates.
10 Sclereids in surface and side views.

CANNABIS

Cannabis sativa L. Cannabaceae

Cannabis, Cannabis Indica, Ganjah, Gauza, Hemp, Indian Hemp

Indian hemp usually occurs as green to brown flattened masses which are hard and resinous. If reduced to a powder the product is brown to greenish-brown with a heavy, characteristic odour and a slight taste.

The diagnostic characters are:

(*a*) The fragments of the *bracts in surface view*. The *upper epidermis* is composed of straight-walled polygonal cells with a faintly striated cuticle; short, conical, unicellular cystolithic trichomes are present and these are very much enlarged at the base, with the calcium carbonate deposits well-defined; a few small glandular trichomes also occur; the cells of the underlying palisade are small and closely packed and an occasional one of these cells contains a cluster crystal of calcium oxalate. The *lower epidermis* is composed of smaller cells than those of the upper epidermis and the walls are distinctly sinuous; very numerous *anomocytic stomata* are present; glandular trichomes are also fairly frequent. Occasional fragments of the *bracts* are also found *in sectional view* showing a single-layered palisade beneath the upper epidermis; the palisade cells which contain calcium oxalate cluster crystals are frequently divided tangentially to form two smaller cells with a crystal in each.

(*b*) The fragments of the *bracteoles in surface view*. The *upper epidermis* is composed of polygonal cells with unevenly thickened and beaded walls. The cells of the *lower epidermis* are smaller than those of the upper epidermis; the walls are more sinuous and only slightly thickened and beaded; anomocytic stomata are present and also numerous short, conical, unicellular covering trichomes which are wide at the base and taper abruptly to a point at the apex. Small cluster crystals of calcium oxalate are present in the mesophyll cells underlying both epidermises.

(*c*) The very abundant *trichomes*; these are found scattered and some of the smaller ones are also found attached to fragments of the epidermises. The *covering trichomes* are of various types; they are all conical and unicellular but some are cystolithic while others do not contain cystoliths. The cystolithic trichomes are either very short and much enlarged at the base (as seen on the upper epidermis of the bract) or large, much elongated, not exceptionally enlarged at the base and having a distinctly warted wall (as seen on the epidermis of the stem); the covering trichomes which do not contain cystoliths are also of two main types, some being fairly short, slightly enlarged at the base and abruptly tapering to the apex whilst others are larger, more elongated with little enlargement at the base and gradually tapering to the apex. All types of covering trichomes are fairly abundant. The *glandular trichomes* are very distinct and characteristic; these also show some variation in form but those which are most abundant are composed of a multicellular, multiseriate stalk with a multicellular head containing from eight to twelve or more radiating cells; the stalks are cylindrical, three to five cells in diameter and the constituent cells are elongated with slightly thickened walls; the stalks are constricted at the apex so that the head may be attached by two cells only; these 'neck' cells usually contain brown pigmented material even in a cleared mount; the cells of the head are thin-walled and have a common cuticle which is raised to form a bladder-like covering but this is rather indistinct and frequently broken; in the powder the heads, including the 'neck' cells, are frequently found detached from the stalks. Other, less commonly occurring, glandular trichomes are much smaller and have a uniseriate stalk composed of one or two cells and a spherical head with from one to four or, occasionally, eight cells.

(*d*) The fragments of the *stigmas* which are fairly abundant; they are orange to reddish-brown and the epidermal cells, which are rather indistinct, are extended to form elongated ***papillae***. These papillae are thin-walled, cylindrical and rounded at the tip; many become detached and are found scattered in the powder.

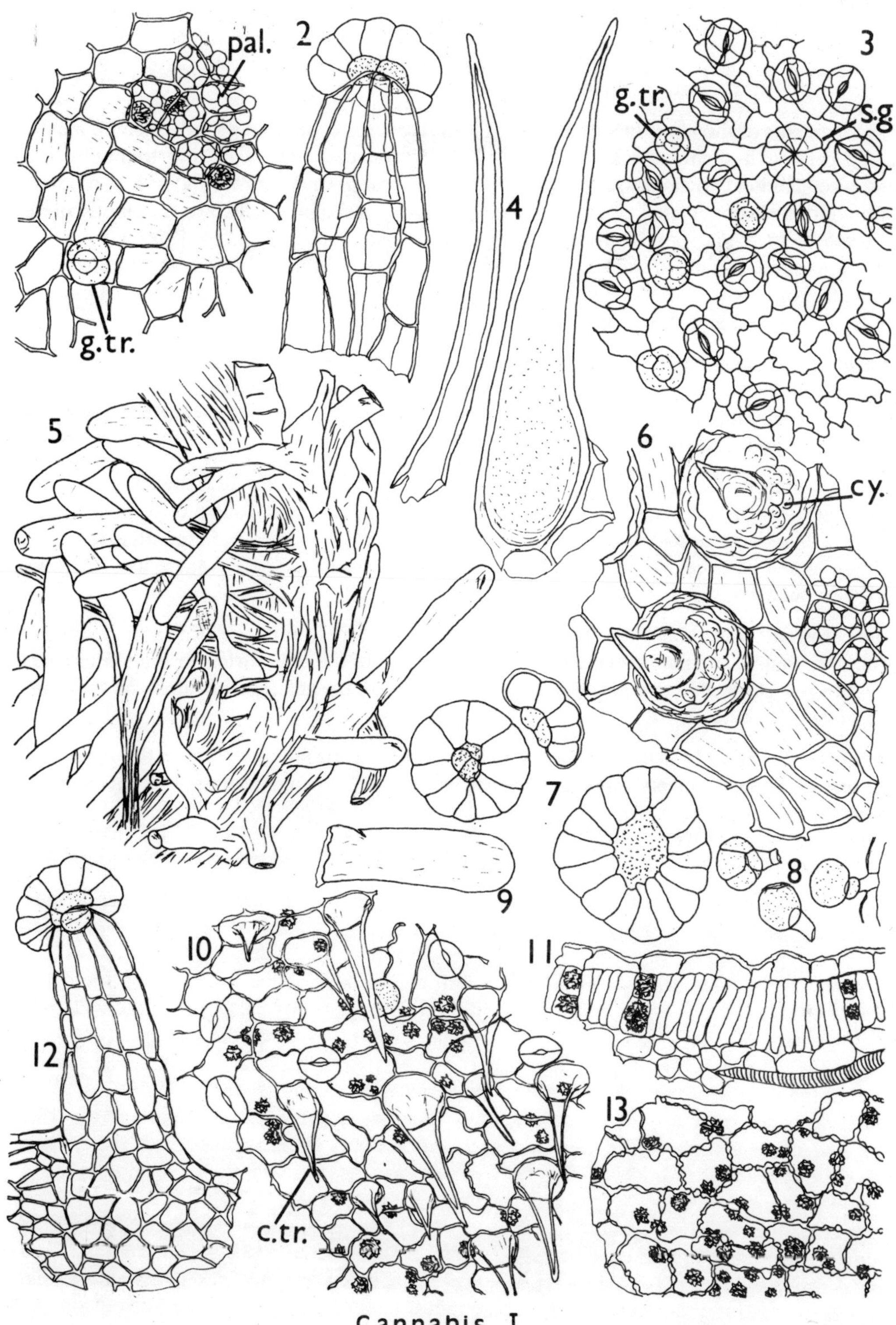

Cannabis I

×330

1 Upper epidermis of a bract in surface view showing faint cuticular striations, a small glandular trichome (g.tr.) and part of the underlying palisade (pal.) with some of the cells containing crystals of calcium oxalate.

2 A multicellular, multiseriate glandular trichome.

3 Lower epidermis of a bract in surface view showing anomocytic stomata, a small glandular trichome (g.tr.) and a sessile gland (s.g.).

4 Covering, non-cystolithic trichomes.

5 Part of a stigma showing papillae.

6 Upper epidermis of a bract in surface view showing covering trichomes containing cystoliths (cy.) and part of the underlying palisade.

7 Detached heads from the multicellular glandular trichomes.

8 Small glandular trichomes.

9 Part of a papilla from a stigma.

10 Lower epidermis of a bracteole in surface view showing anomocytic stomata, covering non-cystolithic trichomes (c.tr.) and calcium oxalate crystals in the underlying mesophyll.

11 Part of a bract in sectional view showing calcium oxalate crystals in the palisade.

12 A multicellular, multiseriate glandular trichome attached to an epidermis.

13 Upper epidermis of a bracteole in surface view showing beaded walls and cluster crystals of calcium oxalate in the underlying mesophyll.

(*e*) The fragments of the *stem*. In surface view the *epidermis* is composed of rather small, axially elongated cells with slightly thickened walls; long, warty, cystolithic covering trichomes are present, also glandular trichomes. Fragments of *parenchyma from the cortex* and *pith* also occur; the cells contain cluster crystals of calcium oxalate which, in the pith cells, are frequently quite large; some of the cells show indistinct pitting on the side walls. Occasional *fibres* from the pericycle are found, usually in small groups; individual fibres are thick-walled with few pits; they are unlignified or only very slightly lignified. The *vessels* are fairly large and occur in small groups; the walls are lignified and show annular or reticulate thickening.

(*f*) The *laticiferous tissue* from the stem and larger veins of the bracts and bracteoles; this consists of elongated, unbranched, thin-walled tubes containing dark orange-brown granular secretion; this tissue is usually found associated with thin-walled parenchyma containing cluster crystals of calcium oxalate and with small, lignified vessels of the xylem.

(*g*) The *sclerenchymatous layer of the pericarp* in surface view. When viewed from above the cells are very thick-walled and markedly sinuous, with striations and numerous pits. When viewed from below there is no apparent lumen and the surface is covered with minute, circular pits; a fairly large lumen becomes visible on focusing slightly downwards. These fragments are brown and not very numerous.

(*h*) The occasional fragments of the *perigone* from the immature fruits in surface view, composed of small, very thin-walled parenchymatous cells. The shape of the cells varies; in some fragments the cells are straight-walled and polygonal, in others they are irregularly elongated and the walls may be markedly sinuous.

(*i*) The *cluster crystals of calcium oxalate*, which are found scattered as well as in the parenchymatous tissues. Some of the crystals show a dense centre with a regular radiating arrangement of the components.

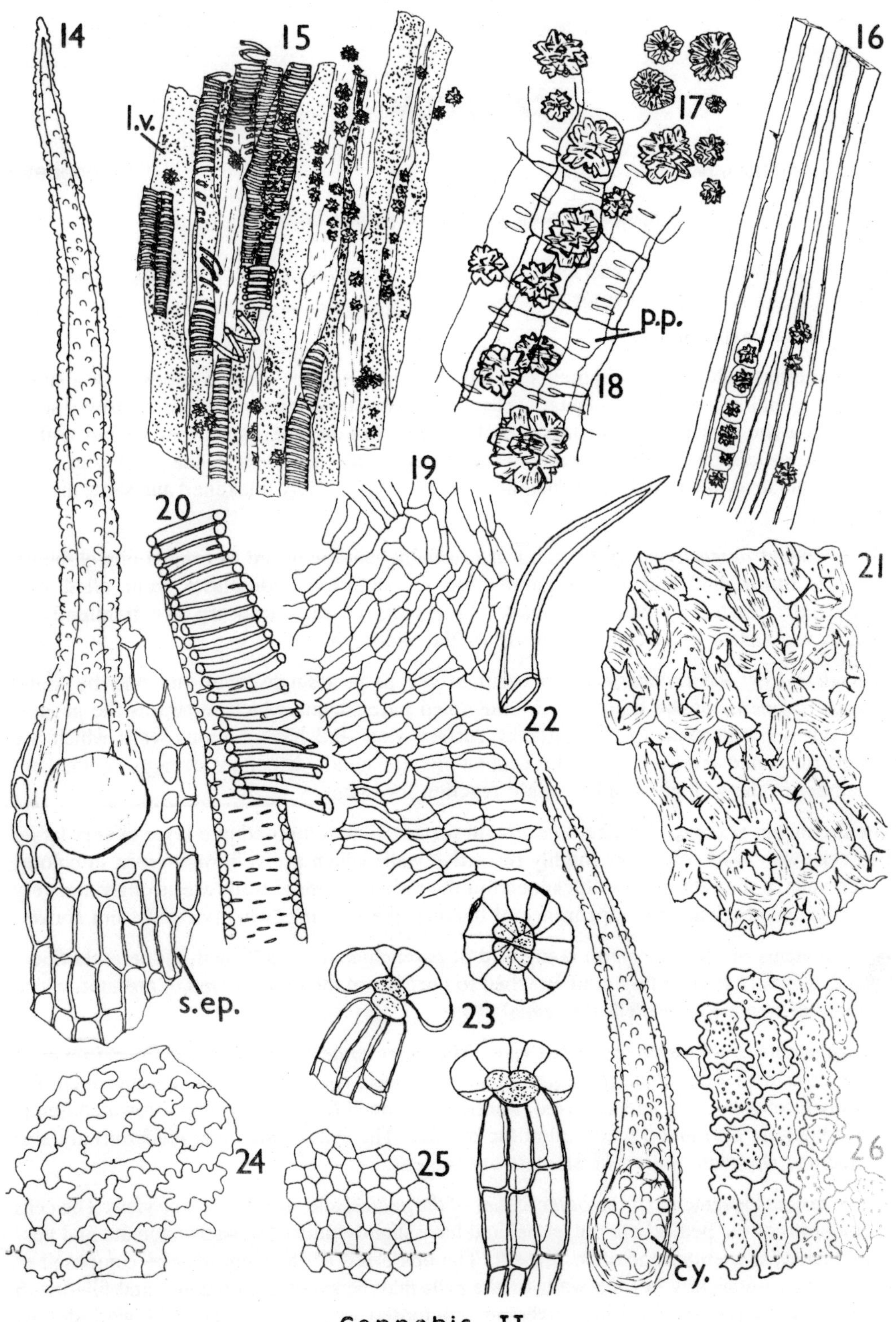

Cannabis II

×330

14 Part of the epidermis of the stem (s.ep.) in surface view with an attached warty-walled covering trichome.

15 Laticiferous tissue (l.v.) from the stem in longitudinal view, with associated vessels and parenchyma containing cluster crystals of calcium oxalate.

16 Part of a group of pericyclic fibres from the stem with associated parenchyma containing cluster crystals of calcium oxalate.

17 Cluster crystals of calcium oxalate.

18 Pith from the stem in longitudinal view showing pitted parenchyma (p.p.) and large cluster crystals of calcium oxalate.

19 Elongated parenchyma of the perigone.

20 Annularly and reticulately thickened vessels from the stem.

21 Sclerenchymatous layer of the pericarp in surface view, from above.

22 Covering trichomes, one warty-walled and containing a cystolith (cy.).

23 Fragments of multicellular, multiseriate glandular trichomes.

24 Sinuous-walled parenchyma of the perigone.

25 Polygonal, straight-walled parenchyma of the perigone.

26 Sclerenchymatous layer of the pericarp in surface view, from below.

CAPSICUM

Capsicum minimum Roxb. Solanaceae

Capsicum Fruits, Cayenne Pepper, Chillies

An orange-red powder with a slight, characteristic odour and a very pungent taste; it is strongly sternutatory and is irritant to the skin and mucous membranes.

The diagnostic characters are:

(*a*) The numerous pale yellow fragments of the *epicarp in surface view*, composed of a single layer of polygonal to slightly elongated cells which are sometimes arranged in rows; some fragments show the presence of a strongly striated *cuticle* but on others striations are not visible. The walls are usually moderately thickened and may be more or less beaded; on occasional fragments (from near the base of the fruit) the walls are considerably thickened and show distinct pits.

(*b*) The abundant *parenchyma of the mesocarp*, usually containing red to orange oily globules; the cells are thin-walled and are frequently broken; occasional idioblasts occur filled with *microsphenoidal crystals of calcium oxalate*. Fragments of the mesocarp are frequently in sectional view attached to part of the epicarp or the endocarp.

(*c*) The *sclereids of the endocarp* which occur in groups in a single layer and may be found attached to fragments of the thin-walled, unlignified parenchyma which separates the groups. The sclereids are polygonal to elongated in surface view and have sinuous walls which are moderately thickened and have numerous distinct pits; the middle lamella is strongly lignified but the remainder of the wall gives only a slight reaction for lignin.

(*d*) The fragments of the *epidermis of the testa* in surface view composed of a layer of very large, lignified cells with markedly wavy, highly refractive walls which are yellowish-green in colour. The outer walls of the cells are not thickened but the radial and inner walls are strongly and very unevenly thickened, giving the appearance of balloon-like swellings when viewed from above.

(*e*) The fragments of the *endosperm* composed of parenchymatous cells with moderately thickened walls; these are frequently found attached to portions of the *parenchyma of the testa*, which is composed of small, thin-walled, polygonal cells.

(*f*) The fragments of the *calyx in surface view*. The *inner epidermis* is composed of thin-walled elongated cells with numerous *glandular trichomes*, each trichome having a unicellular (or occasionally bicellular) stalk and an ovoid, multicellular head filled with yellow-brown contents; these trichomes are also found scattered in the powder. The cells of the *outer epidermis* are also thin-walled and abundant *anisocytic stomata* are present.

(*g*) The occasional fragments of the *outer tissues of the pedicel* and *stem* in surface view. The cells of the epidermis of the pedicel are polygonal and have slightly thickened walls; stomata and very occasional *covering trichomes* may be present. The epidermis of the stem may be composed of elongated cells with slightly beaded walls or the cells may be smaller, polygonal and filled with brown pigment; uniseriate covering trichomes composed of two or three cells with slightly thickened and warty walls are fairly frequent; these trichomes may also be found scattered in the powder.

(*h*) The very occasional rounded *sclereids* from the remains of the thalamus; these are found in groups and have moderately thickened walls and scattered pits.

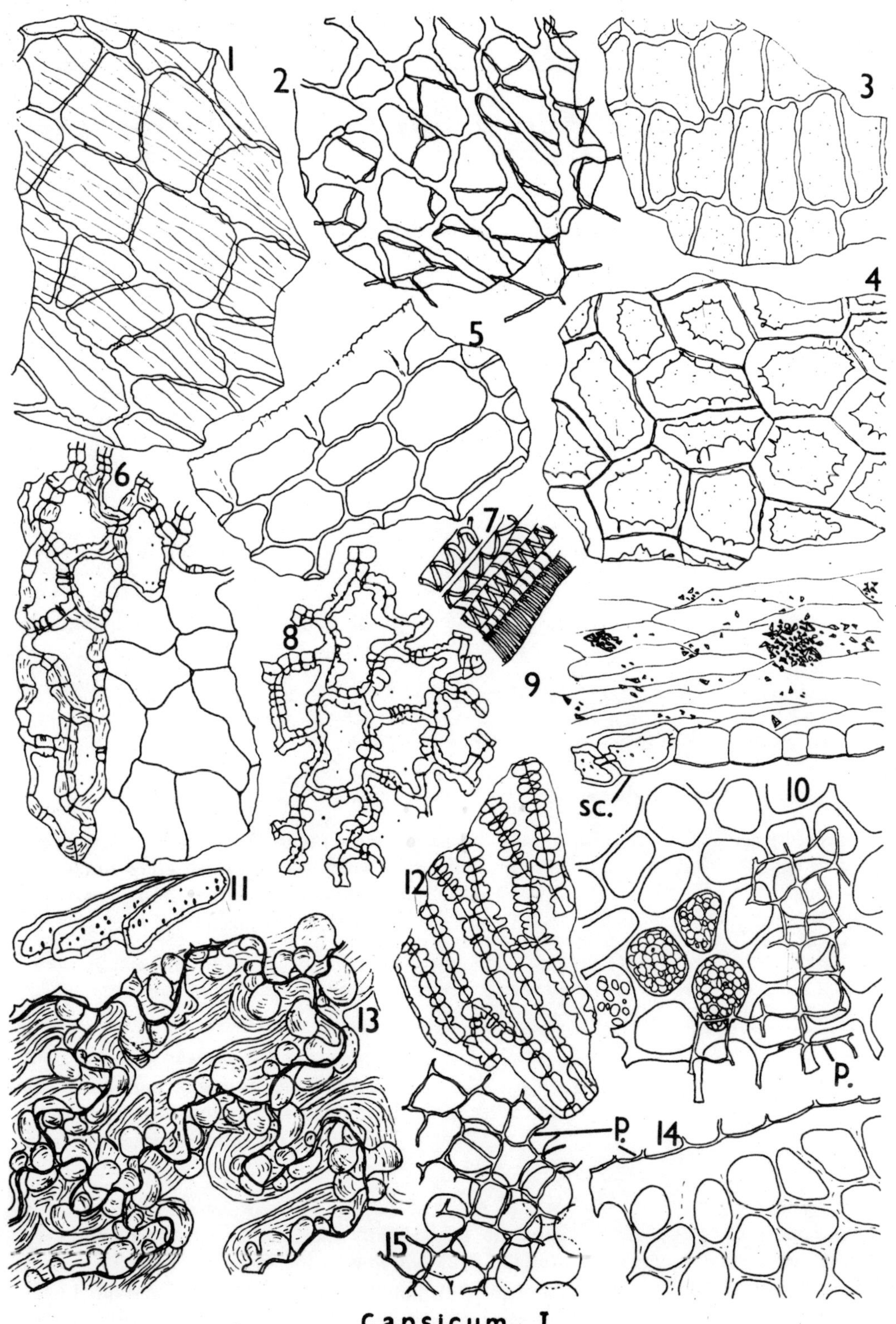

Capsicum I

×330

1 Epicarp in surface view showing cuticular striations.
2 Epicarp and part of the underlying mesocarp in surface view.
3 Epicarp in surface view showing the cells arranged in rows.
4 Epicarp from near the base of the fruit in surface view.
5 Part of the epicarp and underlying mesocarp in sectional view.
6 Sclereids of the endocarp with adjacent parenchyma, in surface view.
7 Part of a group of vessels.
8 Sclereids of the endocarp in surface view.
9 Endocarp and part of the mesocarp in sectional view, showing sclereids (sc.) in the endocarp and cells of the mesocarp containing microsphenoidal crystals of calcium oxalate.
10 Endosperm with part of the overlying parenchyma of the testa (p.) in surface view.
11 Sclereids of the endocarp in oblique longitudinal view.
12 Elongated sclereids of the endocarp in surface view.
13 Epidermis of the testa in surface view.
14 Endosperm and part of the parenchyma of the testa (p.) in sectional view.
15 Parenchyma ot the testa (p.) and underlying endosperm in surface view.

(*i*) The occasional *vessels* and *fibres* from the stem and pedicel. The vessels are small, lignified and spirally or annularly thickened; they occur in small groups. The fibres are thin-walled and only slightly lignified.

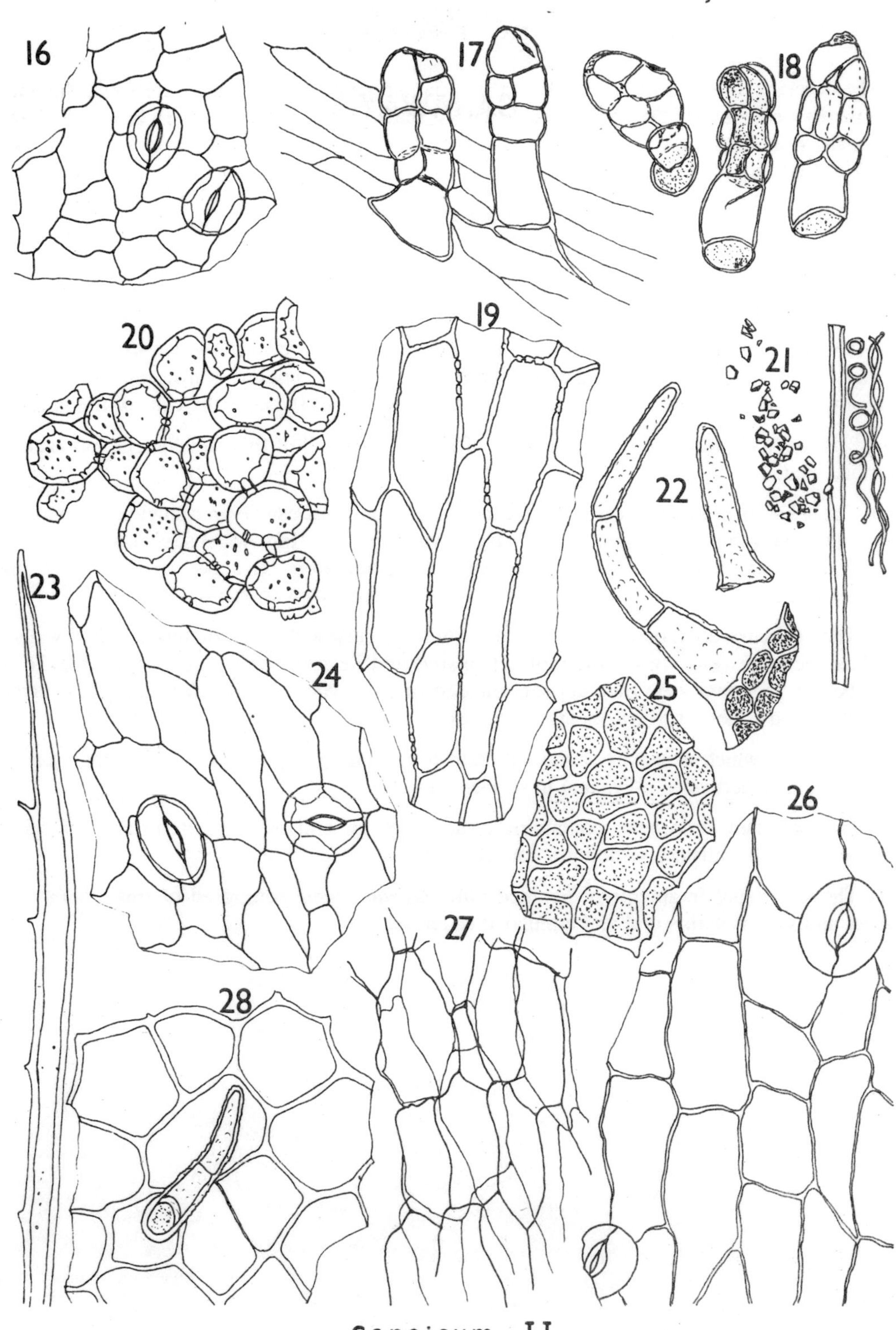

Capsicum II

×330

16 Outer epidermis of the calyx in surface view showing stomata.
17 Inner epidermis of the calyx in surface view showing glandular trichomes.
18 Glandular trichomes from the calyx.
19 Epidermis of the stem in surface view showing elongated cells with beaded walls.
20 Sclereids from the thalamus.
21 Microsphenoidal calcium oxalate crystals and adjacent fibro-vascular tissue from the stem or pedicel.
22 Covering trichomes from the stem.
23 Part of a fibre from the stem or pedicel.
24 Outer epidermis of the calyx in surface view showing stomata.
25 Epidermis of the stem in surface view showing pigmented cells.
26 Epidermis of the pedicel in surface view showing stomata.
27 Parenchyma of the mesocarp in longitudinal view.
28 Epidermis of the pedicel in surface view showing a covering trichome.

CARAWAY

Carum carvi L. Umbelliferae

Caraway Fruits

A dark brown powder with a characteristic, aromatic odour and taste.

The diagnostic characters are:

(*a*) The *epicarp* composed of a layer of rather indistinct, colourless cells with a striated *cuticle*; in surface view the cells are elongated with thin, somewhat sinuous walls; *stomata* are fairly numerous and are orientated with their long axes parallel to those of the cells of the epicarp.

(*b*) The fairly numerous brown fragments of *vittae* composed of thin-walled cells, polygonal in surface view.

(*c*) The *sclereids of the mesocarp* which occur in large groups, usually in a single layer and often associated with thin-walled, unlignified parenchymatous cells. Individual sclereids are rectangular to subrectangular in outline and the walls are moderately thickened in some cells, more heavily thickened in others, with numerous regularly spaced, well marked pits.

(*d*) The *endocarp* composed of a layer of fairly large cells with thin, slightly lignified walls. In surface view the cells are considerably elongated and lie with their long axes parallel to one another; in sectional view they appear rounded or somewhat radially elongated. This layer is usually found adherent to fragments of the testa.

(*e*) The *testa*, which is usually found adherent to the endocarp, composed of a single layer of brown, thin-walled cells, polygonal in surface view.

(*f*) The abundant *endosperm* containing *aleurone grains* and *microrosette crystals of calcium oxalate*; the cell walls are sometimes considerably thickened.

(*g*) The occasional fragments of lignified *fibro-vascular tissue* composed of small, thin-walled fibres and vessels with spiral and annular thickening.

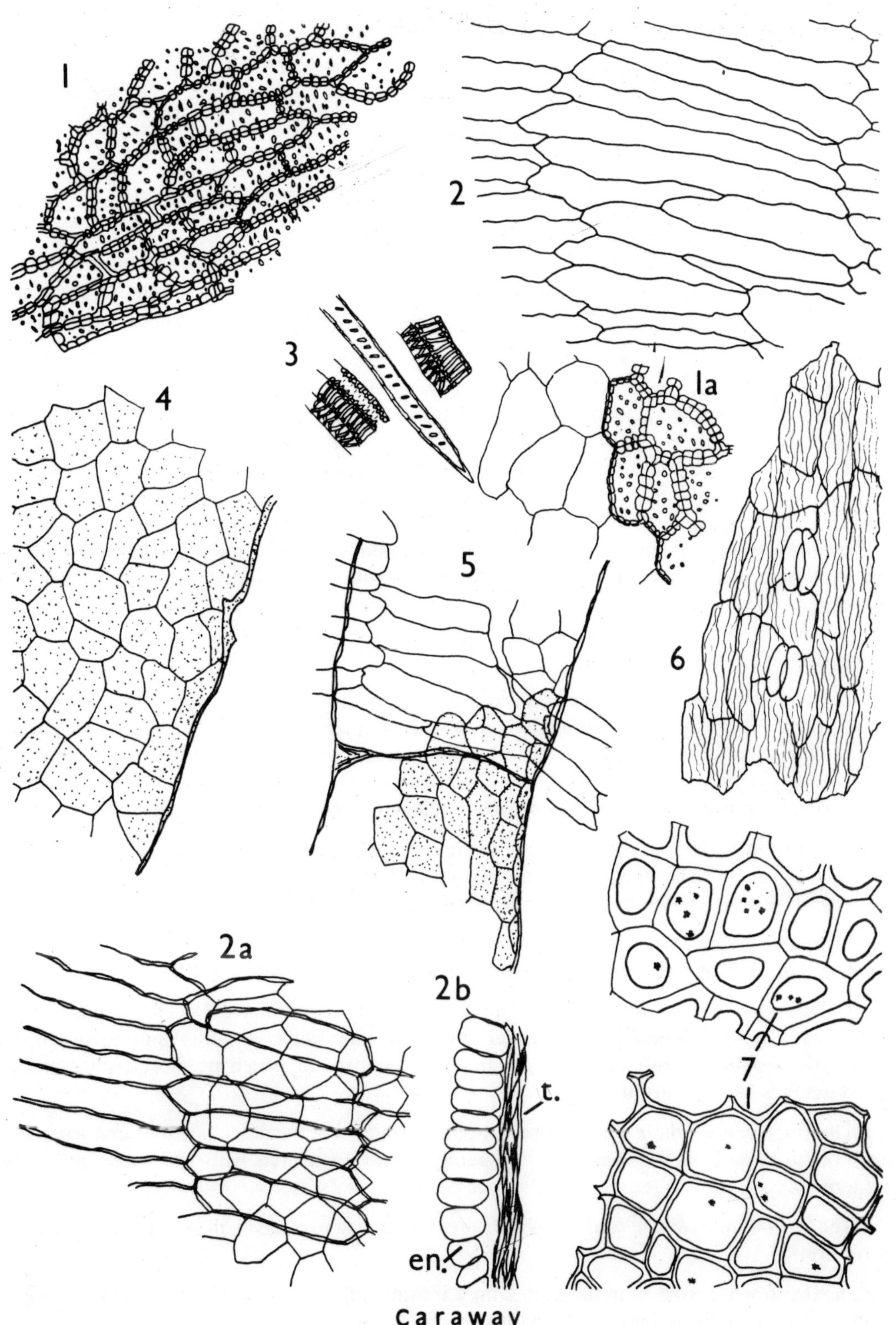

Caraway

×330

1 Part of a group of sclereids from the mesocarp.
1a Thicker-walled sclereids with adjacent thin-walled parenchyma.
2 Endocarp in surface view.
2a Endocarp in surface view with underlying testa.
2b Endocarp (en.) and testa (t.) in sectional view.
3 Elements of the fibro-vascular tissue.
4 Fragment of a vitta.
5 Part of a vitta showing a transverse septum, with underlying endocarp in surface view.
6 Epicarp in surface view showing stomata and striated cuticle.
7 Endosperm containing microrosette crystals of calcium oxalate.

CARDAMOM

Elettaria cardamomum Maton var. *minuscula* Burkill — Zingiberaceae

Cardamom Seeds

A greyish-brown powder with darker brown specks; it is gritty in texture and the odour and taste are aromatic, pleasant and characteristic.

The diagnostic characters are:

(*a*) The very abundant *starch granules*, a few of which are found scattered but the majority occur in dense masses filling the cells of the perisperm. Individual granules are very small and angular; a hilum is not visible.

(*b*) The *sclerenchymatous layer of the testa* composed of a single layer of thick-walled cells which, in a mature seed, are dark reddish-brown in colour; each cell contains a *nodule of silica*. When seen in surface view the cells are polygonal and, if viewed from above, the walls appear only moderately thickened and the silica nodules are clearly visible; when viewed from below the cells appear much thicker-walled and the lumen is somewhat uneven. Occasional fragments of this layer may be found in sectional view showing the cells to be columnar; the inner and radial walls are strongly thickened with the thickening on the radial walls tapering off towards the outside giving a funnel-shaped lumen; the silica nodule almost fills the expanded portion of the lumen at the upper end.

Fragments of this layer from immature seeds are pale brown in colour and in surface view the lumen appears markedly uneven.

(*c*) The abundant fragments of the *epidermis of the testa*, usually seen in surface view, composed of a layer of yellowish-brown prosenchymatous cells with moderately thickened, pitted walls; in sectional view the cells appear more or less isodiametric. Underlying the epidermis, fragments of the *hypodermis* are occasionally seen composed of a single layer of elongated cells with extremely thin walls, lying with their long axes at right angles to those of the epidermal cells.

(*d*) The *oil cells of the testa* consisting of a single layer of large, polygonal to rectangular cells with slightly thickened walls and containing globules of volatile oil. This layer is usually found associated with the epidermis and hypodermis.

(*e*) The *parenchyma of the testa* composed of several layers of small cells, polygonal in surface view, with dark brown contents and slightly thickened, heavily pitted walls.

(*f*) The abundant *parenchyma of the perisperm* and *endosperm* composed of closely packed thin-walled cells. The perisperm cells are densely filled with starch granules and each cell also frequently contains one or more small prisms of calcium oxalate, which are most easily seen after the starch has been removed.

(*g*) The fragments of the *arillus* composed of very thin-walled cells, elongated and irregularly fusiform in surface view. These are frequently found associated with the fragments of the epidermis.

(*h*) The *prisms of calcium oxalate*, which are found scattered as well as in the cells of the perisperm.

(*i*) The occasional *vessels* from the raphe; they are small, lignified, spirally thickened and usually are found in small groups associated with thin-walled parenchyma.

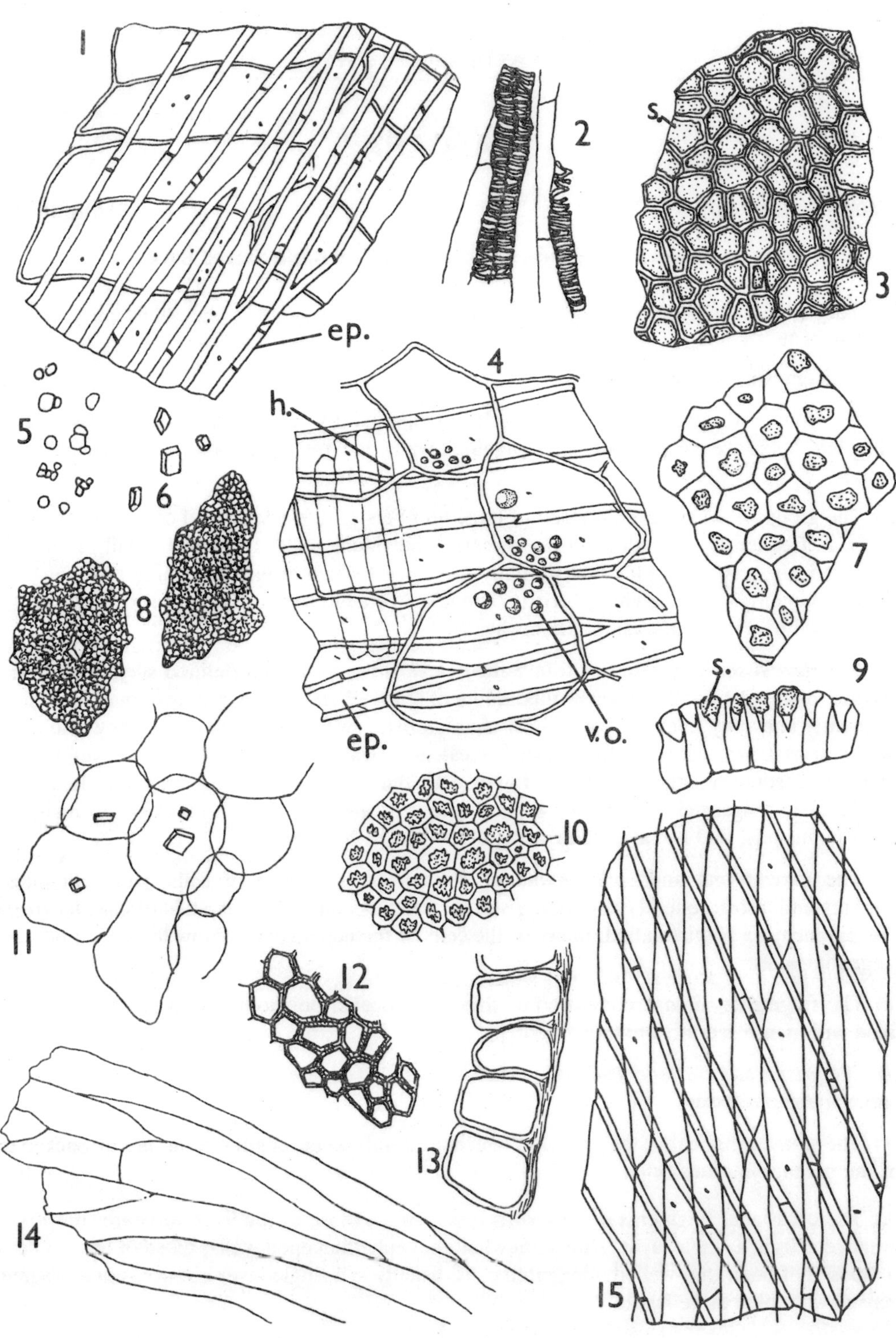

Cardamom

×330

1 Epidermis of the testa (ep.) in surface view with underlying oil cells.

2 A group of spirally thickened vessels and associated parenchyma.

3 Sclerenchymatous layer of the testa in surface view, seen from above, showing silica nodules (s.).

4 Oil cells of the testa in surface view containing globules of volatile oil (v.o.), with underlying hypodermis (h.) and epidermis (ep.).

5 Starch granules.

6 Prisms of calcium oxalate.

7 Sclerenchymatous layer of the testa in surface view, seen from below.

8 Perisperm cells containing starch granules and prisms of calcium oxalate.

9 Part of the sclerenchymatous layer of the testa in sectional view showing silica nodules (s.).

10 Sclerenchymatous layer of the testa from an immature seed, in surface view.

11 Parenchyma of the perisperm from which the starch has been removed, showing prisms of calcium oxalate in some of the cells.

12 Parenchyma of the testa in surface view.

13 Epidermis of the testa in sectional view.

14 Arillus in surface view.

15 Arillus with underlying epidermis of the testa in surface view.

CASCARA

Rhamnus purshianus DC. Rhamnaceae

Cascara Bark, Cascara Sagrada, Chittem Bark, Sacred Bark

A yellowish-brown to reddish-brown powder with a characteristic odour and an intensely bitter and nauseous taste.

The diagnostic characters are:

(*a*) The numerous groups of *fibres*, each surrounded by a calcium oxalate prism sheath; individual fibres are narrow with thick, lignified walls, few pits and a small, often inconspicuous lumen.

(*b*) The groups of *sclereids* composed of large numbers of densely packed cells, the structure of which is frequently very difficult to discern; individual cells are fairly small, rounded to elongated; the walls are thick and partially traversed by numerous, branching pits which open into the lumen giving it a characteristic, irregularly stellate form. The groups of sclereids are surrounded by a calcium oxalate prism sheath.

(*c*) The *sieve tissue* consisting of thin-walled sieve tubes with well defined sieve plates on the oblique end walls, and thicker-walled phloem parenchyma. The parenchymatous cells are frequently unevenly thickened and show characteristic swellings in the walls; they also contain cluster crystals or, occasionally, prisms of calcium oxalate and are filled with yellow-brown contents. *Medullary rays* are usually found with the sieve tissue either in radial longitudinal section or in tangential longitudinal section; the cells are thin-walled, many occasionally show conspicuous pits, and are also filled with yellow-brown contents.

(*d*) The *parenchyma* and *collenchyma* of the cortex composed of cells with yellow-brown contents and also frequently containing starch granules and cluster crystals of calcium oxalate. The parenchyma is thin-walled; many of the cells of the collenchyma show large oval pits in the tangential walls.

(*e*) The fragments of *cork* composed of thin-walled cells, polygonal in surface view; they are filled with dense reddish-brown contents.

(*f*) The *prisms* and *cluster crystals of calcium oxalate*, which are found scattered as well as in the parenchymatous tissues.

(*g*) The small, spherical *starch granules*, which are rarely found scattered but are present in most of the parenchymatous cells.

(*h*) The occasional fragments of *liverworts and mosses*; those of the liverworts are composed of rounded cells in a single layer, with somewhat unevenly thickened walls; those of the mosses are composed of small thin-walled, elongated cells, usually in a single layer but occasional fragments may show two or three layers.

Compare Frangula, page 102.

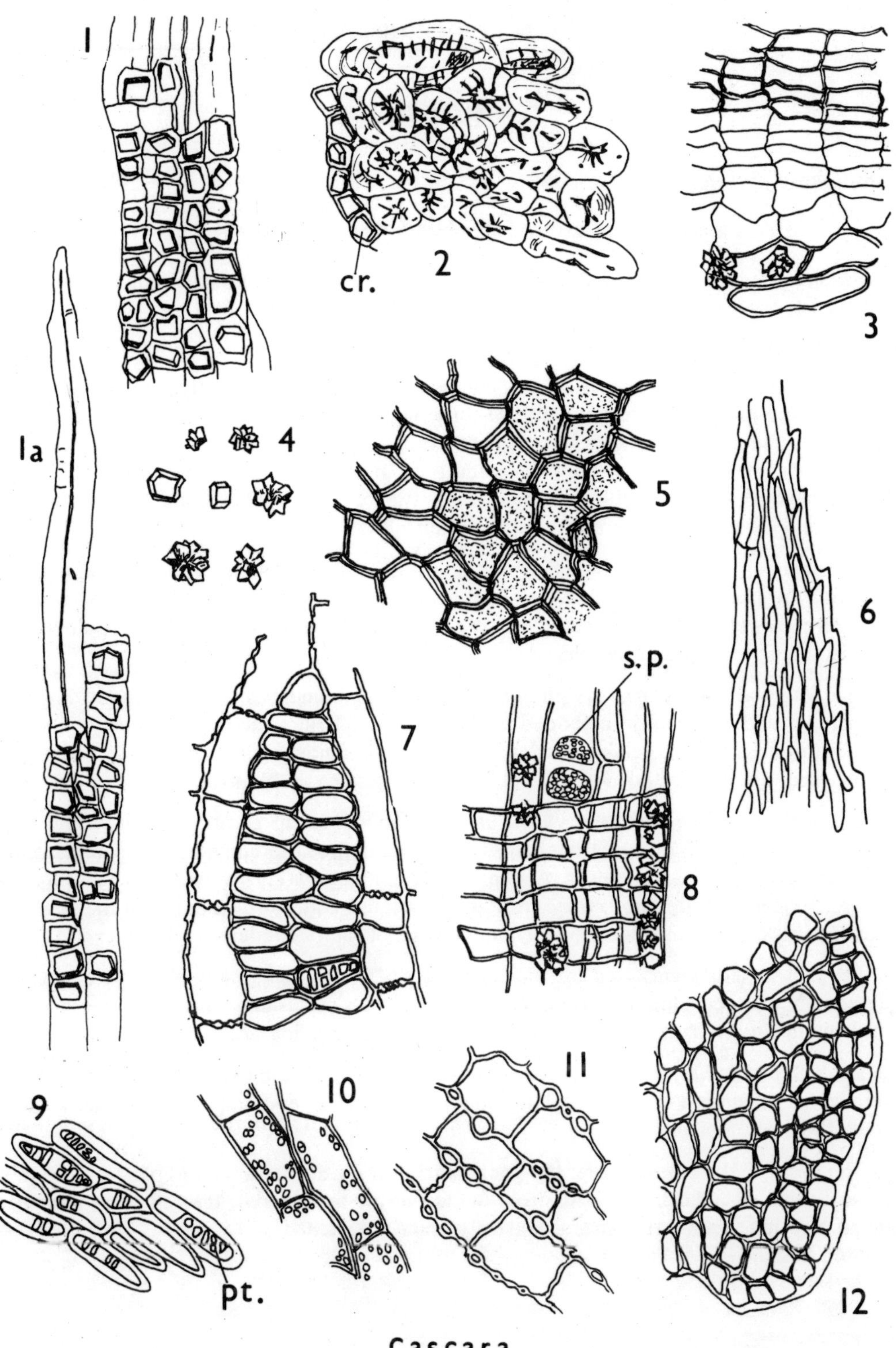

Cascara

×330

1 Part of a group of fibres with calcium oxalate prism sheath.

1a Part of a group of fibres and prism crystal sheath, showing the end of a fibre.

2 Part of a group of sclereids showing a fragment of the crystal sheath (cr.).

3 Part of the cork and cortex in sectional view showing cluster crystals of calcium oxalate in the cortex.

4 Prisms and cluster crystals of calcium oxalate.

5 Cork in surface view.

6 Fragment of a moss.

7 Part of a medullary ray in tangential longitudinal section with associated pitted parenchyma.

8 Part of the phloem in radial longitudinal section showing a sieve tube with sieve plates (s.p.), parenchyma containing cluster crystals of calcium oxalate and a medullary ray.

9 Collenchyma of the cortex showing pits (pt.).

10 Parenchyma containing starch granules.

11 Phloem parenchymatous cells showing swellings in the walls.

12 Fragment of a liverwort.

CASCARILLA

Croton eluteria (L.) W. Wright **Euphorbiaceae**

Cascarilla Bark

A dark, chocolate-brown powder with paler specks; it has an aromatic odour reminiscent of nutmeg and an aromatic, bitter and somewhat pungent taste.

The diagnostic characters are:

(*a*) The very abundant fragments of *cork* composed of lignified cells, polygonal in surface view. The outer and radial walls of the cells are thickened, and adherent to the thin inner walls are numerous small tabular crystals of calcium oxalate; this gives a very characteristic mosaic appearance to the contents of the cells when seen in surface view. Some of the cells contain orange-brown pigment in addition to the calcium oxalate crystals. Occasional fragments are seen in sectional view, but the cells are usually broken.

(*b*) The abundant *secretory tissue*, filled with orange-brown amorphous or, occasionally, granular secretion; the tissue is thin-walled and consists of either single, rounded cells as seen in the phelloderm, or vertical files of rectangular cells as seen in longitudinal views of the phloem; single cells also occur scattered in the phloem.

(*c*) The *fibres*, which occur in the phloem and are fairly numerous; they are found singly or in small groups and are usually embedded in other phloem tissue. The walls are lignified and vary considerably in thickness, being sometimes so thick as to almost occlude the lumen; striations are well marked, but pits are not visible. The ends are rounded or bluntly pointed.

(*d*) The *calcium oxalate crystals*, which are very abundant; in addition to the small *tabular* crystals in the cork cells other, larger *prisms* are found both scattered and in the parenchymatous cells of the phelloderm and phloem. Also present are numerous *cluster crystals* which vary in size and are frequently quite large; they are found scattered and, more usually, in the cells of the medullary rays; a few also occur in the parenchyma of the phelloderm.

(*e*) The thin-walled *parenchyma* and *medullary rays* of the phloem; many of the parenchymatous cells contain orange-yellow secretion. The medullary rays are usually uniseriate and most of the cells contain cluster crystals of calcium oxalate, a few containing granular secretion.

(*f*) The *starch granules*, which are not very abundant; they are mostly simple and spherical to ovoid with a slit-shaped or stellate hilum sometimes visible; a few compound granules occur with two or three components.

(*g*) The occasional *trichomes* from the young bark; they are very large and peltate in form with numerous thin-walled cells radiating from the top of the central axis; the cells are pigmented in the inner region. These trichomes are usually found fragmented.

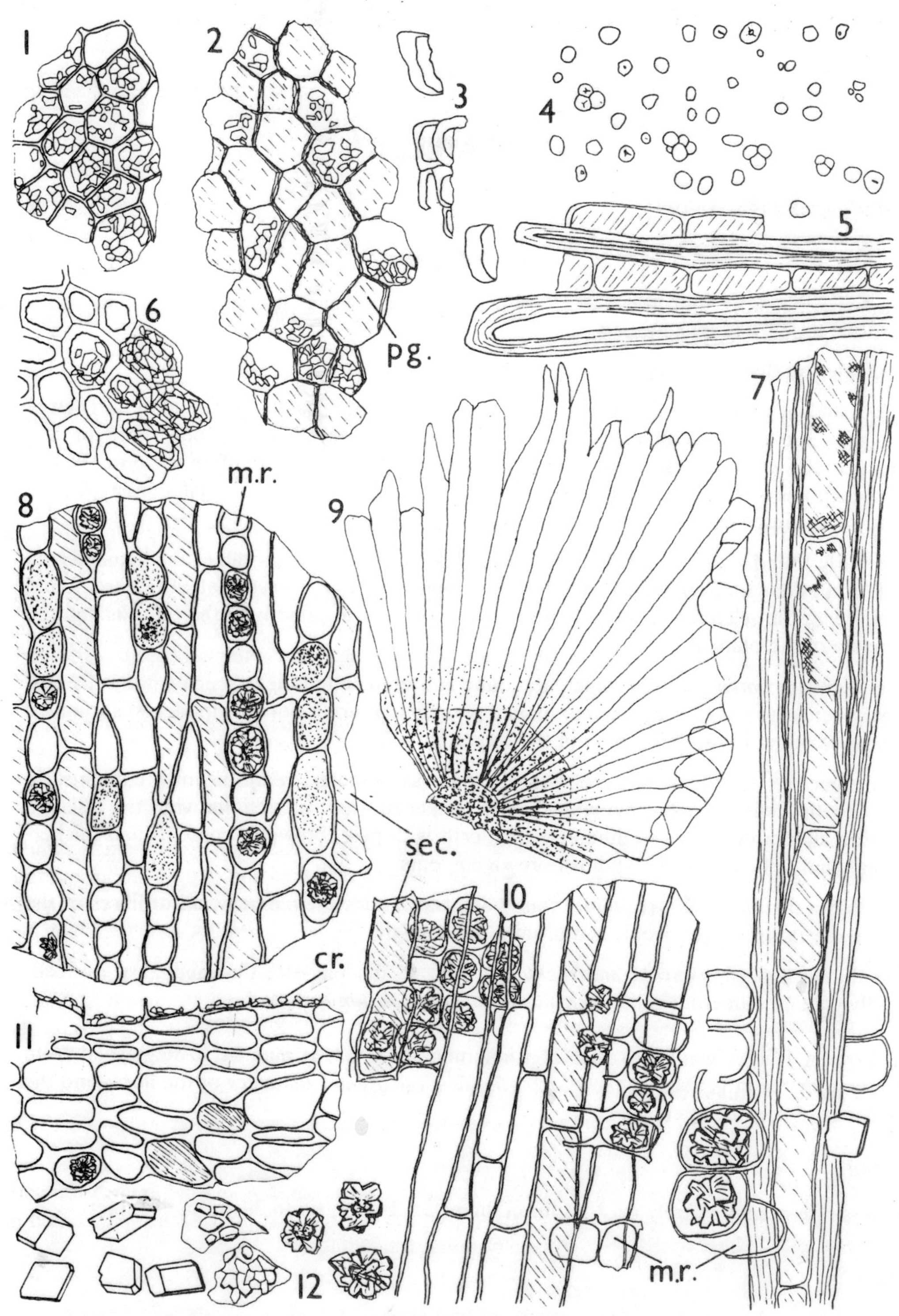

Cascarilla

×330

1 Cork in surface view, inner wall uppermost, with tabular crystals of calcium oxalate.
2 Cork in surface view showing pigment (pg.) in some cells, crystals in others.
3 Fragments of cork cells in sectional view.
4 Starch granules.
5 Parts of two fibres and a file of secretion cells.
6 Cork in surface view, outer wall uppermost, showing the thickened walls and calcium oxalate crystals in some of the cells.
7 Part of a group of fibres with overlying secretion tissue, and part of a medullary ray (m.r.) in radial longitudinal section, some cells containing cluster crystals of calcium oxalate.
8 Phloem in tangential longitudinal section showing secretion tissue (sec.) and uniseriate medullary rays (m.r.) containing secretion and cluster crystals of calcium oxalate.
9 Part of a peltate trichome.
10 Phloem in radial longitudinal section, showing secretion tissues (sec.) and medullary ray cells (m.r.) containing cluster crystals of calcium oxalate.
11 Phelloderm in sectional view showing adherent fragments of cork with tabular crystals (cr.).
12 Prisms and cluster crystals of calcium oxalate and fragments of cork cells containing tabular crystals.

CASSIA

Cinnamomum cassia Blume — Lauraceae

Cassia Bark, Chinese Cinnamon, Cassia Lignea

A reddish-brown powder with a characteristic, pleasant odour similar to that of Cinnamon and a characteristic, slightly mucilaginous taste.

The diagnostic characters are:

(*a*) The abundant *sclereids*, which usually occur singly but more usually are found in fairly large groups; they show considerable variation in size and shape but are usually more or less isodiametric; the walls of most of the cells are moderately thickened and often the outer wall is less thickened than the others; occasional cells have very thick walls with a small lumen; pits are numerous and conspicuous, and striations are usually visible.

(*b*) The fairly abundant *fibres*, which usually occur singly; they are thick-walled and lignified with a small, somewhat uneven lumen and few inconspicuous pits. Occasional fibres are found associated with the sclereids of the pericycle; others occur associated with the oil cells and the parenchyma of the phloem.

(*c*) The abundant *starch granules*, which are found scattered and in the parenchymatous tissues; they are spherical to ovoid, simple or compound with up to four or more components; a rounded or slit-shaped hilum is visible in some of the larger granules.

(*d*) The numerous fragments of *cork* with conspicuous granular, reddish-brown contents. In surface view the cells are polygonal with slightly thickened walls; in sectional view the cells are arranged in alternating layers of thinner-walled cells with pale, brownish contents and thicker-walled lignified cells with dense, reddish-brown contents.

(*e*) The thin-walled *oil cells*, frequently found associated with the parenchyma or fibres of the phloem; the cells are large, ovoid, and usually occur singly.

(*f*) The thin-walled *parenchyma* and *medullary rays* of the phloem; the medullary ray cells frequently contain numerous small, *acicular crystals of calcium oxalate*.

This powder is very similar to that of Cinnamon, page 62; it may be distinguished from Cinnamon by the larger size of the starch granules, the greater diameter of the fibres and the abundance of cork fragments.

Cinnamon

Starch, single granules rarely over 10 μm in diameter. Fibres, up to 30 μm in diameter.

Cassia

Starch, single granules often more than 10 μm in diameter. Fibres, up to 40 μm in diameter.

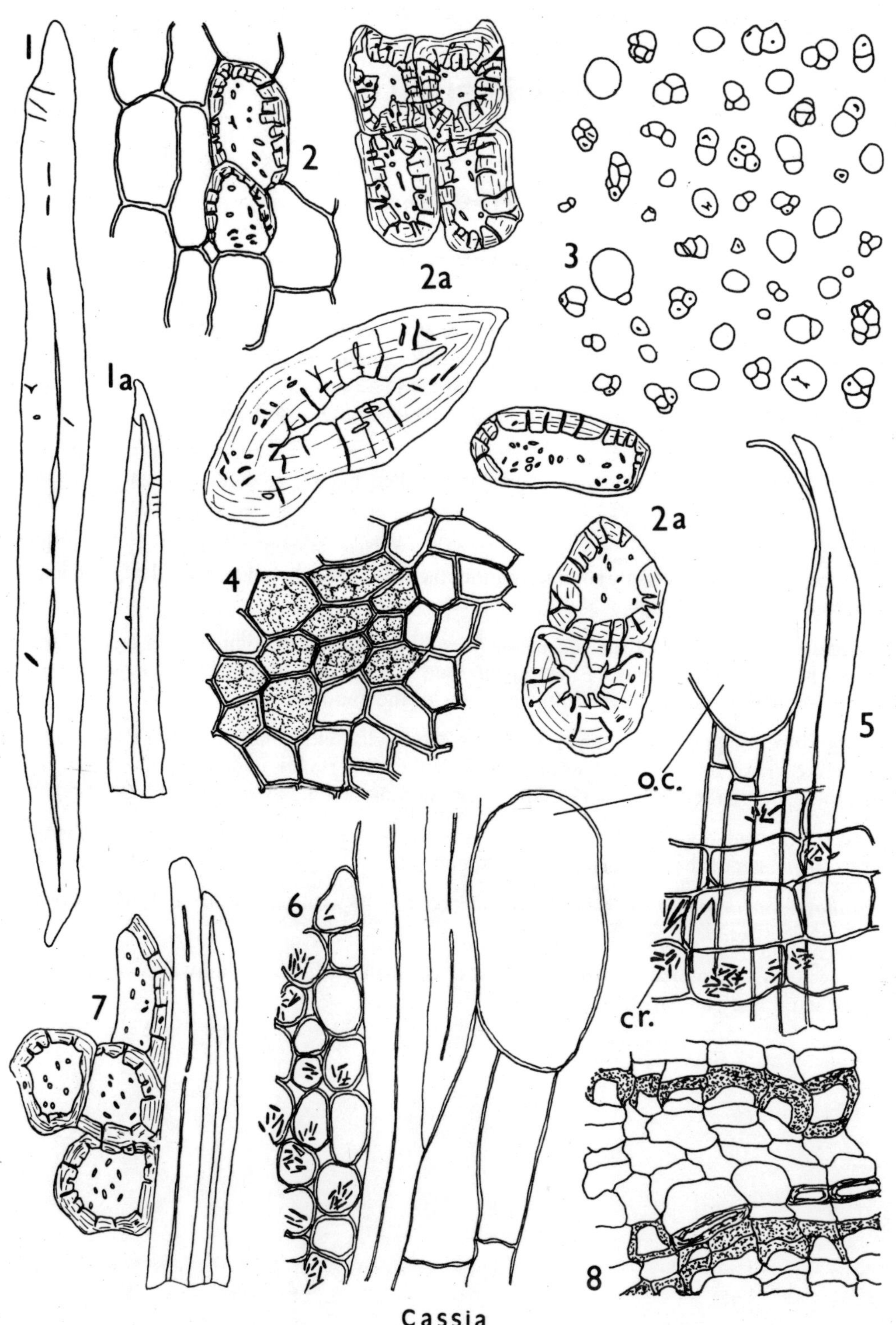

Cassia

×330

1 A single fibre.
1a Part of a fibre.
2 Sclereids with associated parenchymatous cells.
2a Sclereids.
3 Starch granules.
4 Cork in surface view.
5 Part of the phloem in radial longitudinal section showing a fibre, part of an oil cell (o.c.), parenchyma, and a medullary ray with some of the cells containing acicular crystals of calcium oxalate (cr.).
6 Part of the phloem in tangential longitudinal section showing an oil cell (o.c.) with associated fibres and parenchyma, and part of a medullary ray with some of the cells containing acicular crystals of calcium oxalate.
7 Sclereids and fibres of the pericycle.
8 Part of the cork in sectional view showing the alternating layers of thin-walled and thicker-walled cells.

CELERY FRUIT

Apium graveolens L. Umbelliferae

Apium, Celery

A dark brown powder with a characteristic, aromatic odour and taste.

The diagnostic characters are:

(*a*) The *epicarp* composed of a layer of rather indistinct, colourless cells with an irregularly striated *cuticle*; in surface view the cells are somewhat elongated with thin, slightly sinuous walls; *stomata* are fairly frequent and almost circular in outline. The surface of the fruit is uneven and bears small protuberances which are seen on fragments of the epicarp in side view.

(*b*) The fairly numerous dark brown fragments of the *vittae* composed of fairly large cells, polygonal in surface view; the cells are mainly thin-walled but show slight thickening at the corners.

(*c*) The *sclereids of the mesocarp*, which are rather irregularly shaped, varying from ovoid to elongated rectangular with a slightly sinuous outline; the walls are only moderately thickened and have numerous well marked pits.

(*d*) The occasional fragments of the *innermost layer of the mesocarp* composed of large, dark brown parenchymatous cells, elongated rectangular in surface view with slightly thickened walls. This layer is frequently found adherent to fragments of the endocarp.

(*e*) The *endocarp* composed of a layer of thin-walled cells, elongated in surface view and arranged in groups of about six or more cells with their long axes parallel to one another; frequently there are marked differences in the orientation of the long axes of the groups of cells.

(*f*) The *testa* composed of a single layer of brown, thin-walled cells, usually seen in sectional view attached to fragments of the pericarp and endosperm.

(*g*) The *endosperm* composed of thick-walled cells containing *aleurone grains* and *microrosette crystals of calcium oxalate*.

(*h*) The fragments of lignified *fibro-vascular tissue* consisting of small, thin-walled fibres and vessels with spiral and annular thickening.

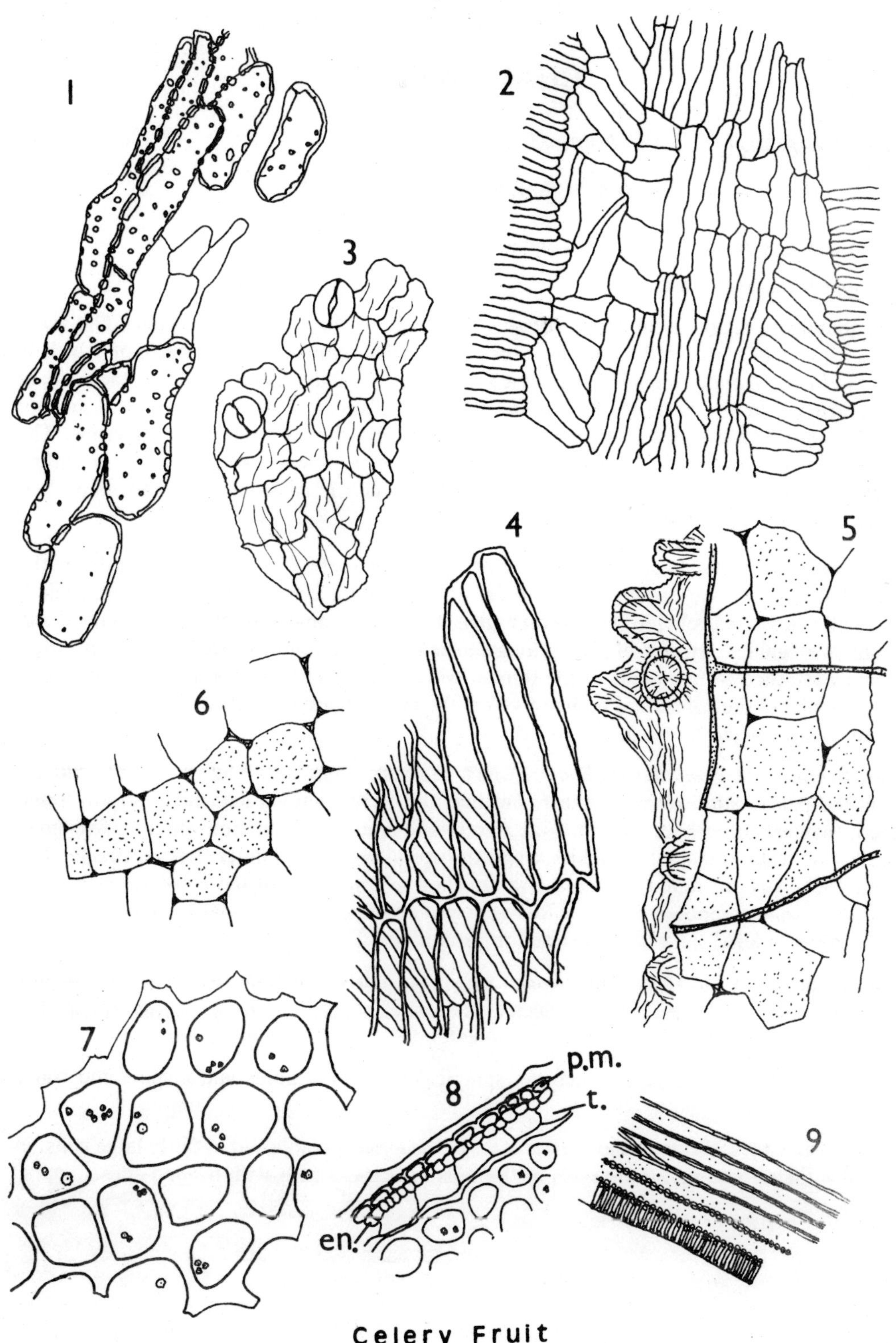

Celery Fruit

×330

1 Sclereids of the mesocarp.
2 Endocarp in surface view.
3 Epicarp in surface view showing stomata and striated cuticle.
4 Part of the innermost layer of the mesocarp in surface view with underlying endocarp.
5 Part of the epicarp in side view with protuberances, and part of a vitta showing transverse septa.
6 Fragment of a vitta.
7 Endosperm containing microrosette crystals of calcium oxalate.
8 Part of the pericarp and seed in sectional view showing the innermost layer of the mesocarp (p.m.), the endocarp (en.), the testa (t.) and the endosperm.
9 Part of a group of fibro-vascular tissue.

CHAMOMILE

Chamaemelum nobile (L.) All. (*Anthemis nobile* L.) Compositae

Chamomile Flowers, Roman Chamomile

A pale buff powder with an aromatic odour and a bitter and aromatic taste.

The diagnostic characters are:

(*a*) The abundant fragments of the *corollas of the ligulate florets in surface view*. The *inner epidermis* is mainly composed of fairly large, thin-walled polygonal cells each of which is extended to form a *papilla* which in surface view appears as a large, distinct circle on each cell; in fragments from near the base of the corolla the cells are smaller, thicker-walled and are not papillose; glandular trichomes occur in the basal region but they are not very numerous. The *outer epidermis* is composed of thin-walled cells which are usually markedly sinuous in outline although straighter-walled cells occur near the base; the *cuticle* is strongly striated; numerous glandular trichomes are present.

(*b*) The fragments of the *paleae* and *involucral bracts in surface view*. Fragments from the margins of the paleae are usually only one cell thick and are composed of very thin-walled, longitudinally elongated cells; in the central region the cells become considerably thickened and pitted and are lignified; groups of these elongated *sclereids* are found scattered in the powder, occasionally attached to fragments of the thinner-walled cells from the margins. The involucral bracts are similar to the paleae but fragments from the basal region frequently show the presence of numerous *anomocytic stomata*.

(*c*) The *covering* and *glandular trichomes*, which are very abundant. The covering trichomes occur on the paleae and involucral bracts but they are nearly always detached and are found scattered; they are uniseriate, conical, with a very long apical cell and from three to five small basal cells; the walls are slightly thickened and the apical cell has a faintly striated cuticle. The glandular trichomes are found scattered and attached to fragments of the corollas; each has a short biseriate stalk composed of two or four cells and a biseriate head, usually composed of two cells; around each head the cuticle is raised to form a bladder-like covering.

(*d*) The fragments of the *styles* and *stigmas*, which are fairly abundant; the styles are mainly composed of thin-walled cells, many of which contain small *cluster crystals of calcium oxalate*; the epidermal cells of the apices of the stigmas are extended to form elongated *papillae*.

(*e*) The occasional *pollen grains*, which are spherical with three pores and a spiny and warty exine.

(*f*) The occasional fragments of the *fibrous layer of the anthers* composed of fairly large cells; in surface view the thickening on the walls of the cells appears as rods with beaded ends.

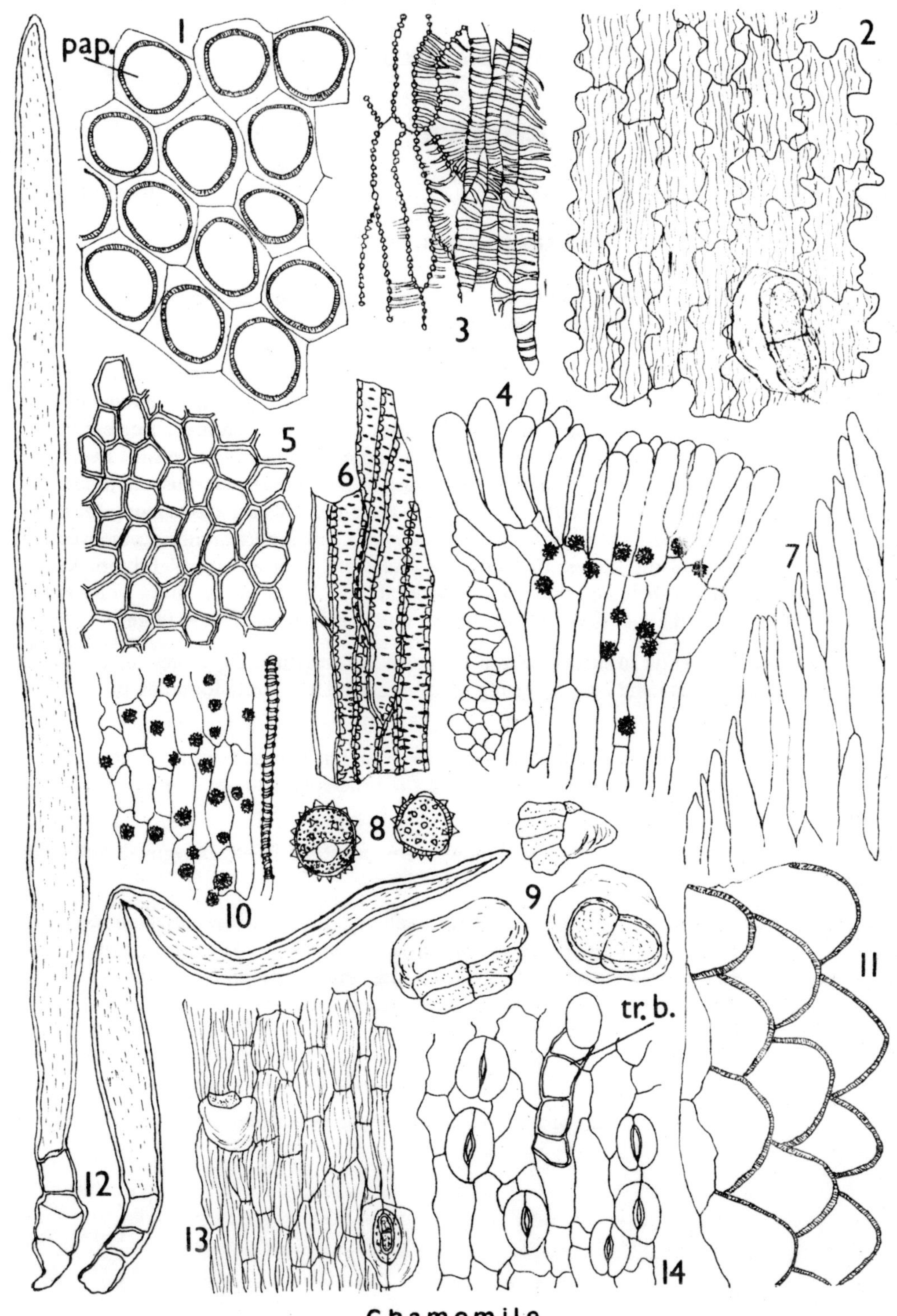

Chamomile

×330

1 Inner epidermis of the corolla in surface view showing papillae (pap.).
2 Outer epidermis of the corolla in surface view showing striations and a glandular trichome.
3 Fibrous layer of the anther in surface view.
4 Papillose stigma and part of the style in surface view with associated cluster crystals of calcium oxalate.
5 Inner epidermis near the base of the corolla in surface view.
6 Sclereids from the central region of a bract or palea.
7 Part of the margin of a palea in surface view.
8 Pollen grains.
9 Glandular trichomes.
10 Part of the inner tissue of the style with cluster crystals of calcium oxalate and part of an annularly thickened vessel.
11 Inner epidermis of the corolla in oblique surface view.
12 Covering trichomes.
13 Outer epidermis near the base of the corolla in surface view.
14 Epidermis from the basal region of a bract in surface view showing stomata and the base of a covering trichome (tr.b.).

CHERVIL

Anthriscus cerefolium (L.) Hoffm. Umbelliferae

Garden Chervil

Usually consists of the fresh leaves and flowering tops. When dried consists of small, bright green fragments of the leaves and inflorescences. Odour and taste slightly aromatic.

The diagnostic characters are:

(*a*) The *upper epidermis of the leaf lamina* composed of cells with thin, slightly sinuous walls in surface view; occasional cells have yellowish-brown amorphous contents; stomata are absent; the underlying palisade cells are irregular in size and fairly loosely packed. The cells of the *lower epidermis* are smaller and slightly more sinuous than those of the upper epidermis and numerous *anomocytic stomata* are present; in the regions over the veins the cells are larger, longitudinally elongated and straight-walled with a faintly striated *cuticle*. *Covering trichomes* occur over the veins and on the margins of the leaves; they are unicellular and conical with slightly thickened walls and a faintly striated cuticle and they vary considerably in length, those on the veins being quite long while those on the leaf margins are shorter and sometimes occur as teeth.

(*b*) The *epidermis of the petiole* in surface view is composed of longitudinally elongated cells with scattered anomocytic stomata and long, covering trichomes similar to those found on the veins of the leaf.

(*c*) *Covering trichomes* also occur on the *bracteoles*; they are fairly long, uniseriate, conical and composed of one or two cells. The epidermal cells of the bracteoles are small and have slightly sinuous anticlinal walls.

(*d*) The *epidermis of the peduncle* in surface view is composed of small, polygonal cells with moderately thickened walls.

(*e*) The cells of the *outer epidermis of the corolla* are small with thin, sinuous anticlinal walls and occasional stomata; those of the *inner epidermis* are distinctly *papillose*. The *fibrous layer of the anther*, in surface view, shows typical beading on the side walls. The *pollen grains* are small, irregularly ovoid to oblong with two pores and a finely pitted exine.

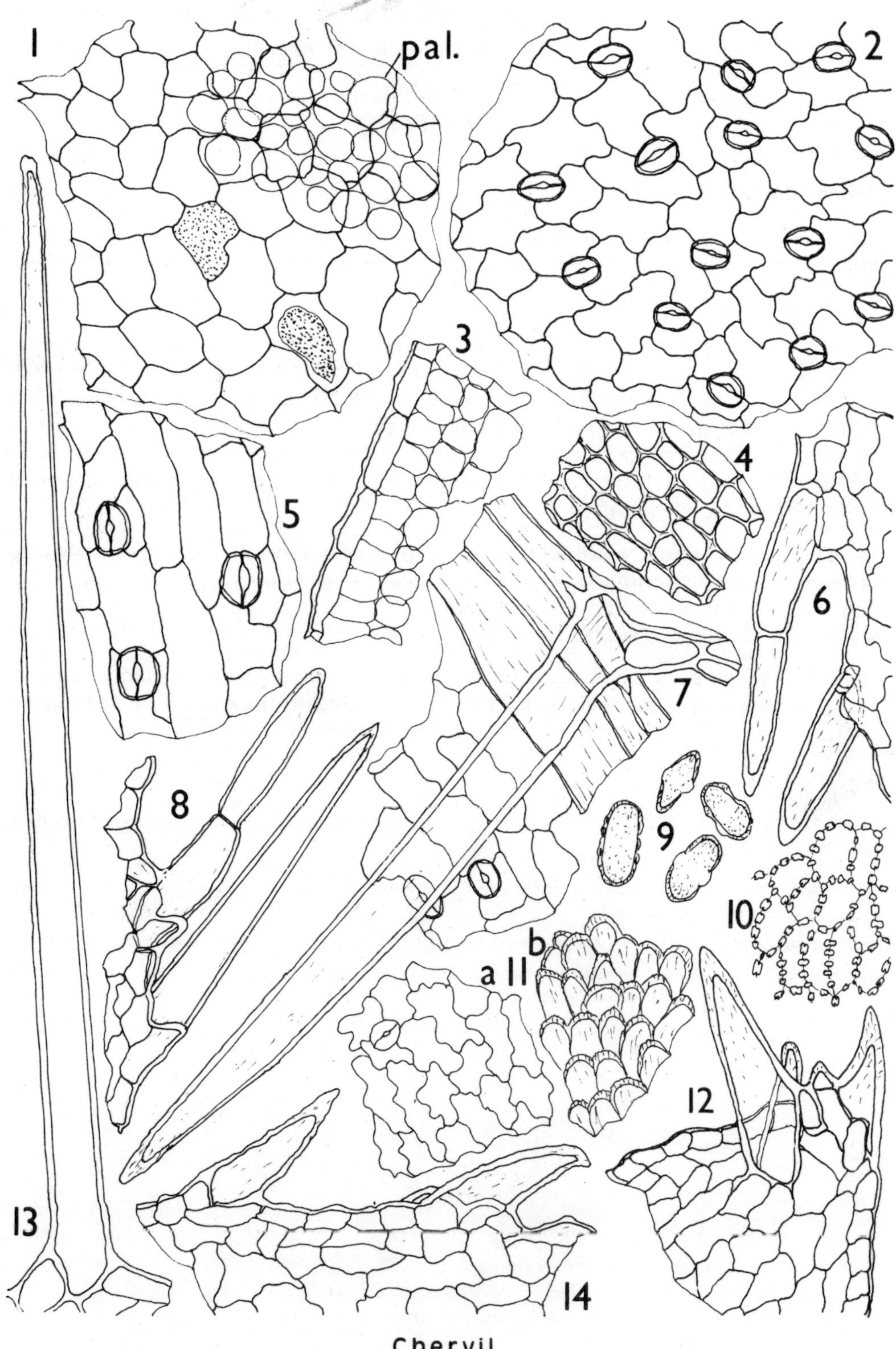

Chervil

×330

1 Upper epidermis of the leaf lamina in surface view showing two cells containing amorphous deposit and part of the underlying palisade (pal.).
2 Lower epidermis of the leaf lamina in surface view showing numerous anomocytic stomata.
3 Part of the lamina in sectional view.
4 Epidermis of the peduncle in surface view.
5 Epidermis of the petiole in surface view.
6 Part of the margin of a bracteole showing covering trichomes.
7 Lower epidermis of the leaf in surface view, including part of a vein with a covering trichome.
8 Part of the margin of a bracteole showing covering trichomes and small teeth.
9 Pollen grains.
10 Fibrous layer of the anther in surface view.
11 (a) outer epidermis and (b) inner epidermis of the corolla in surface view.
12 Tip of a leaf segment showing covering trichomes and small teeth.
13 Covering trichome from the petiole.
14 Part of the leaf margin showing covering trichomes.

CHIVES

Allium schoenoprasum L. Liliaceae

The fresh leaves are cylindrical, hollow and dark green; the dried, commercial material consists of thin, flattened, more or less transverse slices, much paler in colour. Odour and taste faintly alliaceous.

The diagnostic characters are:

(*a*) The *epidermis* composed of thin-walled, narrow, much elongated cells, squared at the ends; where stomata occur, the end walls of the adjacent epidermal cells are slightly swollen and thickened. The *stomata* are large, rounded to ovoid, and they sometimes occur in the same position in alternate rows of epidermal cells, forming transverse lines in surface view; in other areas they are randomly distributed. In *sectional view* the epidermal cells are seen to be long and tabular with a moderately thick *cuticle*. The underlying palisade mesophyll cells vary considerably in size and are loosely arranged.

(*b*) The lignified *vessels*, which show great variation in size and are frequently quite large; they are usually associated with thin-walled, elongated parenchymatous cells of the mesophyll. The vessels are spirally or annularly thickened and in some of the larger elements the thickenings are widely spaced and may become separated.

(*c*) The *secretion ducts* which occur in the mesophyll and may be associated with the vascular tissue; they are simple, much elongated structures with slightly thickened walls and pale yellowish contents; thin, transverse septa occur at infrequent intervals.

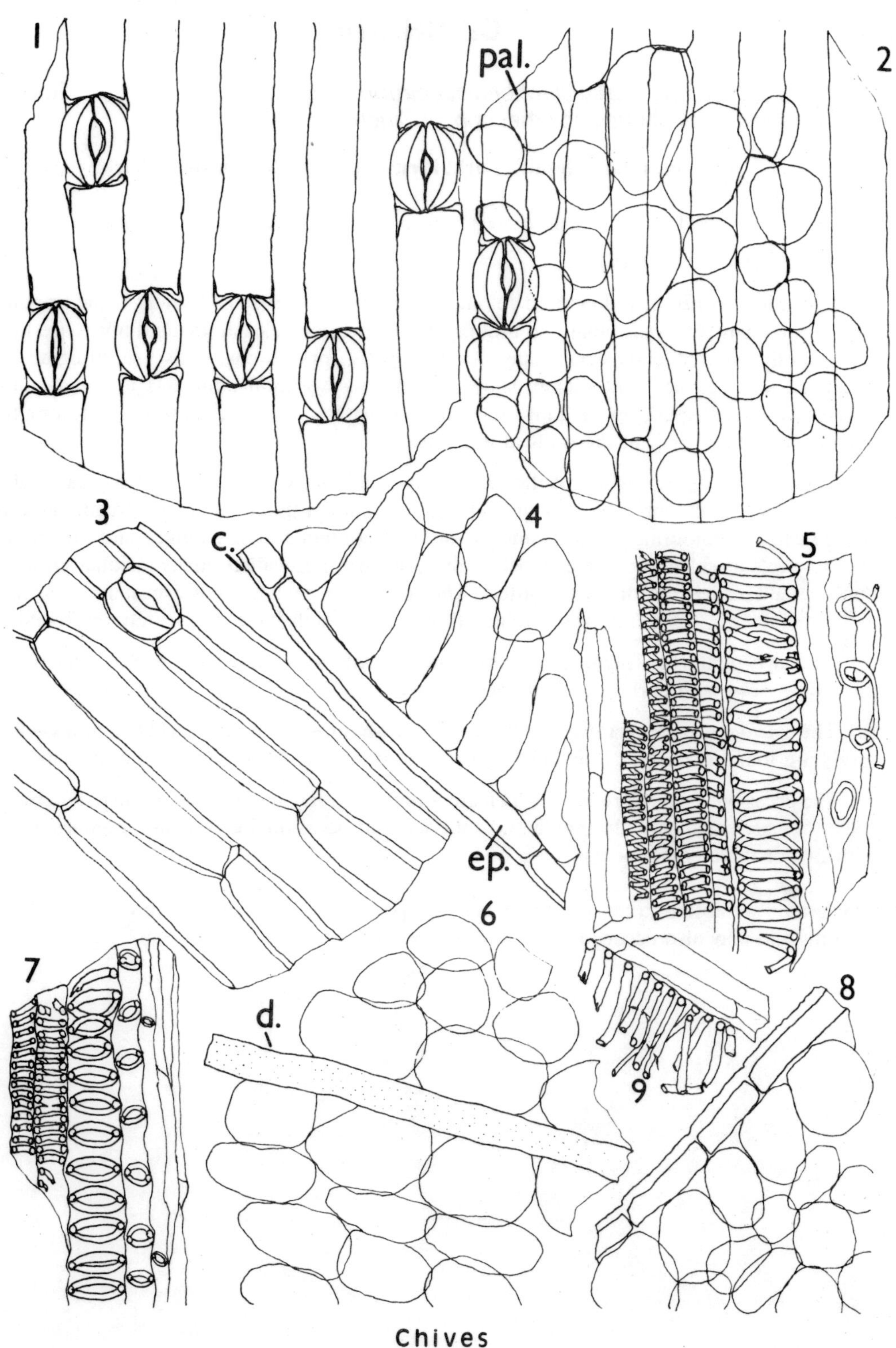

Chives

×330

1 Epidermis in surface view with numerous stomata.
2 Epidermis in surface view showing underlying cells of the palisade mesophyll (pal.).
3 Epidermis in oblique surface view.
4 Part of the lamina in longitudinal sectional view showing the cuticle (c.), epidermis (ep.) and part of the underlying mesophyll.
5 Elements of the xylem.
6 Part of the mesophyll showing a duct (d.).
7 Smaller elements of the xylem.
8 Part of the lamina in transverse sectional view.

CINCHONA

Cinchona pubescens Vahl. (*Cinchona succirubra* Pavon) or its varieties and hybrids and other spp. of *Cinchona* — Rubiaceae

Cinchona Bark, Jesuit's Bark, Peruvian Bark, Red Cinchona Bark

A reddish-brown powder with a slight, characteristic odour and a bitter and astringent taste.

The diagnostic characters are:

(*a*) The abundant *fibres*, yellowish in colour, which are very large and usually found fragmented; they occur singly or, occasionally, in groups of two or three cells. Individual fibres are fusiform with bluntly pointed ends which may be indistinctly forked; the walls are straight, heavily thickened and lignified and usually show conspicuous striations; the pits are numerous and distinctly funnel-shaped, opening into the lumen which is somewhat uneven; short, longitudinal fissures also often occur in the walls at intervals.

(*b*) The abundant *parenchyma* of the phloem and medullary rays, varying from pale yellow to reddish-brown in colour. Many of the cells of the phloem parenchyma are fragmented and in addition to the colouring matter some of the cells contain starch granules and others contain microcrystals of calcium oxalate; most of the cells are thin-walled but occasional groups have thicker walls which are distinctly pitted. The medullary rays are more usually seen in radial longitudinal view, frequently associated with fibres; the cells have moderately thickened walls.

(*c*) The fairly numerous fragments of *cork* composed of moderately thick-walled cells, polygonal in surface view, with dark red to brown contents.

(*d*) The *calcium oxalate crystals*, which occur in masses in some of the parenchymatous cells; they rarely are found scattered. Individual crystals are very small and are irregular in shape.

(*e*) The occasional *starch granules*, which are found scattered and in some of the parenchymatous cells; they are small, usually simple and spherical but occasional compound granules are found with two or three components.

Sclereids are absent in most of the *Cinchona* species. They are present in *Cinchona lancifolia* Mutis and may also occur in some of the other species and hybrids.

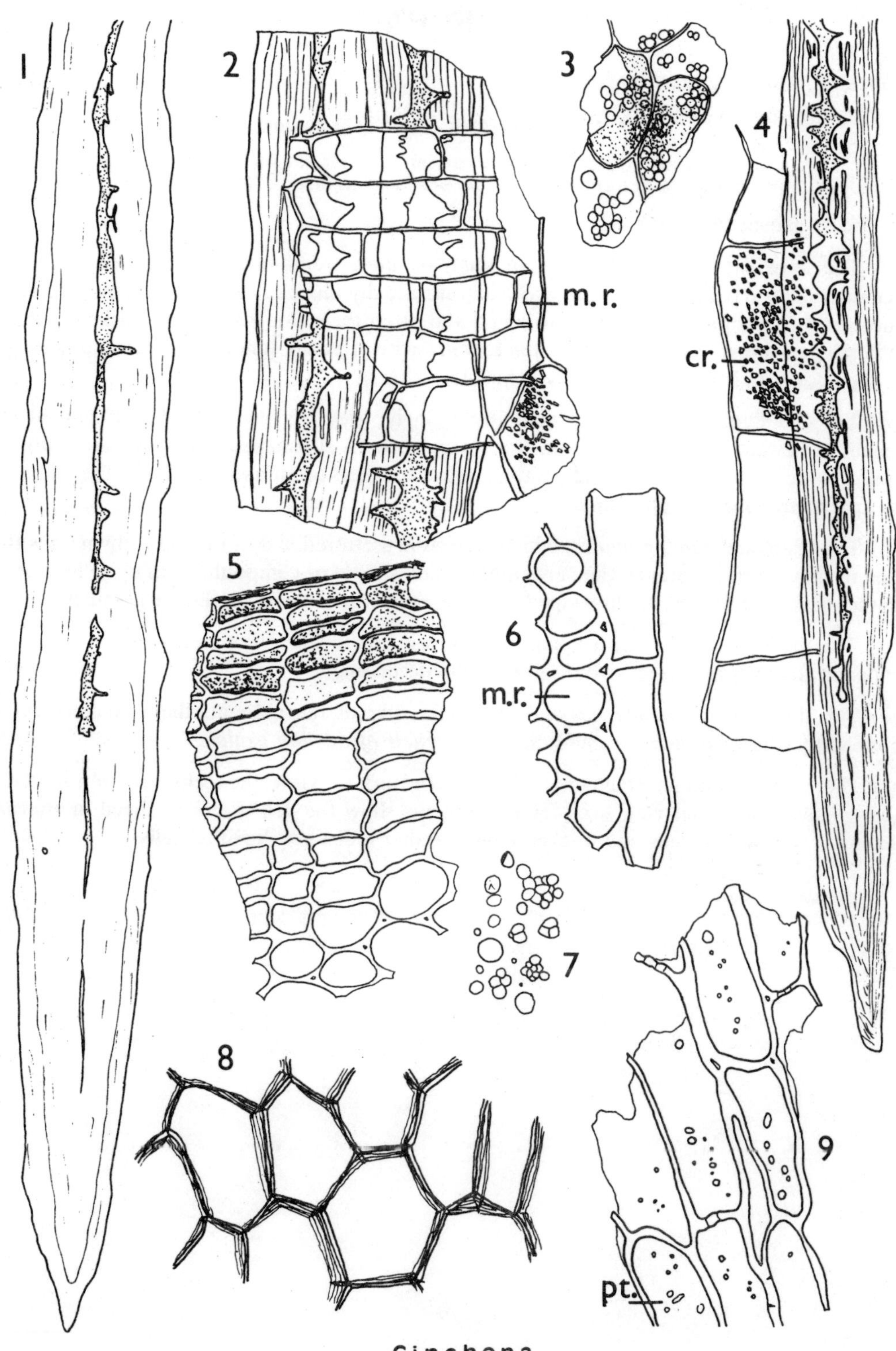

Cinchona

×330

1 Part of a single fibre.
2 Part of a group of fibres and phloem parenchyma with overlying medullary ray (m.r.) in radial longitudinal section.
3 Parenchymatous cells containing starch granules and brown pigment.
4 Part of a fibre with phloem parenchyma, one cell containing calcium oxalate microcrystals (cr.).
5 Cork and phelloderm in sectional view.
6 Phloem parenchyma and part of a medullary ray (m.r.) in tangential longitudinal section.
7 Starch granules.
8 Cork in surface view.
9 Phloem parenchyma with pits (pt.).

CINNAMON

Cinnamomum zeylanicum Nees **Lauraceae**

Cinnamon Bark, Ceylon Cinnamon

A reddish-brown powder with a characteristic, pleasant and aromatic odour and taste.

The diagnostic characters are:

(*a*) The abundant *sclereids*, which occur singly or, more frequently, in small groups; they show considerable variation in size and shape but are usually more or less isodiametric; the walls of most of the cells are moderately thickened and often the outer wall is less thickened than the others; occasional cells have very thick walls with a small lumen; pits are numerous and conspicuous, and striations are usually visible.

(*b*) The abundant *fibres*, which usually occur singly; they are thick-walled and lignified with a small, somewhat uneven lumen and few, inconspicuous slit-shaped pits. Occasional fibres are found associated with the sclereids of the pericycle; others occur associated with the oil cells and the parenchyma of the phloem.

(*c*) The abundant *starch granules*, which are found scattered and in the parenchymatous tissues and in some of the sclereids; they are rather small, simple or compound with up to four or more components; a rounded or slit-shaped hilum is visible in some of the larger granules.

(*d*) The thin-walled *oil cells*, frequently found associated with the parenchyma or fibres of the phloem; the cells are large, ovoid, and usually occur singly.

(*e*) The thin-walled *parenchyma* and *medullary rays* of the phloem; the medullary ray cells frequently contain numerous small, *acicular crystals of calcium oxalate*.

(*f*) The very occasional fragments of *cork*. In surface view the cells are thin-walled and polygonal; in sectional view occasional fragments show the cell layers arranged in alternating bands of thin-walled cells and thicker-walled, rather indistinct, lignified cells.

Compare Cassia, page 50.

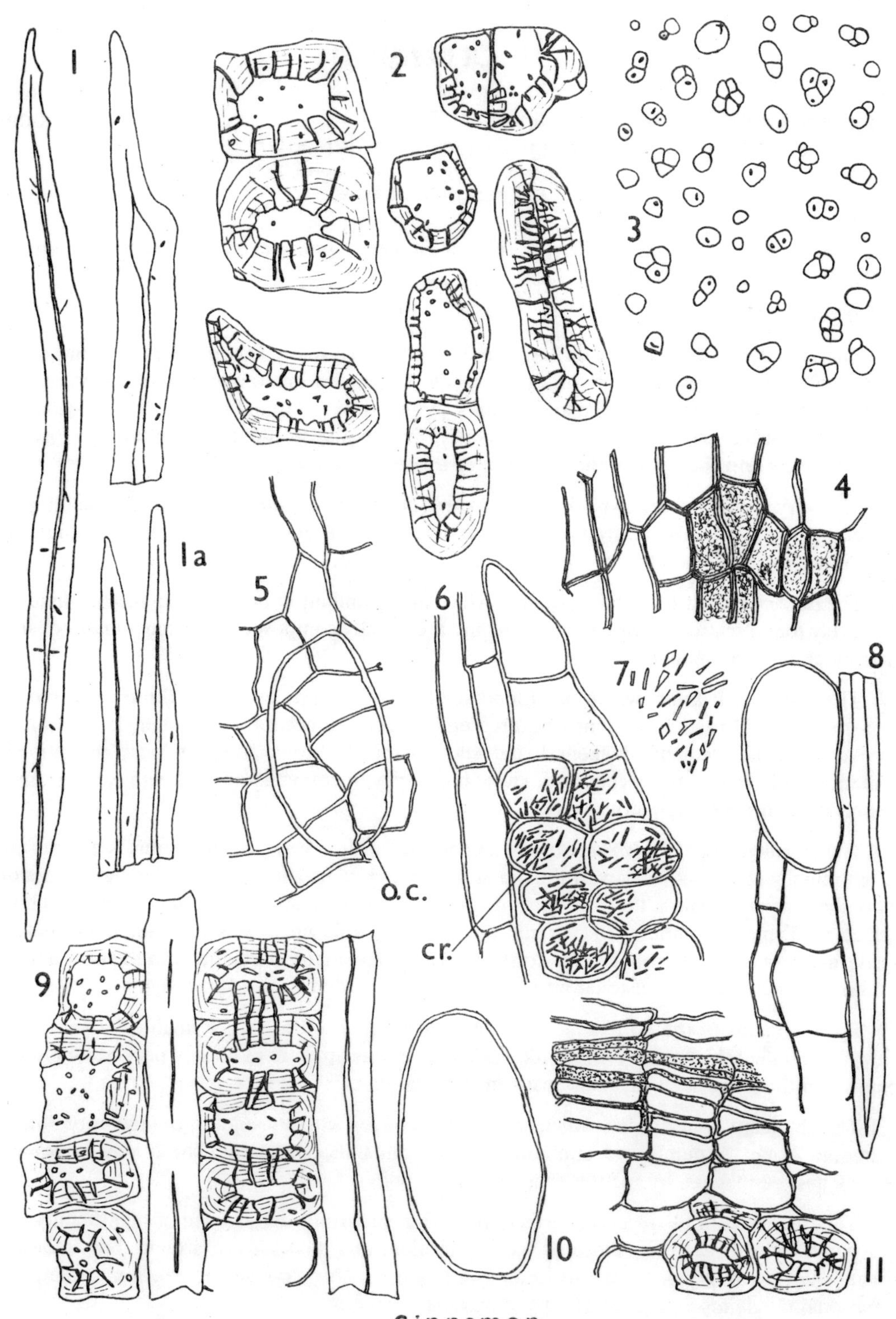

Cinnamon

×330

1 Fibres.
1a Part of a small group of fibres.
2 Sclereids.
3 Starch granules.
4 Cork in surface view.
5 Phloem parenchyma and an oil cell (o.c.).
6 Part of a medullary ray with some of the cells containing acicular crystals of calcium oxalate (cr.), and associated phloem parenchyma in tangential longitudinal section.
7 Calcium oxalate crystals.
8 Part of a fibre with an associated oil cell and phloem parenchyma.
9 Part of a group of fibres and sclereids from the pericycle.
10 A single oil cell.
11 Part of the cork and cortex in sectional view.

CLOVE

Syzygium aromaticum (L.) Merrill and L.M. Perry Myrtaceae
[(*Eugenia caryophyllus*) (C. Spreng.) Bullock and Harrison]

Caryophyllum, Cloves

A dark brown powder with a characteristic, spicy odour and an aromatic, pungent and slightly astringent taste.

The diagnostic characters are:

(*a*) The abundant fragments of the *hypanthium in surface view*. The *epidermis* is composed of small, polygonal cells with slightly thickened walls; large, almost circular *anomocytic stomata* are fairly numerous; the underlying tissue contains abundant, very large, brown, ovoid *oil glands* and occasional cluster crystals of calcium oxalate. Fragments of the hypanthium also occur in sectional view and these show the presence of a very thick *cuticle*.

(*b*) The very abundant yellowish-brown *parenchyma of the hypanthium* in which the oil glands are embedded; the cells are frequently unevenly thickened and appear collenchymatous; they contain numerous small cluster crystals of calcium oxalate.

(*c*) The *cluster crystals of calcium oxalate*, which are abundant in the parenchymatous tissue but are rarely found scattered; they vary in size and are usually composed of a large number of small, sharply pointed components.

(*d*) The occasional *fibres*, which are found singly or in groups of two or three cells; they are rather short and broad with bluntly pointed ends which are occasionally notched; the walls are lignified, usually strongly thickened and show faint striations and few pits; the lumen is sometimes filled with brown contents. These fibres may be found associated with small groups of vessels or with parenchymatous cells.

(*e*) The fragments of the *filaments of the anthers*. In surface view the epidermis is composed of longitudinally elongated cells with thin, slightly sinuous walls and a striated cuticle. In sectional view the fragments show the presence of a central vascular strand containing small, lignified *vessels* with spiral or annular thickening; the thin-walled parenchymatous tissue underlying the epidermis contains numerous cluster crystals of calcium oxalate, particularly in the cells adjacent to the vascular strand; occasional oil glands occur embedded in the parenchyma.

(*f*) The fragments of the *fibrous layer of the anther* composed of rather small cells; in sectional view the lignified thickening on the side walls of the cells appears as closely packed longitudinal bands and these are seen as small beads in surface view.

(*g*) The abundant *pollen grains* which are small, biconvex with a rounded, triangular outline and a smooth exine. A number of immature pollen grains also occur and these may be found in closely packed masses, frequently enclosed in the pollen sacs.

(*h*) The fragments of the *petals in surface view*. The epidermis is composed of slightly thickened, polygonal cells, larger than those of the hypanthium and stomata are absent. The underlying tissue consists of parenchymatous cells containing cluster crystals of calcium oxalate with occasional oil glands and small groups of vascular elements.

(*i*) The occasional fragments of the *aerenchyma of the hypanthium* composed of chains of two or three parenchymatous cells with moderately thickened walls; the contiguous walls of adjacent cells are traversed by numerous very small pits.

(*j*) The very occasional *sclereids* from the stalk; they are oval to subrectangular in outline with strongly thickened and striated walls which have numerous simple or branched pits; the lumen is frequently filled with brown contents.

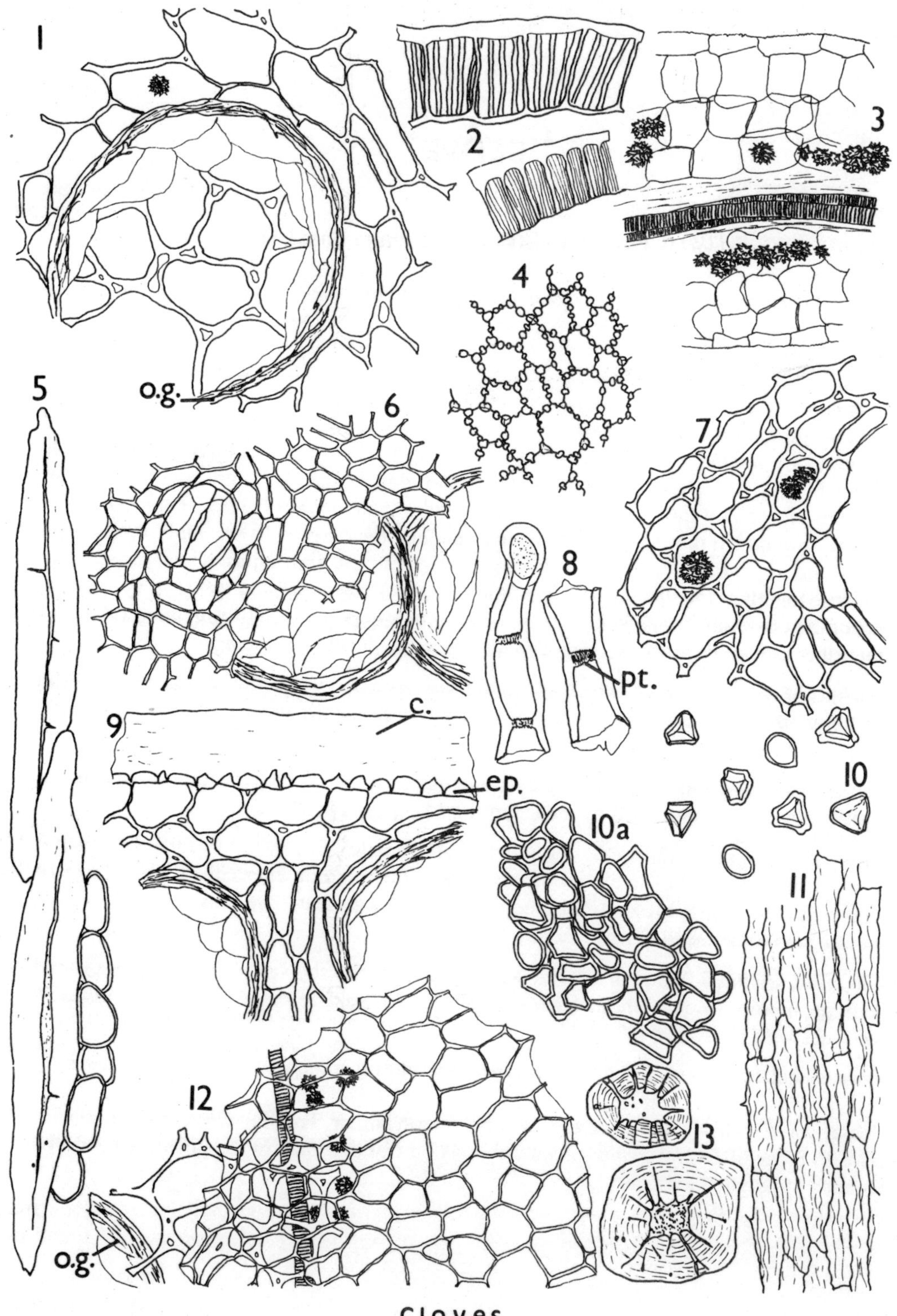

Cloves

×330

1 Parenchyma of the hypanthium showing an oil gland (o.g.).
2 Fibrous layer of the anther in sectional view.
3 Part of the filament of the anther in longitudinal section, showing the central vascular strand and parenchymatous cells containing cluster crystals of calcium oxalate.
4 Fibrous layer of the anther in surface view.
5 Fibres and associated parenchymatous cells.
6 Epidermis of the hypanthium in surface view showing a stoma and underlying oil glands.
7 Parenchyma of the hypanthium with cluster crystals of calcium oxalate.
8 Fragments of aerenchyma from the hypanthium showing pits (pt.).
9 Part of the hypanthium in sectional view showing the thick cuticle (c.), epidermis (ep.) and underlying parenchyma with oil glands.
10 Mature pollen grains.
10a Part of a group of immature pollen grains.
11 Epidermis of the filament of the anther in surface view.
12 Epidermis of a petal in surface view with underlying tissue composed of parenchymatous cells containing cluster crystals of calcium oxalate, part of an oil gland (o.g.) and part of a vascular strand.
13 Sclereids from the stalk.

COCA

Erythroxylum coca Lam. Erythroxylaceae

Coca Leaves, Bolivian Coca Leaves, Huanuco Coca Leaves

A dull greenish-brown powder with a faint odour and a slightly bitter taste, slowly giving a sensation of numbness.

The diagnostic characters are:

(*a*) The abundant fragments of the *lamina in surface view*. The *upper epidermis* is composed of fairly large, polygonal cells with moderately thickened walls which show irregular beading and pitting; stomata are absent; prisms of calcium oxalate occur very occasionally, usually as single crystals in each of two adjacent smaller cells; the underlying palisade cells are small and rather closely packed. The cells of the *lower epidermis* are smaller than those of the upper epidermis and slightly thinner-walled but they also show irregular beading; the outer walls are *papillose* giving in surface view the appearance of a circle in each cell, those on two adjacent cells frequently appearing close together; the subsidiary cells of the numerous *paracytic stomata* are not papillose. Fragments of the epidermis from over the veins also occur composed of subrectangular cells with moderately thickened and distinctly beaded walls; they are devoid of stomata.

(*b*) The *prisms of calcium oxalate*, which are found scattered and frequently associated with the groups of fibres; they vary considerably in size and are occasionally quite large and irregularly shaped.

(*c*) *The fibres*, which are found in groups; they are lignified and thick-walled with a narrow lumen and few pits; they are accompanied by a calcium oxalate prism sheath.

(*d*) Occasional fragments of the *epidermis and underlying mesophyll* occur *in sectional view* but complete sections through the lamina are not common; the palisade is usually a single layer of thin-walled cells. The spongy mesophyll is composed of thin-walled stellate cells and fragments of this tissue are sometimes seen in surface view.

(*e*) The lignified *idioblasts*, some of which occur associated with the veins and others are found scattered in the mesophyll; they are frequently somewhat irregular in shape and have moderately thickened walls with numerous pits.

(*f*) The occasional fragments of *collenchyma* from the midrib composed of fairly large cells.

The leaves of *Erythroxylum truxillense* Rusby (Peruvian or Truxillo Coca) are similar in structure to those of *Erythroxylum coca*; they may be distinguished in the powdered form by the absence of lignified idioblasts.

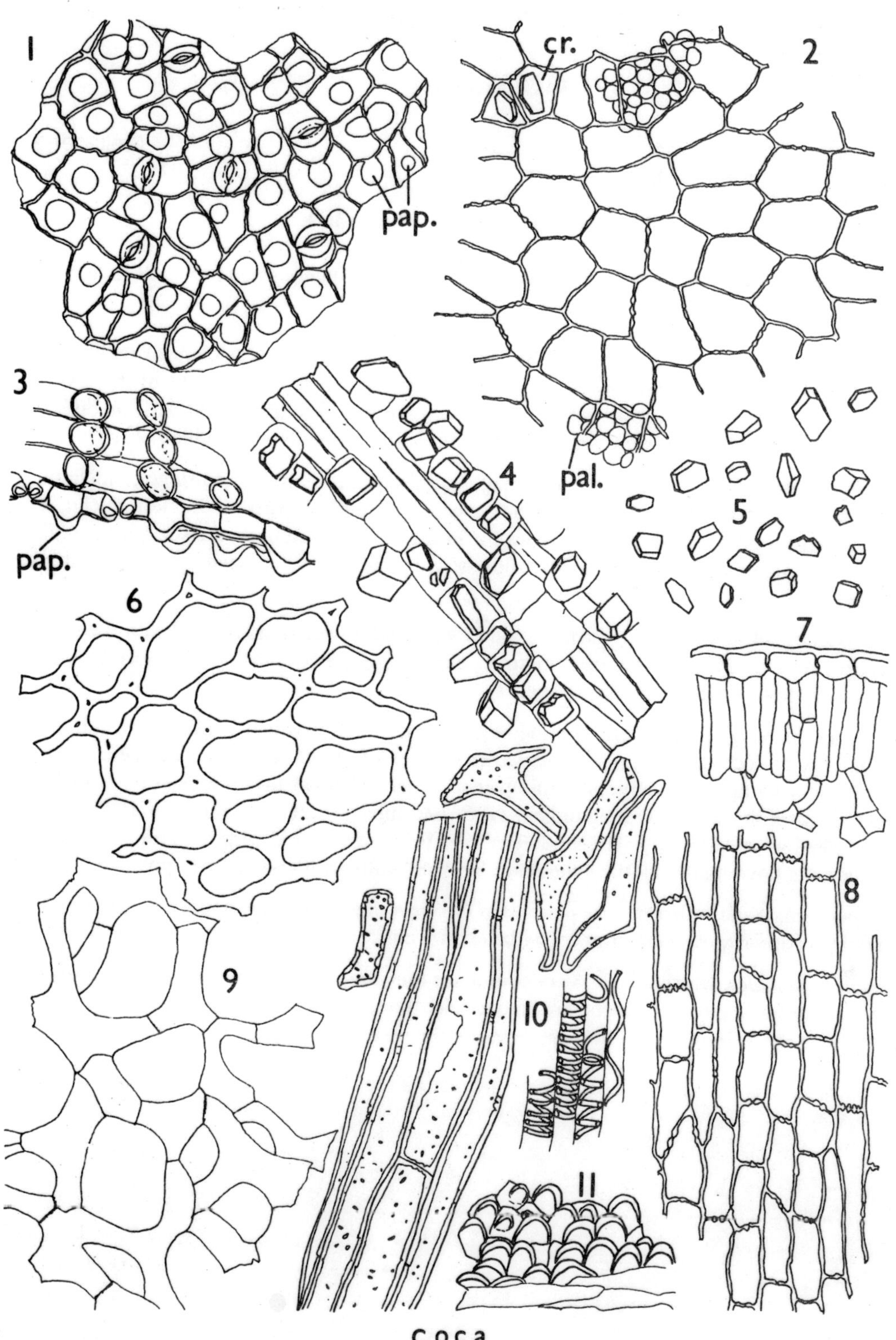

coca

×330

1 Lower epidermis in surface view showing papillae (pap.) and paracytic stomata.
2 Upper epidermis in surface view, with prisms of calcium oxalate (cr.) and underlying palisade (pal.).
3 Part of the lamina in sectional view showing the lower epidermis with papillae (pap.), stomata and cells of the spongy mesophyll.
4 Fibres with part of a calcium oxalate prism sheath.
5 Calcium oxalate prisms.
6 Collenchyma in transverse section.
7 Part of the lamina in sectional view showing the upper epidermis, palisade and part of the spongy mesophyll.
8 Epidermis from over a vein in surface view.
9 Spongy mesophyll in surface view.
10 Lignified idioblasts and xylem vessels.
11 Lower epidermis in oblique surface view showing papillae.

COCILLANA

Guarea guidonia (L.) Sleumer
[*Guarea rusbyi* (Britton) Rusby]

Meliaceae

Cocillana Bark, Grape Bark, Guapi Bark

A light brown powder with a characteristic, spicy odour and a slightly pungent and astringent taste.

The diagnostic characters are:

(*a*) The very abundant *fibres*, which occur in groups accompanied by a calcium oxalate prism sheath; they are thick-walled and strongly lignified and the parenchymatous cells of the crystal sheath are also lignified. The groups of fibres are frequently found associated with medullary rays, in tangential longitudinal view, in which some or all of the cells are lignified.

(*b*) The very abundant *sclereids*, usually in groups but also occasionally found singly; individual cells are rectangular to elongated or somewhat irregular in outline with moderately thickened walls and numerous pits; faint striations are visible in the walls and some of the sclereids contain yellowish-brown pigment. The groups of sclereids are frequently associated with parenchymatous cells containing prisms of calcium oxalate.

(*c*) The *prisms of calcium oxalate*, which are found scattered as well as associated with the fibres and sclereids; they vary in size and are sometimes quite large, particularly when associated with the sclereids. A few *twinned crystals* also occur.

(*d*) The *parenchyma* of the phloem and medullary rays, most of which is filled with reddish-brown contents or, occasionally, with compacted masses of starch granules. The cells of the phloem parenchyma are fairly large and thin-walled. The medullary rays are from one to three cells wide, as seen in tangential longitudinal view, and most of the cells are moderately thin-walled and filled with pigment; in the medullary rays found associated with the groups of fibres some of the cells have markedly thickened and lignified walls with conspicuous pits.

(*e*) The fragments of dark brown *cork* composed of thin-walled cells, polygonal in surface view; fragments in sectional view show four to six layers of cells.

(*f*) The *starch granules*, which are not very abundant; they are found scattered but more usually are seen in masses in some of the parenchymatous cells. The granules are simple and spherical, or compound with up to four (or possibly more) components; a point hilum is sometimes visible.

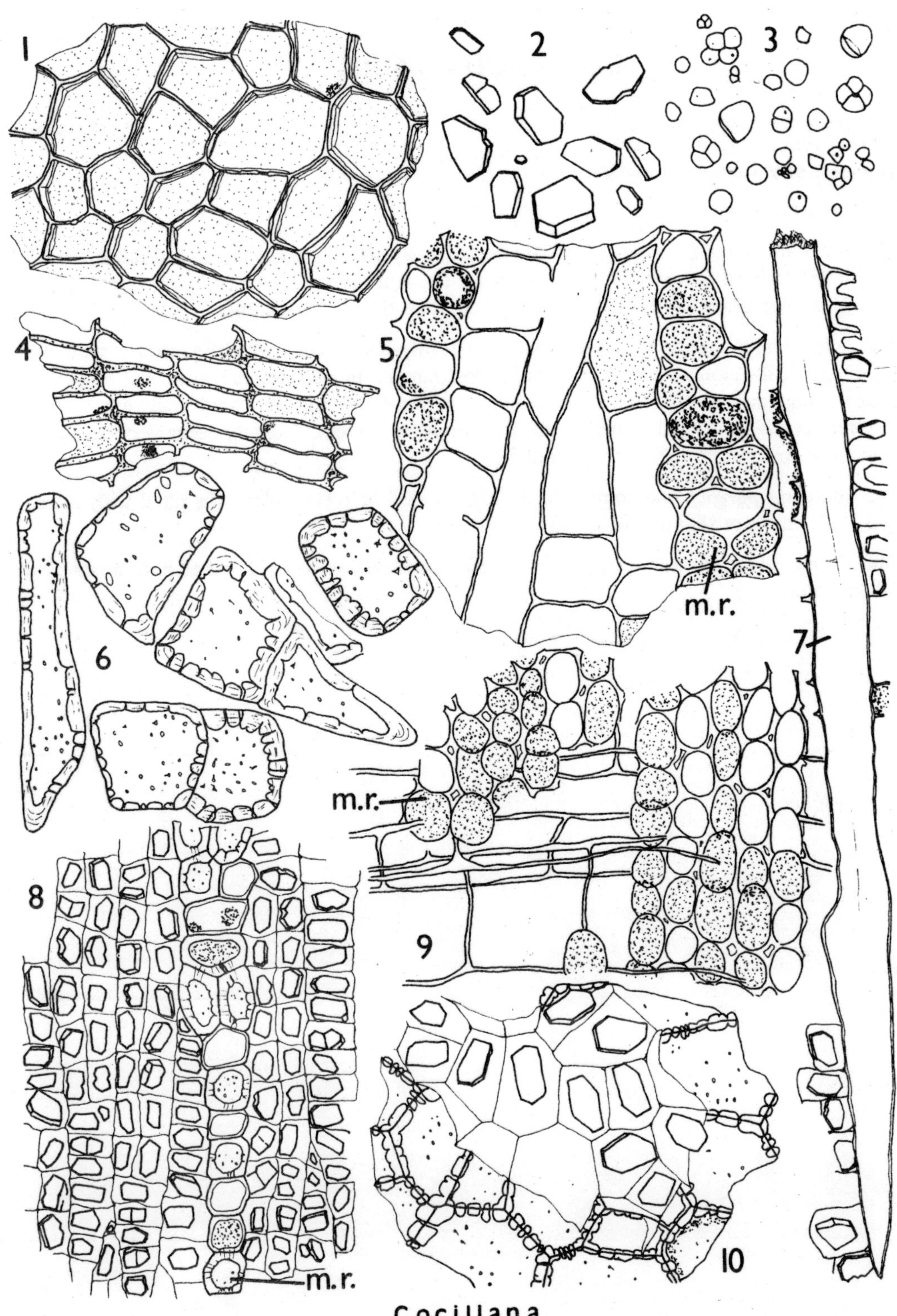

Cocillana

×330

1 Cork in surface view.
2 Calçium oxalate prisms and twinned crystals.
3 Starch granules.
4 Cork in sectional view.
5 Part of the phloem in tangential longitudinal section showing medullary ray cells (m.r.) containing pigment.
6 Sclereids.
7 Part of a single fibre with remains of the crystal sheath.
8 Part of a group of fibres with calcium oxalate prism sheath and part of a medullary ray (m.r.) in tangential longitudinal section.
9 Part of the phloem in radial longitudinal section showing medullary ray cells (m.r.) and phloem parenchyma.
10 Part of a group of sclereids with associated parenchymatous cells containing calcium oxalate prisms.

COLCHICUM CORM

Colchicum autumnale L. **Liliaceae**

A pale grey to buff powder with no odour and a bitter, starchy taste.

The diagnostic characters are:

(*a*) The abundant *starch granules*, which are occasionally simple and spherical but more usually compound with two to four or more components. The central, well marked hilum is irregularly oval in the smaller granules and triangular to stellate in the larger granules.

(*b*) The *epidermis* consisting of a single layer of tawny-brown cells which in surface view are usually tangentially elongated but may be almost square in outline; the anticlinal walls are frequently irregularly thickened with characteristic swellings; the periclinal walls are usually smooth but occasional irregular surface markings may be present. *Stomata* occur very occasionally, but these are rarely seen in the powder.

(*c*) The abundant *parenchyma* composed of large, ovoid or rectangular cells filled with starch granules; the walls are slightly and evenly thickened.

(*d*) The *vessels*, which are found singly or in small groups; the walls are lignified and show spiral or annular thickening.

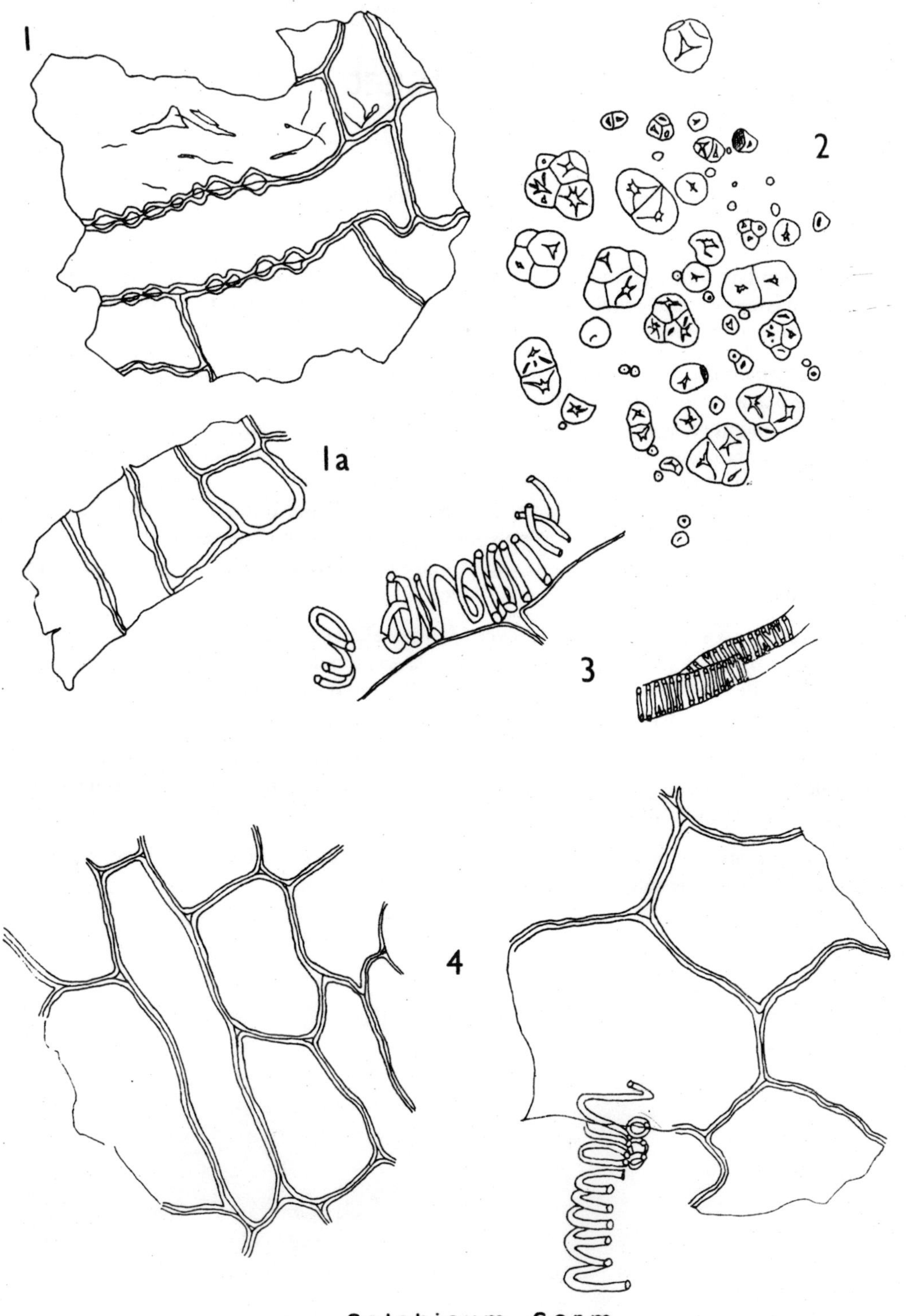

Colchicum Corm

×330

1 Epidermis in surface view showing characteristic swellings on the anticlinal walls and markings on the periclinal walls.

1a Epidermis in surface view showing cells with more uniformly thickened walls.

2 Starch granules.

3 Fragments of vessels with spiral and annular thickening.

4 Parenchyma and part of a spirally thickened vessel.

COLCHICUM SEED

Colchicum autumnale L. Liliaceae

A mid-brown powder with no odour and a very bitter and unpleasant taste.

The diagnostic characters are:

(*a*) The fairly abundant *starch granules*, mostly simple although the smaller granules tend to form tightly packed masses; an occasional compound granule occurs with two components. Individual granules are spherical to polyhedral and usually have a fairly distinct cleft or radiate hilum.

(*b*) The *parenchymatous layers of the testa* in surface view composed of cells with brown walls. The cells of the *outer layer* are rectangular to polygonal and fairly large, with moderately thick walls; they are frequently fragmented. The cells of the *middle layer* are slightly smaller than those of the outer layer and they are more rounded; the walls are unevenly thickened and usually show conspicuous beading; characteristic, rounded intercellular spaces occur. The *inner layer* is composed of thin-walled cells which are smaller than those of the outer layers and are more regularly arranged; they are rectangular to polygonal and there are no intercellular spaces. Each of these layers is usually found adherent to one or more of the other layers, and the inner layer may also be found associated with the pigment layer.

(*c*) The *pigment layer* composed of a single layer of thin-walled cells, rectangular in surface view and slightly larger than the parenchyma of the inner layer; the cells are filled with dark brown pigment but the walls are colourless. This layer is usually found associated with either the outer layers of the endosperm or with the inner parenchymatous layer of the testa.

(*d*) The abundant fragments of the *endosperm* composed of large, rectangular cells with thick walls perforated by very large pits which appear circular or oval in surface view; the pitting is less frequent in the cells of the outer layers.

(*e*) The thin-walled *parenchyma of the strophiole* filled with starch granules; the cells are rounded to rectangular with irregular intercellular spaces.

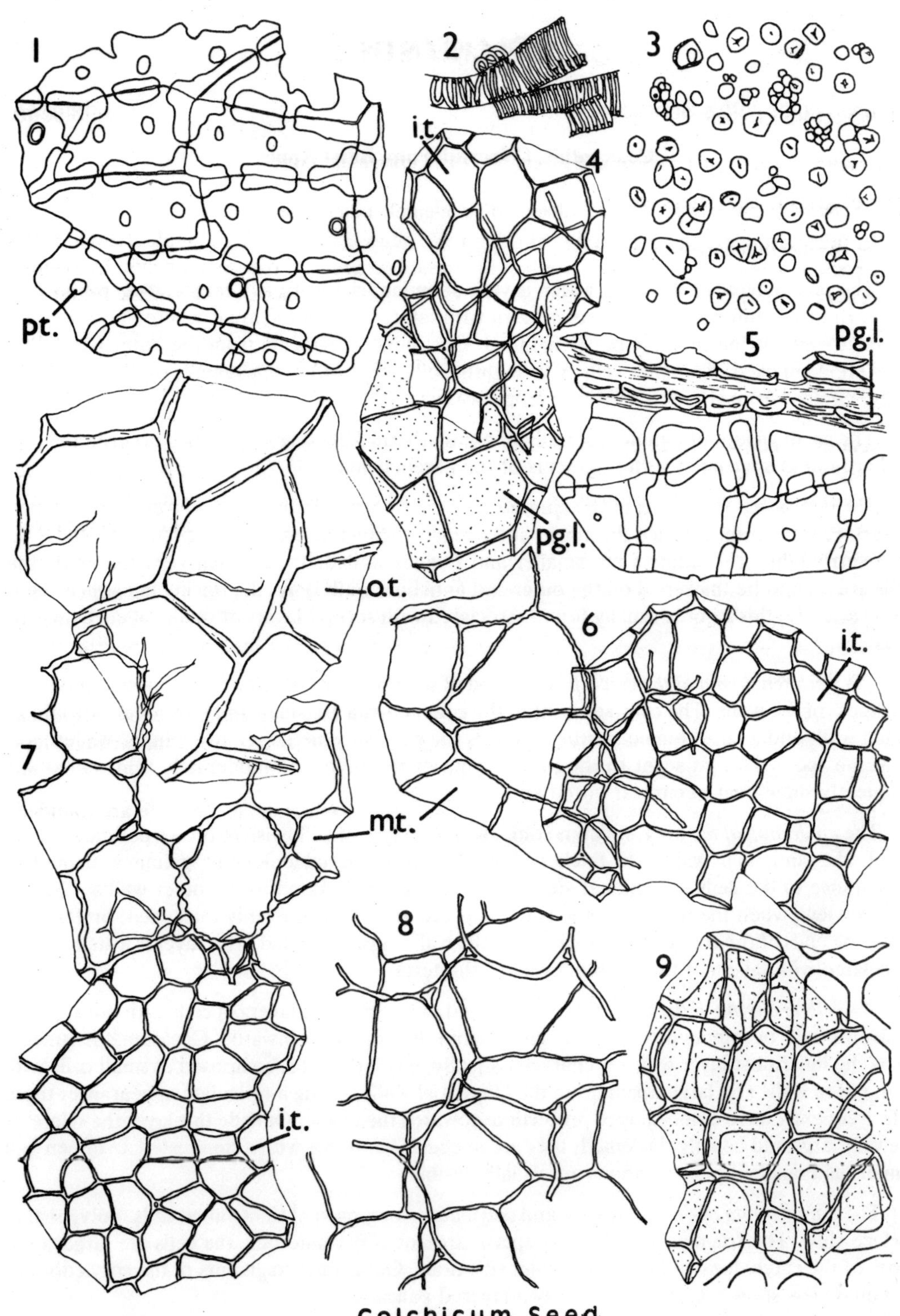

Colchicum Seed

×330

1 Part of the endosperm showing pits (pt.).
2 Part of a group of vessels from the raphe.
3 Starch granules.
4 Inner parenchymatous layer of the testa (i.t.) with underlying pigment layer (pg.l.) in surface view.
5 Part of the parenchyma, pigment layer (pg.l.) and endosperm in sectional view.
6 Middle layer of the testa (m.t.) and underlying inner parenchymatous layer (i.t.) in surface view.
7 Outer (o.t.), middle (m.t.) and inner (i.t.) parenchymatous layers of the testa in surface view.
8 Thin-walled parenchyma of the strophiole.
9 Pigment layer in surface view with underlying endosperm cells.

COLOCYNTH

Citrullus colocynthis Schrader — Cucurbitaceae

Colocynthis, Colocynth Pulp, Bitter Apple

A pale yellowish-buff powder with no odour and an intensely bitter taste.

The diagnostic characters are:

(*a*) The *parenchyma of the pulp*, which is very abundant but is usually fragmented; parts of the large, rounded thin-walled cells may be seen with faint, finely pitted areas where the cells are in contact; some of the cells are partly lignified. Occasional fragments from the outer part of the pulp are composed of smaller cells with slightly collenchymatous thickening; on these cells the large, circular to oval pitted areas are more distinct.

(*b*) The small groups of lignified, spirally or annularly thickened *vessels*, which occur in the pulp and are found associated with fragments of the parenchyma.

(*c*) The occasional fragments of the *epidermis of the epicarp* composed of a layer of cells which, in surface view, appear much thickened and irregular with scattered large, circular *stomata*; the cells surrounding the stomata are smaller and thinner-walled. In sectional view the epidermal cells are seen to be thickened on the outer and anticlinal walls only, the thickening appearing as an inverted U; this layer is usually found associated with several layers of small collenchymatous cells.

(*d*) The *sclerenchyma of the epicarp* composed of several layers of cells varying in size and in the thickness of the walls. The cells adjacent to the collenchyma are small and polygonal, with thick, pitted walls and a small lumen; farther inwards the cells become larger and thinner-walled, and those on the inside, adjacent to the parenchyma of the pulp, are moderately thin-walled and frequently show oval to circular pitted areas.

(*e*) The *epidermis of the testa*, which is composed of a layer of yellowish to brown palisade cells in which the anticlinal walls are thickened with rods of variable length, giving a flame-like appearance to the cells in sectional view; these rods do not extend to the outer wall so that, in surface view, when the top of the cell is in focus the walls appear evenly thickened; on focusing down the ends of the rods come into view and the walls appear beaded. This layer is usually found associated with layers of the sclerenchyma of the testa.

(*f*) The *sclerenchyma of the testa*; this is composed of a number of layers of cells with thick, pitted walls, the cells becoming progressively larger from the epidermis inwards. Occasional fragments show the innermost layer which is characteristically developed; it is composed of small cells with thin, pitted walls and large openings in the tangential walls, giving a reticulate appearance; these cells frequently have dome-shaped projections towards the inside. Outside this layer the sclereids are very large and heavily thickened; they are irregular in outline with a small, stellate lumen and numerous branched pits; striations are usually visible.

(*g*) The *parenchyma of the endosperm* and *cotyledons* composed of thin-walled cells, polygonal in surface view. The fragments of the endosperm are not very numerous; the cells are larger than those of the cotyledons and may show faint striations. Occasional fragments of the cotyledons in sectional view show the presence of a two-layered palisade.

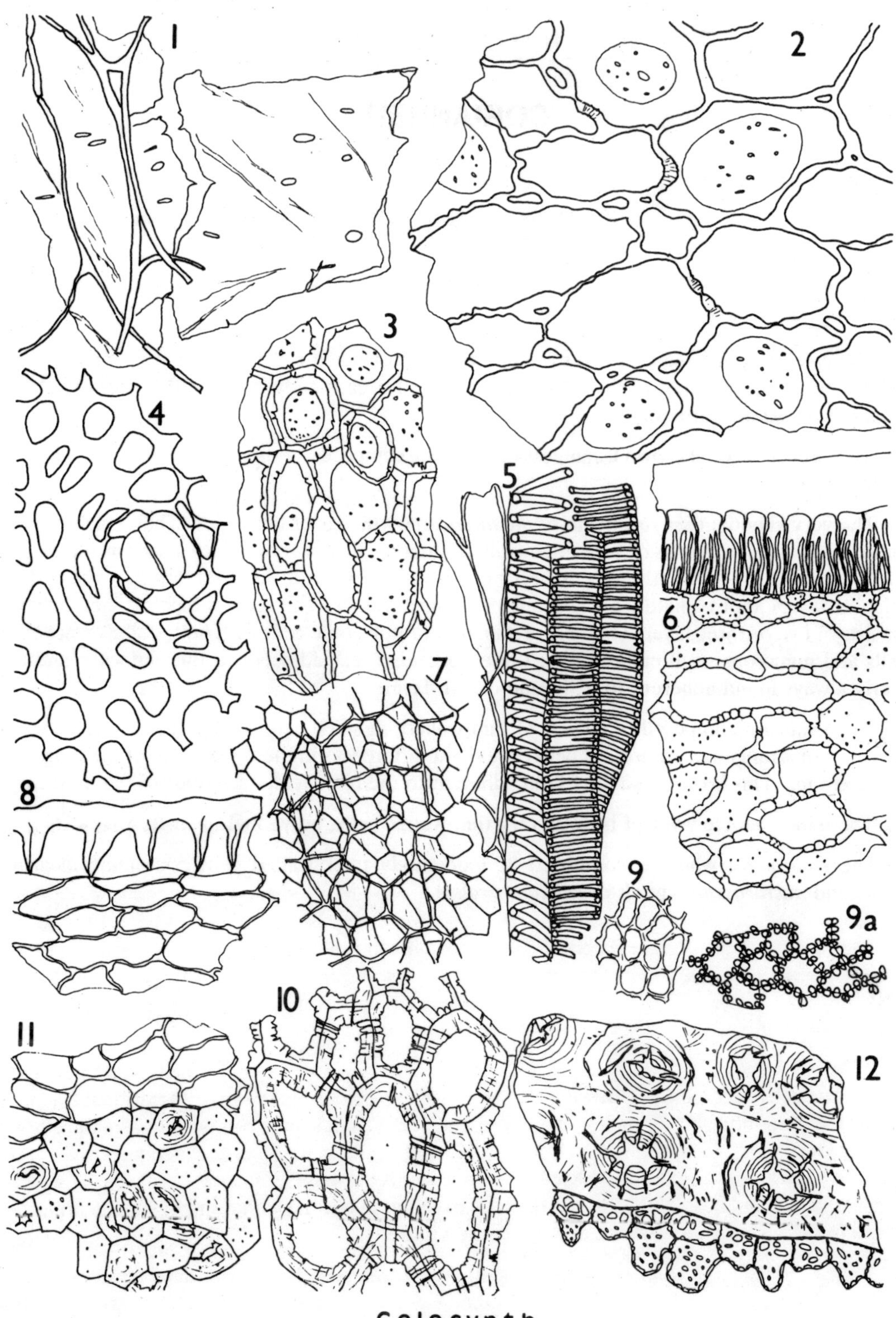

Colocynth

×330

1 Parenchyma of the pulp.
2 Collenchyma of the outer part of the pulp showing pitted areas on some of the cells.
3 Sclerenchyma of the epicarp showing pitted areas.
4 Epidermis of the epicarp in surface view showing a stoma.
5 A group of spirally and annularly thickened vessels.
6 Outer part of the testa in sectional view showing the epidermis (flame cells) and adjacent layers of the sclerenchyma.
7 Parenchyma of the endosperm with underlying parenchyma of the cotyledons.
8 Epidermis of the epicarp in sectional view with part of the adjacent collenchyma.
9 Epidermis of the testa from above.
9a Epidermis of the testa on focusing down to show the beaded anticlinal walls.
10 Sclerenchyma of the testa.
11 Sclerenchyma of the epicarp, with adjacent collenchyma.
12 Innermost layers of the sclerenchyma of the testa showing the heavily thickened sclereids with branched pits and the small, reticulately thickened cells with dome-shaped projections.

CORIANDER

Coriandrum sativum L. Umbelliferae

Coriander Fruits

A medium brown powder with a characteristic, aromatic odour and a spicy taste.

The diagnostic characters are:

(*a*) The *epicarp* composed of a layer of colourless, thin-walled cells, polygonal in surface view, with a smooth cuticle; most of the cells contain one, or occasionally two, small *prisms of calcium oxalate; stomata* are infrequent.

(*b*) The very occasional brown fragments of the *vittae* composed of thin-walled cells, polygonal in surface view.

(*c*) The very abundant *sclerenchyma of the mesocarp*, which is of two types. That which is more abundant consists of masses of very thick-walled, sinuous, fusiform cells with a narrow lumen and few, rather indistinct pits; these cells occur in several layers with the orientation of the cells in adjacent layers approximately at right angles to one another. The second type of sclerenchyma consists of two or three layers of large, rectangular or polygonal cells with only slightly thickened walls and numerous, well-marked pits; these sclereids occur adjacent to the endocarp and are nearly always found adherent to it, in one or two layers.

(*d*) The *endocarp* composed of a layer of thin-walled, lignified cells, elongated in surface view; the cells are arranged in groups but with only slight differences in the orientation of the long axes of the groups. This layer is usually found adherent to the rectangular sclereids of the mesocarp.

(*e*) The *testa*, a single layer of brown, very thin-walled cells, polygonal in surface view.

(*f*) The *endosperm* which is composed of moderately thick-walled cells containing *aleurone grains* and *microrosette crystals of calcium oxalate*.

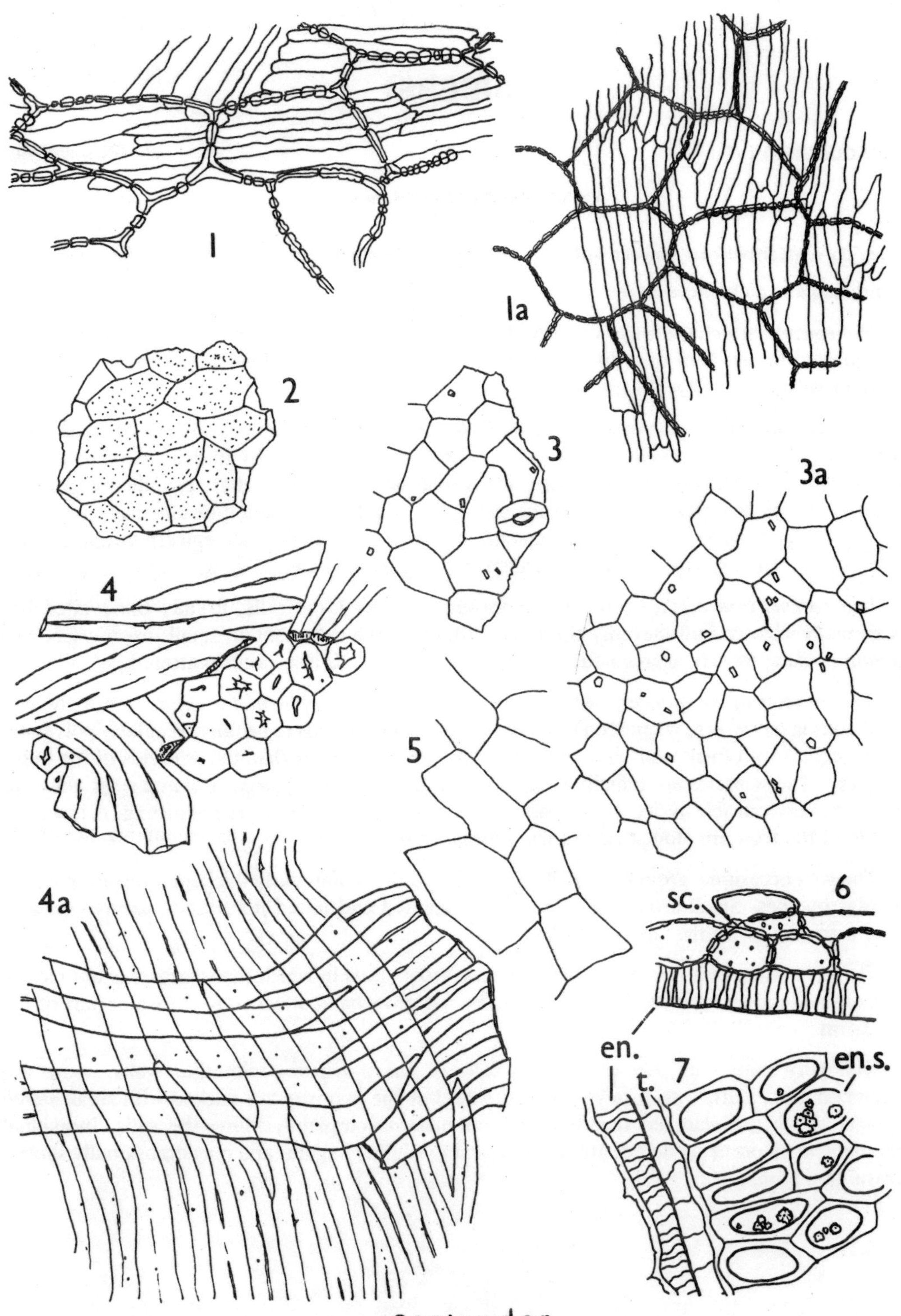

Coriander

×330

1 Rectangular sclereids of the mesocarp with underlying endocarp in surface view.
1a As 1, showing thinner-walled sclereids.
2 Fragment of a vitta.
3 Epicarp in surface view showing a stoma and calcium oxalate prisms in some of the cells.
3a Epicarp in surface view.
4 Groups of fusiform sclereids of the mesocarp, some in sectional view.
4a Groups of fusiform sclereids of the mesocarp showing two layers orientated at right angles to one another.
5 Testa in surface view.
6 Rectangular sclereids of the mesocarp (sc.) and cells of the endocarp (en.) in sectional view.
7 Part of the pericarp and seed in sectional view showing the endocarp (en.), testa (t.) and endosperm (en.s.) containing microrosette crystals of calcium oxalate.

CUBEBS

Piper cubeba L. Piperaceae

Cubeb Berries, Tailed Pepper

A very dark reddish-brown powder with an aromatic odour and a spicy, rather bitter and lingering taste.

The diagnostic characters are:

(*a*) The *epicarp*, which is always adherent to the outermost sclerenchyma of the mesocarp and is distinguished by areas of dark brown pigment in which are embedded small *prism crystals of calcium oxalate*; the cell walls are not easily discerned.

(*b*) The *sclereids of the outer mesocarp*, which do not form continuous layers but occur in small groups, sometimes composed of only two or three cells separated by ill-defined parenchyma; frequently there are two layers. The sclereids vary in size and shape but are usually polygonal to rectangular with strongly thickened walls and fairly numerous rounded or slit-shaped pits; all have dark brown contents. They are frequently found associated with the epicarp but may occur isolated or in small groups attached to fragments of parenchymatous tissue.

(*c*) The *parenchyma of the mesocarp* composed of fairly large cells, usually thin-walled but occasionally slightly and unevenly thickened. Many of the cells contain small *prism crystals of calcium oxalate*, loosely aggregated. Occasional large *oil cells* also occur scattered.

(*d*) The *sclereids of the endocarp*, which are very abundant. They form one or, more usually, two continuous layers which, when seen in *surface view*, show the cells to be fairly regularly polygonal to rectangular with thick walls and numerous pits; they are larger than the sclereids of the outer mesocarp. The sclereids are radially elongated and they frequently occur isolated when they are seen to be very variable in size, shape and wall thickness and also in degree of pitting. A few from the tail of the fruit are elongated to form *fibrous sclereids*.

(*e*) The very occasional groups of small, lignified, spirally or annularly thickened *vessels* from the vascular bundles. Small groups of thin-walled, lignified and pitted *fibres* and *parenchyma* also occur associated with the vascular tissue.

(*f*) The very infrequent fragments of the yellow-brown *testa* in which the structure is not clearly defined; in sectional view the layer is seen to be a narrow band attached to the outer part of the perisperm.

(*g*) The very numerous parenchymatous cells of the *perisperm* with thin walls; some are developed as *oil cells*, with pale yellow contents, but the majority are packed with small *starch granules* which are clumped together to form masses completely filling the cells. Individual granules, which occur scattered, are subspherical to slightly angular and may occasionally show a central point hilum.

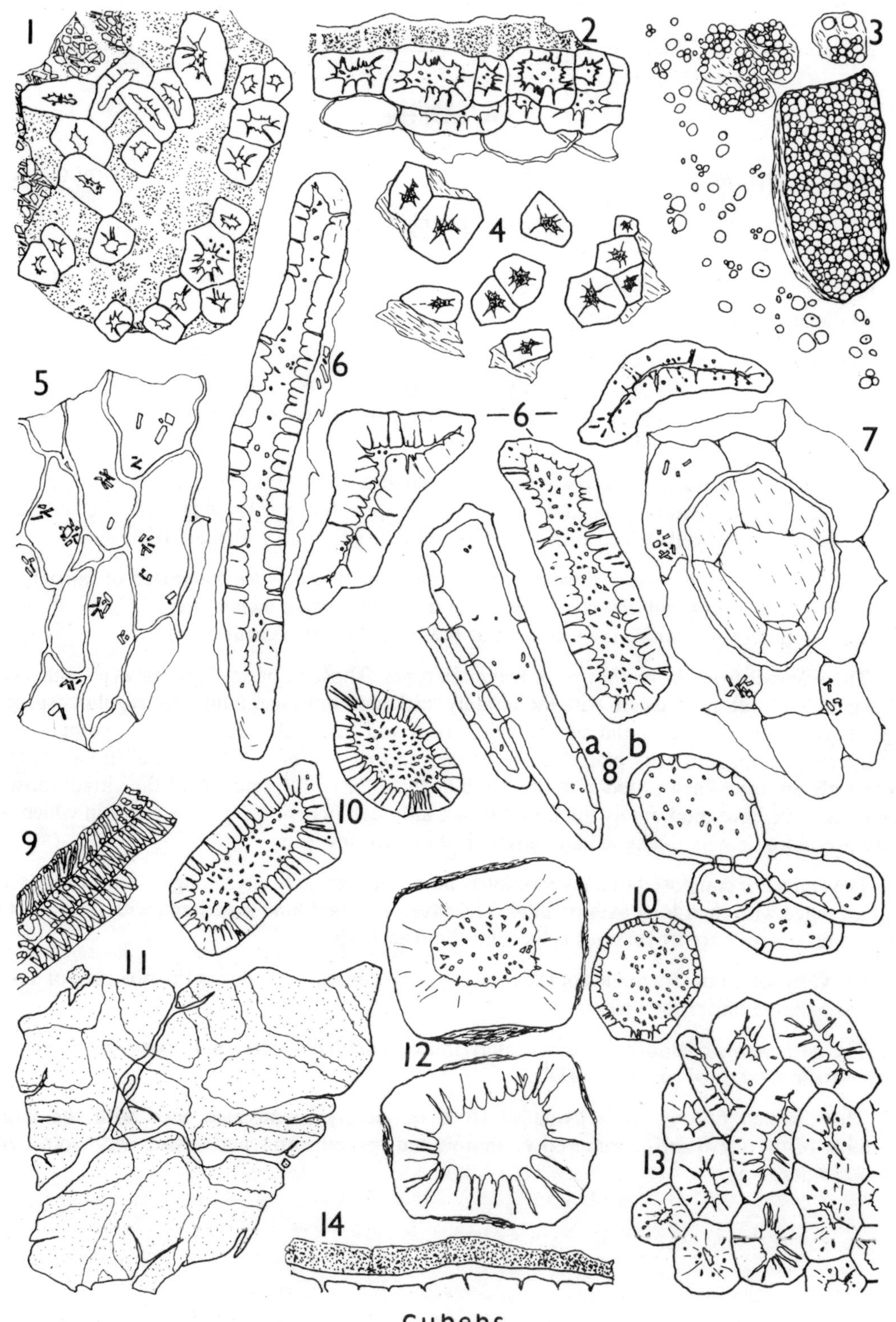

Cubebs

×330

1 Two layers of sclereids of the outer mesocarp with adhering epicarp containing pigment and calcium oxalate crystals, in surface view.
2 Outer part of the pericarp in sectional view showing the epicarp and underlying sclereids and parenchyma of the mesocarp.
3 Perisperm cells containing densely compacted masses of starch granules and some loose granules.
4 Isolated sclereids of the outer mesocarp, some attached to fragments of indistinct parenchyma.
5 Parenchymatous cells of the mesocarp containing prism crystals of calcium oxalate.
6 Elongated sclereids from the endocarp.
7 Parenchyma and an oil cell of the mesocarp.
8 (a) fibres and (b) sclereids from the vascular tissue.
9 A group of vessels from a vascular strand.
10 Isolated sclereids from the endocarp.
11 Testa in surface view.
12 A sclereid from the endocarp in two planes of focus.
13 Part of a layer of sclereids of the endocarp in surface view.
14 Testa in sectional view with part of the outermost layer of the perisperm.

CUMMIN

Cuminum cyminum L. **Umbelliferae**

Cumin, Cummin Fruits

A yellowish-brown powder with a characteristic, aromatic, slightly camphoraceous odour and taste.

The diagnostic characters are:

(*a*) The *epicarp* composed of a layer of colourless cells, polygonal in surface view with thin, sinuous walls and a faintly and irregularly striated *cuticle; stomata* are fairly frequent and, very occasionally, *cicatrices* may be present. Underlying the epicarp the thin-walled cells of the palisade are sometimes visible.

(*b*) The *covering trichomes*, which are usually found attached to small fragments of the epicarp; they are pluricellular, multiseriate and rounded at the apex; they vary in length and are composed of fairly thick-walled cells which sometimes show faint, scattered cuticular striations.

(*c*) The fairly numerous pale yellowish-brown fragments of the *vittae* composed of fairly large, thin-walled cells, polygonal in surface view. The fragments which include the whole width of the vittae show them to be wider than in most of the other Umbelliferous fruits.

(*d*) The *sclereids from the mesocarp*, of two main types. Those of one type occur as a single layer of longitudinally elongated cells with moderately thickened walls and numerous regularly spaced, well marked pits. Those of the second type are found in small groups and are composed of considerably elongated cells placed more or less end to end in a longitudinal direction; they frequently are found associated with the vascular tissue or with fragments of the vittae; most of these sclereids have moderately thickened walls, although occasional groups occur in which the walls are more heavily thickened and striated; there are few pits.

(*e*) The *endocarp* composed of a layer of fairly large, thin-walled cells, elongated in surface view and arranged with their long axes parallel. This layer may be found associated with fragments of the vittae or with parenchymatous cells from the mesocarp.

(*f*) The very occasional fragments of the *pericarp in sectional view* showing the presence of a two-layered palisade under the epicarp.

(*g*) The *endosperm* composed of moderately thick-walled cells containing *aleurone grains* and *microrosette crystals of calcium oxalate*.

(*h*) The lignified *fibro-vascular tissue* which is frequently found associated with the larger sclereids of the mesocarp, composed of thin-walled, pitted fibres and vessels with spiral and annular thickening.

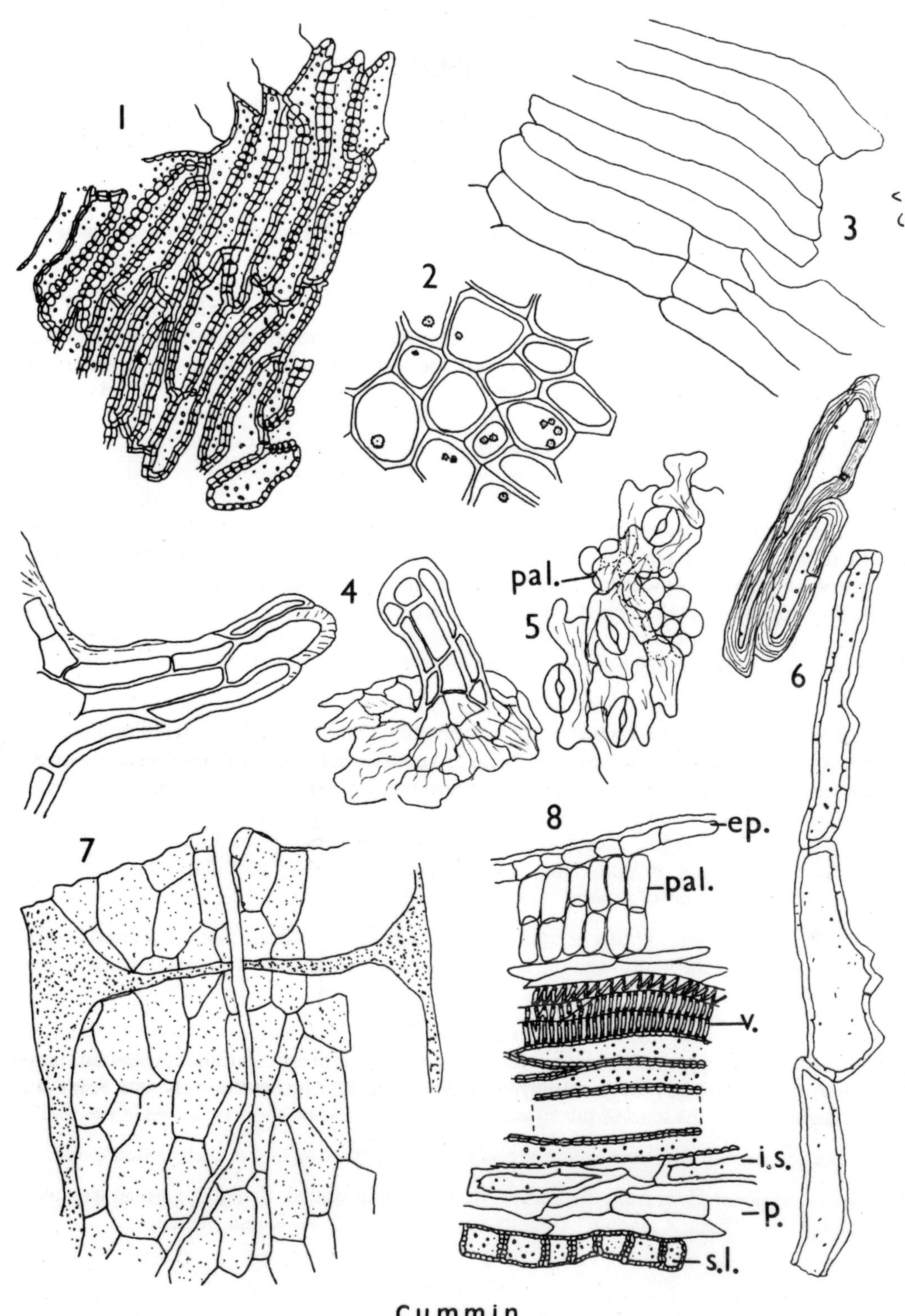

Cummin

×330

1 A group of sclereids from the sclerenchymatous layer of the mesocarp.
2 Endosperm containing microrosette crystals of calcium oxalate.
3 Endocarp in surface view.
4 Covering trichomes attached to fragments of the epicarp in surface view.
5 Epicarp in surface view showing stomata, striated cuticle and part of the underlying palisade (pal.).
6 Groups of sclereids from the mesocarp.
7 Fragment of a vitta showing a transverse septum.
8 Part of the pericarp in sectional view showing the epicarp (ep.), two-layered palisade (pal.), vascular tissue (v.), isolated sclereids (i.s.), parenchyma (p.) and the sclerenchymatous layer (s.l.).

DAMIANA

Turnera diffusa Willd. var. *aphrodisiaca* (Ward.) Urb. Turneraceae

Damiana Leaf, Turnera

A bright yellowish-green powder with a characteristic, aromatic odour and a slightly bitter and pungent taste.

The diagnostic characters are:

(*a*) The fragments of the *lamina in surface view*. The *upper epidermis* is composed of cells with straight or slightly sinuous walls; the majority are thin-walled but at fairly frequent intervals single cells, or small groups of cells, occur which are strongly and unevenly thickened and usually contain a yellowish-brown secretion; stomata are absent; the underlying palisade cells are fairly small and closely packed. The cells of the *lower epidermis* are rather more sinuous in outline and, as in the upper epidermis, occasional cells are unevenly thickened and contain secretion; *stomata* are numerous, usually *paracytic* but frequently the arrangement of the subsidiary cells is irregular; the leaf is isobilateral and the palisade cells underlying the lower epidermis are frequently somewhat larger and more loosely packed than those underlying the upper epidermis. Both the upper and lower epidermis show numerous *cicatrices* where covering trichomes were attached; they appear as small, almost circular scars around which the epidermal cells occur in a radiating arrangement. Cicatrices are particularly abundant on the epidermis of the larger veins; the epidermal cells in these regions are rectangular, slightly striated and have evenly thickened, yellowish-brown walls.

(*b*) The slender *covering trichomes* which are very abundant and are found scattered or attached to fragments of the epidermis; they are unicellular, sometimes somewhat twisted and convoluted and taper gradually towards the apex; they vary considerably in length and are frequently very long. The base may be enlarged and curved; the slightly warted walls are very thick and frequently a lumen is not visible except at the base; the basal region gives a reaction for lignin.

Very occasional *glandular trichomes* may be found; they have a short unicellular stalk and large multicellular head composed of several very thin-walled cells.

(*c*) The numerous fairly large *cluster crystals of calcium oxalate* which are found scattered and in the cells of the cortex of the midrib and the larger veins; a few smaller cluster crystals occur in the mesophyll and in some of the palisade cells.

(*d*) The fragments of the *lamina in sectional view* showing the thick cuticle over both epidermises and the presence of an upper and lower palisade. The yellowish-brown secretion present in some of the epidermal cells is seen to occur mainly in the outer region. The lignified trichome bases are depressed slightly below the level of the adjacent epidermal cells and show striations in the walls.

(*e*) The occasional small spherical *pollen grains* with three furrows and a finely pitted exine.

(*f*) The very occasional *fibres* from the midrib; they are thick-walled, lignified, with an irregular lumen and few pits. A small amount of lignified *pitted parenchyma* is also present.

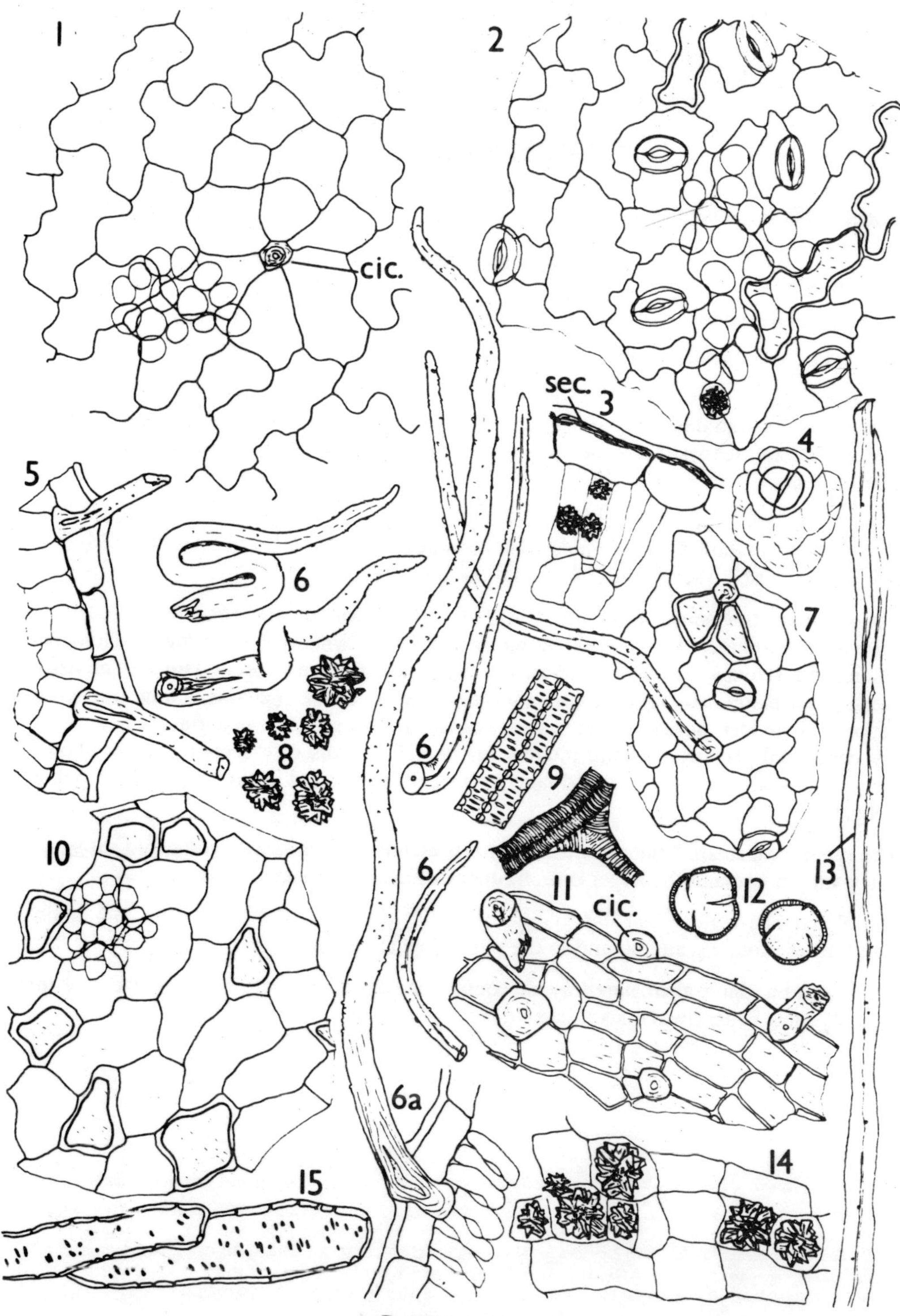

Damiana

×330

1 Upper epidermis in surface view showing a cicatrix (cic.) and part of the underlying palisade.

2 Lower epidermis in surface view with numerous stomata, occasional thick-walled cells containing secretion, and part of the underlying palisade.

3 Part of the lamina in sectional view showing the secretion (sec.) in the epidermal cells, and underlying palisade containing cluster crystals of calcium oxalate.

4 An isolated glandular trichome, seen from below.

5 Part of the lamina in sectional view showing trichome bases.

6 Covering trichomes.

7 Lower epidermis in surface view with a cicatrix and an attached trichome.

8 Calcium oxalate cluster crystals.

9 Fragments of vascular tissue.

10 Upper epidermis in surface view showing scattered thick-walled cells containing secretion.

11 Epidermis from the midrib or one of the larger veins in surface view showing striations and numerous cicatrices (cic.).

12 Pollen grains.

13 Part of a group of fibres.

14 Parenchyma of the cortex of one of the larger veins containing cluster crystals of calcium oxalate.

15 Pitted parenchyma from the midrib.

DANDELION ROOT

Taraxacum officinale Weber — Compositae

Taraxacum Root

A pale fawn to brown powder with a faint odour and a bland, slightly sweet taste.

The diagnostic characters are:

(*a*) The fragments of *cork*, which are fairly abundant; they are dull brown and the outermost layers are indistinct and darker in colour. In surface view the cells are polygonal and somewhat variable in size, and the walls may be moderately thickened; they frequently have dark brown, granular contents.

(*b*) The *covering trichomes* from the crown of the root. These are colourless to light brown, very long, uniseriate, composed of a number of thin-walled cells which are frequently twisted and more or less collapsed; they are usually found fragmented.

(*c*) The abundant fragments of *phloem tissue*, many of which contain *laticiferous vessels*. The greater part of the phloem is composed of thin-walled parenchymatous cells which are longitudinally elongated. Groups of narrow, regularly arranged sieve tubes also occur with very indistinct, transverse sieve plates. The laticiferous vessels are pale yellowish in colour and in longitudinal view appear as slender, anastomosing strands containing fine granular material.

Very occasional fragments of the phloem are found in transverse sectional view, showing patches of small-celled sieve tubes and laticiferous cells embedded in the larger-celled phloem parenchyma.

(*d*) The *vessels*, which are lignified and usually reticulately thickened with elongated slit-shaped pits; they vary in size and the larger ones frequently have oblique end walls.

(*e*) The abundant irregular, angular masses of *inulin*, which are only visible in non-aqueous mounts; they are found scattered and in the parenchymatous cells.

(*f*) The abundant thin-walled *parenchyma* containing inulin; the cells vary in size and may occasionally show collenchymatous thickening.

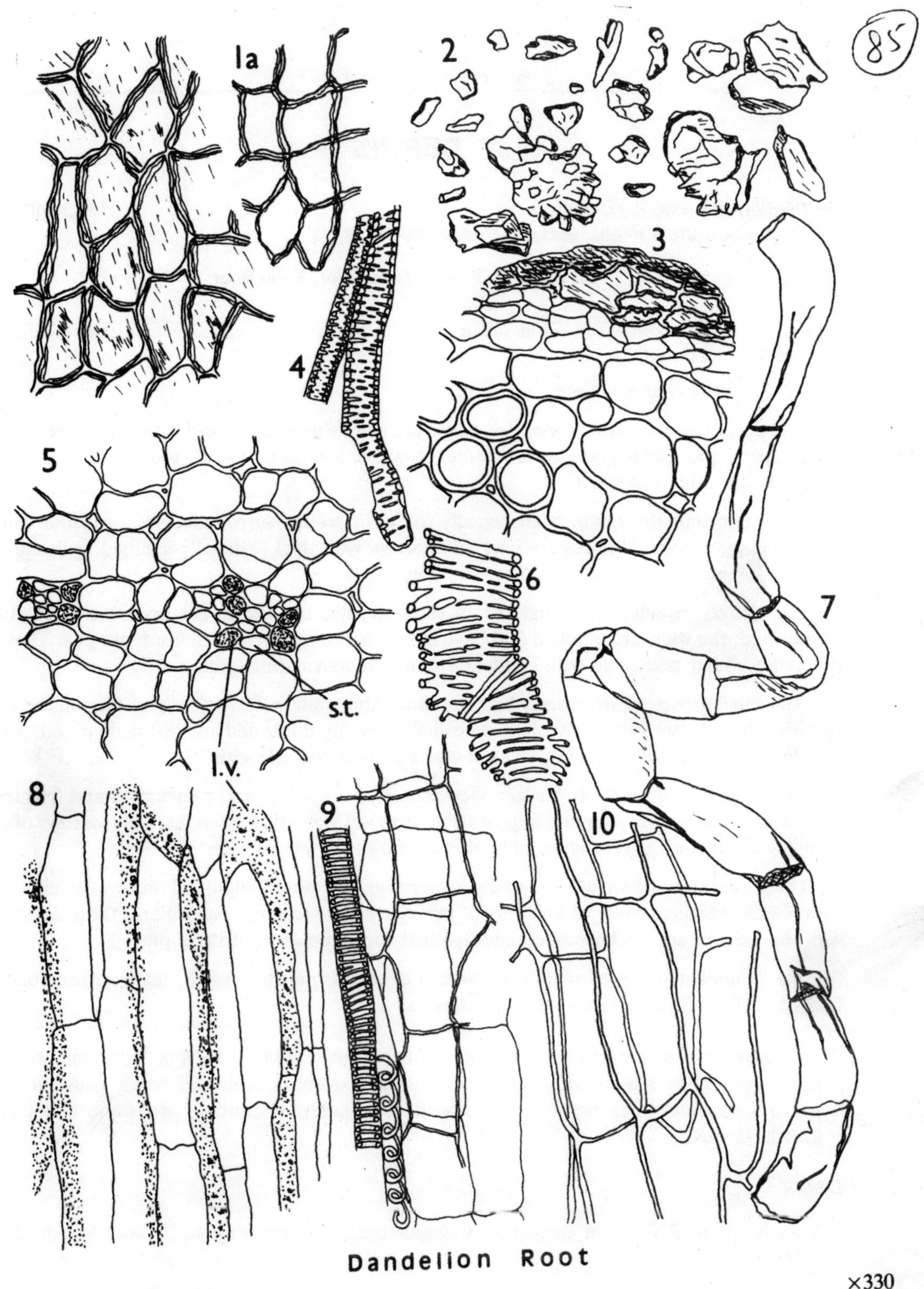

Dandelion Root

×330

1 Larger, thicker-walled cork cells in surface view.
1a Smaller, thinner-walled cork cells in surface view.
2 Masses of inulin in an Alcohol mount.
3 Part of the outer tissues in sectional view.
4 Small, reticulately thickened vessels.
5 Part of the phloem in transverse section showing small patches of sieve tissue (s.t.) and laticiferous vessels (l.v.) embedded in phloem parenchyma.
6 Part of a larger reticulately thickened vessel.
7 Part of a trichome.
8 Phloem tissue in longitudinal view showing anastomosing laticiferous vessels (l.v.).
9 Vessels with spiral and annular thickening and adjacent thin-walled parenchyma of the pith, in longitudinal view.
10 Thicker-walled parenchymatous cells in longitudinal view.

DERRIS

Derris elliptica (Roxb.) Benth. Leguminosae
Derris malaccensis Prain, and other species of *Derris*

Derris Root, Touba, Tuba Root, Tube Root

A pale brown to buff powder with a faint odour and a bitter taste causing a persistent sensation of numbness in the mouth and throat.

The diagnostic characters are:

(*a*) The fairly abundant *starch granules*, which are simple and compound with two, three or more components. Individual granules are rather small, spherical or ovoid; the hilum is small and rounded and rather indistinct.

(*b*) The abundant *fibres*, which are usually found in groups surrounded by a calcium oxalate prism sheath. Individual fibres are long and narrow with thick, partially lignified walls and few pits; the lumen is small and often discontinuous.

(*c*) The *vessels*, which occur singly or in small groups and the larger ones are often found fragmented; the walls are lignified and have numerous closely arranged bordered pits. They are frequently found associated with lignified xylem parenchymatous cells.

(*d*) The small groups of *sclereids*, which are more abundant in *D. malaccensis* than in the other species. The cells are subrectangular, somewhat unevenly thickened and distinctly pitted; prisms of calcium oxalate are frequently found associated with the sclereids.

(*e*) The fragments of *cork*. In surface view the cells are polygonal, thin-walled and frequently filled with dense brown contents; fragments in sectional view show from three to five rows of cork cells associated with parenchyma and collenchyma of the phelloderm.

(*f*) The *parenchyma of the xylem* and *medullary rays*, composed mainly of thin-walled cells filled with starch granules; some of the cells of the xylem parenchyma, particularly those associated with the vessels, are thicker-walled and lignified with numerous, distinct pits.

(*g*) The abundant scattered *prisms of calcium oxalate* from the crystal sheath surrounding the fibres and the cells associated with the sclereids.

This powder is similar to that of Lonchocarpus, page 148; it may be distinguished from Lonchocarpus by the size of the vessels, calcium oxalate crystals and starch granules, all of which are smaller in Derris than they are in Lonchocarpus. Starch is also more abundant in Lonchocarpus.

Derris

Vessels up to 220 μm in diameter. Calcium oxalate prisms up to 20 μm. Starch, single granules 3–**6–12**–20 μm in diameter.

Lonchocarpus

Vessels up to 500 μm in diameter. Calcium oxalate prisms 20 to 30 μm. Starch, single granules 6–**15–20**–25 μm in diameter.

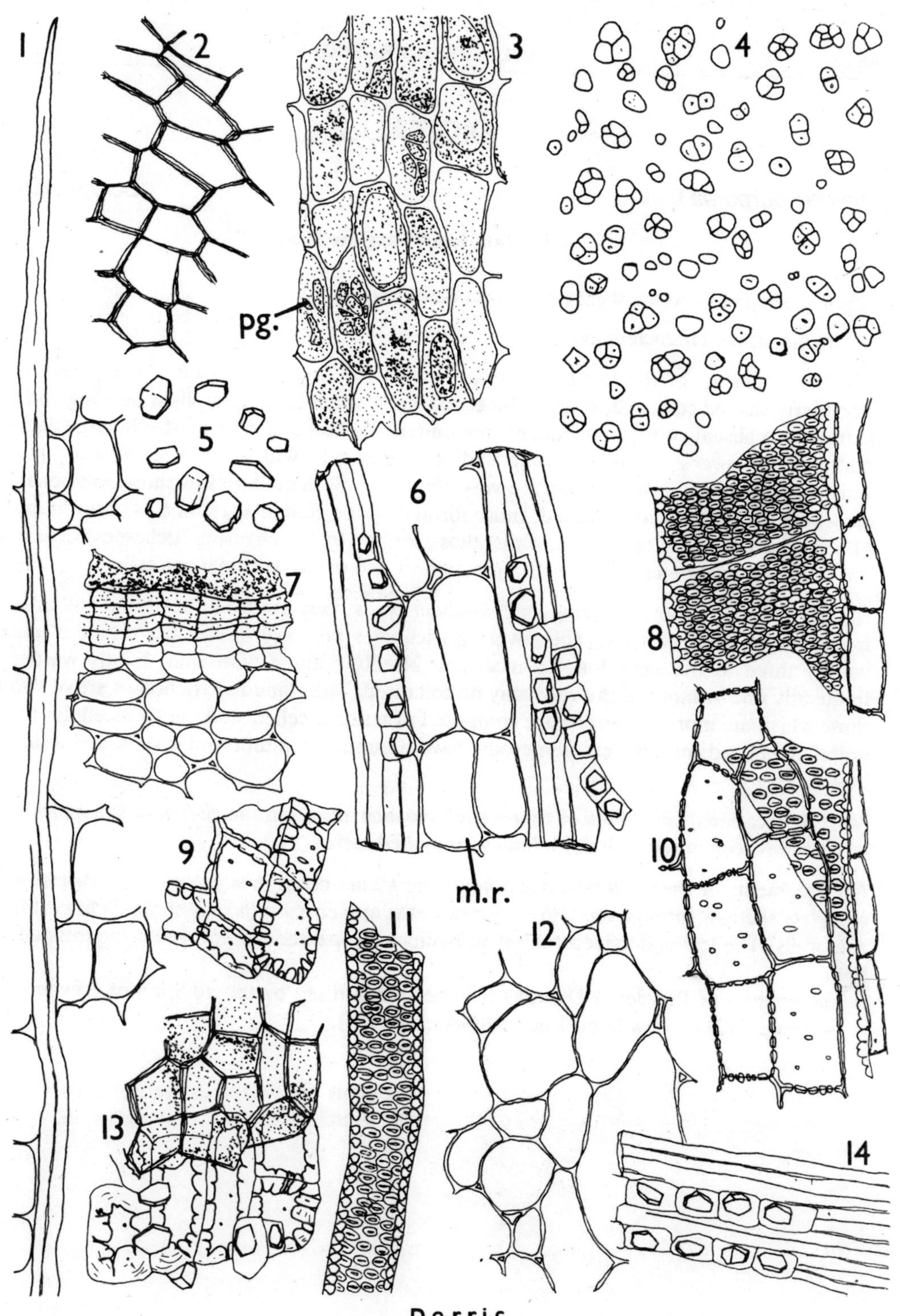

Derris

×330

1 Part of a single fibre with associated parenchyma.
2 Cork in surface view.
3 Cork in surface view showing pigment (pg.).
4 Starch granules.
5 Calcium oxalate prisms.
6 Parts of two groups of fibres with associated calcium oxalate prism sheaths, enclosing part of a medullary ray (m.r.) in tangential longitudinal section.
7 Cork and phelloderm in sectional view.
8 Part of a bordered pitted vessel with associated lignified xylem parenchyma.
9 Part of a group of sclereids.
10 Lignified xylem parenchyma with part of a bordered pitted vessel.
11 A smaller bordered pitted vessel.
12 Parenchyma.
13 Cork cells containing pigment, in surface view, with underlying sclereids and associated calcium oxalate prisms.
14 Part of a group of fibres with associated calcium oxalate prism sheath.

DIGITALIS

Digitalis purpurea L. Scrophulariaceae

Digitalis Leaf, Foxglove Leaf

A pale green powder with a slight odour and a bitter taste.

The diagnostic characters are:

(*a*) The fragments of the *lamina in surface view*. The *upper epidermis* is composed of rather irregularly shaped cells with slightly thickened walls which may show slight beading and pitting; stomata are absent or very infrequent; the underlying palisade cells are fairly large and loosely packed. The *lower epidermis* is composed of smaller cells with thinner, conspicuously sinuous walls; circular *anomocytic stomata* are very abundant. Both epidermises show occasional *cicatrices* where trichomes were attached; those formed by the glandular trichomes occur in the centre of a smaller cell in the epidermis, whilst those formed by the covering trichomes occur either in the centre of a single cell or over the junction of two or more epidermal cells.

(*b*) The *trichomes*, both *covering* and *glandular* types; they are found scattered and attached to fragments of the epidermis. The covering trichomes are very numerous; they are uniseriate, usually three to five cells long, conical and bluntly pointed with thin, faintly warted walls; frequently one or more of the cells may be collapsed. The glandular trichomes are of two types; those which are more numerous are composed of a single-celled stalk and a bicellular (or rarely unicellular) head; others, less numerous, have a uniseriate multicellular stalk and a unicellular head.

(*c*) The occasional fragments of thin-walled *parenchyma* from the cortex of the midrib and the larger veins, composed of longitudinally elongated cells.

(*d*) Fragments of the *epidermis and underlying tissues* occasionally occur *in sectional view* but complete sections through the lamina are rare; the epidermal cells may show slight pitting on the side walls. The leaf is dorsiventral but sometimes the palisade is not well differentiated.

The potency of Powdered Digitalis may be standardised by the addition of Powdered Grass (see page 112) or Powdered Lucerne (see page 150).

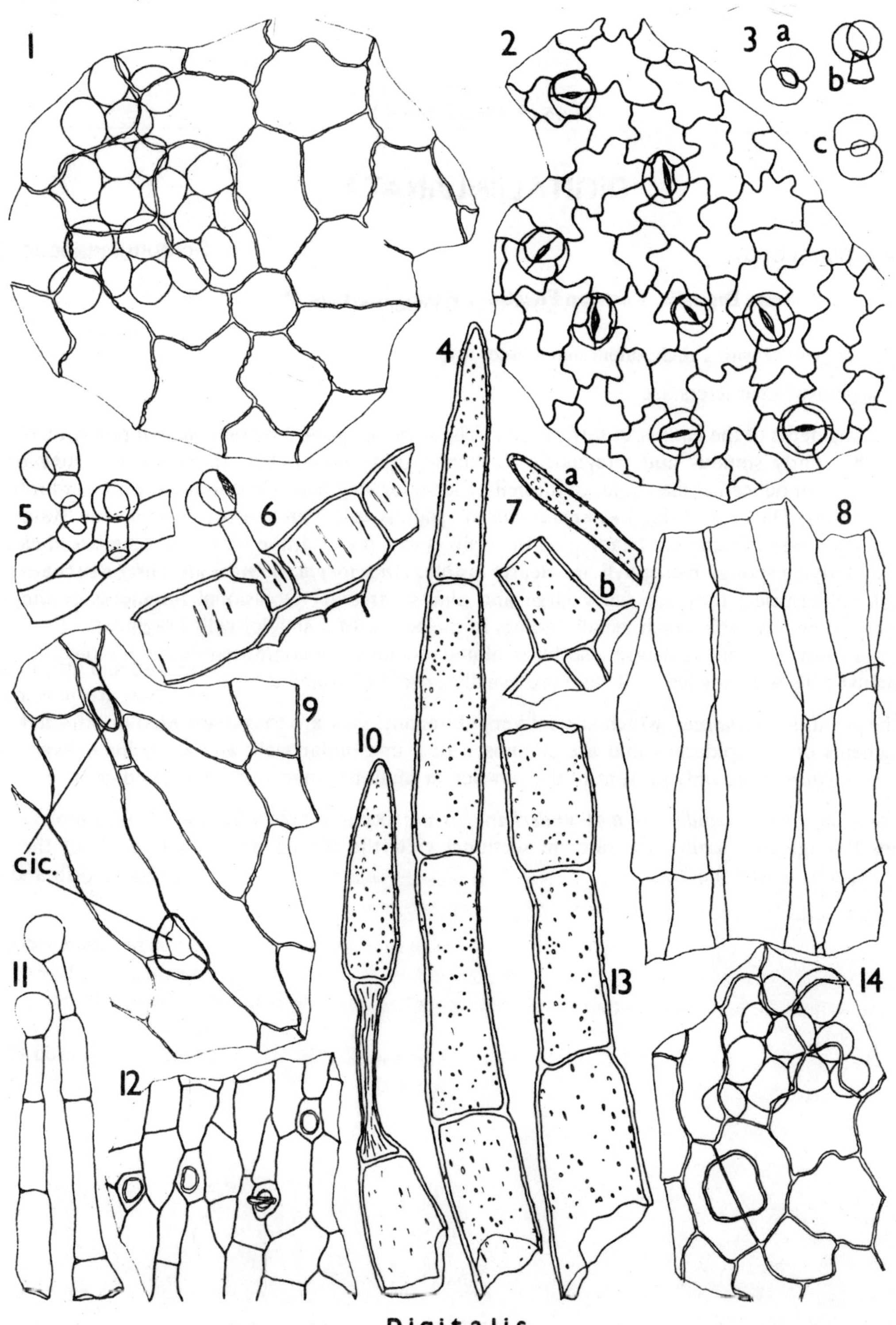

Digitalis

×330

1 Upper epidermis in surface view with underlying palisade cells.
2 Lower epidermis in surface view with anomocytic stomata.
3 Glandular trichome with bicellular heads seen (a) from below (b) from the side and (c) from above.
4 Part of a covering trichome.
5 Glandular trichomes attached to a fragment of the epidermis.
6 Epidermis in sectional view showing pitting in the walls and a glandular trichome.
7 Fragments of covering trichomes: (a) apical cell and (b) basal cell attached to a fragment of epidermis.
8 Cortical parenchyma in longitudinal view.
9 Epidermis in surface view showing cicatrices (cic.).
10 Part of a covering trichome showing a collapsed cell.
11 Glandular trichomes with uniseriate stalks and unicellular heads.
12 Epidermis from over a vein in surface view, showing cicatrices.
13 Fragment of a large covering trichome.
14 Upper epidermis in surface view showing a cicatrix and underlying palisade cells.

DIGITALIS LANATA

Digitalis lanata Ehrh. Scrophulariaceae

Austrian Digitalis, Austrian Foxglove, Woolly Digitalis, Woolly Foxglove

A pale green powder with a slight odour and a bitter taste.

The diagnostic characters are:

(*a*) The fragments of the *lamina in surface view*. The *upper epidermis* is composed of rectangular cells with slightly sinuous and irregularly thickened or beaded walls, the thickening being particularly pronounced at the angles of the cells; the underlying palisade cells are fairly large and loosely packed. The cells of the *lower epidermis* are slightly larger and more irregular than those of the upper epidermis and the beading on the walls is well marked; the thin-walled stellate cells of the underlying spongy mesophyll are clearly visible. *Anomocytic stomata* are fairly abundant on both epidermises; they are fairly large and almost circular. Occasional fragments of the epidermis show a *cicatrix* which usually occurs in the centre of a smaller cell. Fragments of the epidermis from over the veins are also fairly abundant; they are composed of much elongated rectangular cells with beaded walls and are usually devoid of stomata.

(*b*) The *glandular trichomes*, which are not very abundant; they are found scattered or attached to fragments of the epidermis and are composed of a unicellular stalk and a bicellular head. *Covering trichomes* are only present in the powder as small fragments of thin-walled cells.

(*c*) Fragments of the *epidermis and underlying tissues* occur *in sectional view* but complete sections through the lamina are rare; in sectional view the pitting on the side walls of the epidermal cells is well marked.

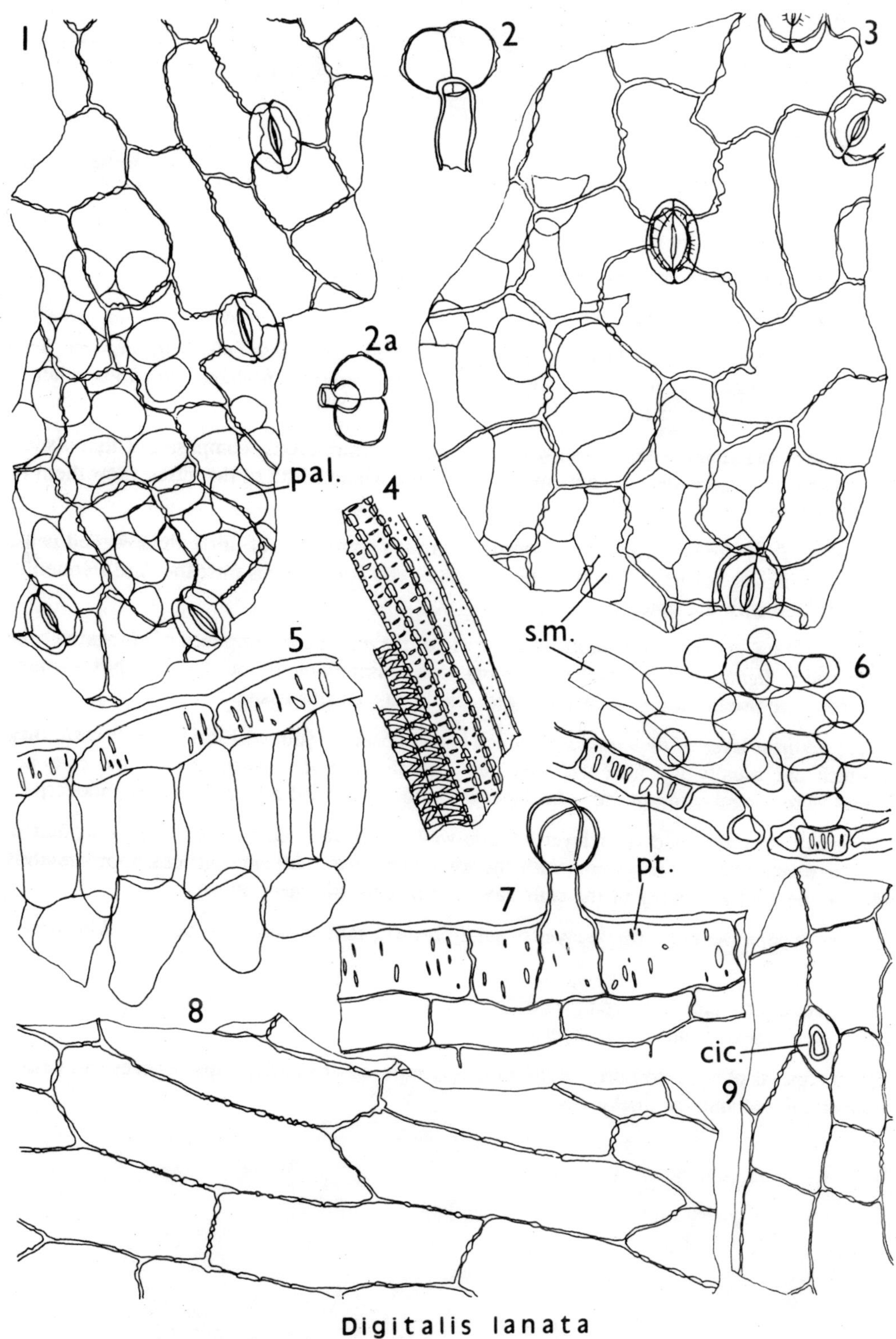

Digitalis lanata

×330

1 Upper epidermis in surface view showing anomocytic stomata and underlying palisade (pal.).
2 Glandular trichome in side view.
2a Glandular trichome from above.
3 Lower epidermis in surface view with anomocytic stomata and underlying spongy mesophyll (s.m.).
4 Vascular tissue from a larger vein.
5 Upper epidermis and palisade in sectional view.
6 Lower epidermis with pits (pt.) and spongy mesophyll (s.m.) in sectional view.
7 Epidermis over a vein in sectional view with pits (pt.) and a glandular trichome.
8 Epidermis from over a vein in surface view.
9 Epidermis in surface view showing a cicatrix (cic.).

DILL FRUIT

Anethum graveolens L. Umbelliferae

Dill

A dark brown powder with a characteristic, aromatic odour and taste.

The diagnostic characters are:

(*a*) The *epicarp* composed of a layer of fairly well-defined, colourless cells with uniform, well marked *cuticular striations*; in surface view the cells are variable in shape with thin, slightly sinuous walls; *stomata* are infrequent.

(*b*) The brown fragments of the *vittae*, which are not very numerous, composed of thin-walled cells, polygonal in surface view. Fragments including the whole width of the vittae show them to be rather narrow.

(*c*) The *sclereids of the mesocarp*; these occur in groups composed of fairly thick-walled cells, square to rectangular in outline, with numerous small and conspicuous pits; they are frequently found associated with the epicarp.

(*d*) The occasional groups of *reticulate parenchyma of the mesocarp* composed of elongated cells with fairly thick, lignified walls traversed by numerous conspicuous, rounded to oval pits. Groups of these cells are usually found associated with the fibro-vascular tissue.

(*e*) The *innermost layer of the mesocarp*, which is composed of yellowish-brown cells with thick walls which are usually lignified and have few, indistinct pits; in surface view the cells are polygonal to rectangular in outline. This layer is frequently found adherent to the endocarp.

(*f*) The *endocarp* composed of a layer of thin-walled, lignified cells which are elongated in surface view and arranged in groups with the long axes of the adjacent groups approximately parallel to one another; many of the cells have a markedly sinuous outline.

(*g*) The *testa*, composed of a single layer of small, brown, thin-walled cells, polygonal in surface view.

(*h*) The abundant *endosperm* composed of thick-walled cells containing *aleurone grains* and *microrosette crystals of calcium oxalate*.

(*i*) The fragments of lignified *fibro-vascular tissue* composed of small groups of fibres and vessels showing spiral and annular thickening.

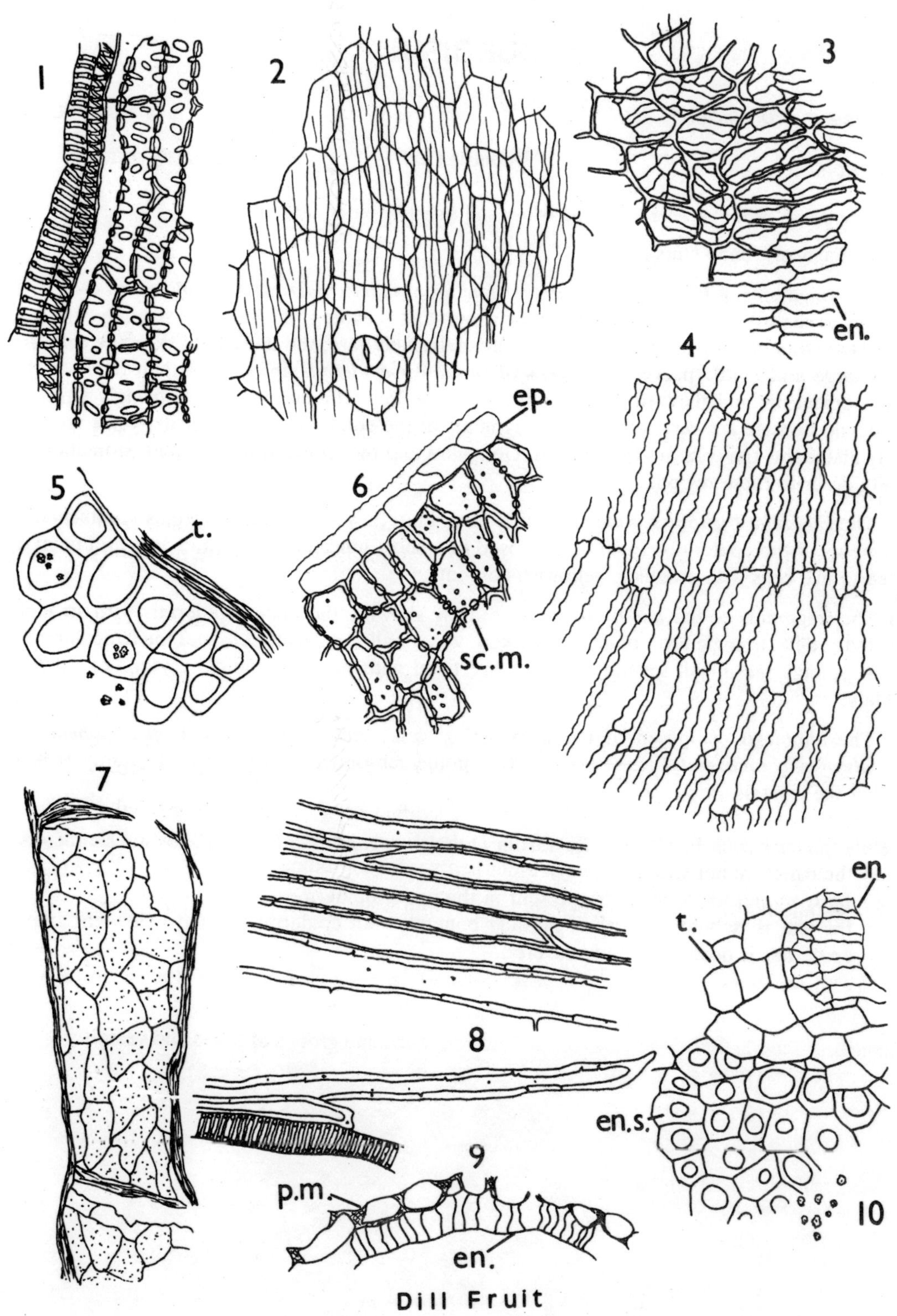

Dill Fruit

×330

1 Vascular tissue and associated reticulate parenchyma of the mesocarp.
2 Epicarp in surface view showing a stoma and striated cuticle.
3 The innermost layer of the mesocarp with underlying endocarp (en.) in surface view.
4 Endocarp in surface view.
5 Part of the endosperm containing microrosette crystals of calcium oxalate, and the testa (t.) in sectional view.
6 Epicarp (ep.) and sclereids of the mesocarp (sc.m.) in sectional view.
7 Part of a vitta showing transverse septa.
8 Elements of the fibro-vascular tissue.
9 Innermost layer of the mesocarp (p.m.) and the endocarp (en.) in sectional view.
10 Endosperm (en.s.), with associated cells of the testa (t.) and endocarp (en.) in surface view.

DUBOISIA

Duboisia myoporoides R. Br. — Solanaceae

Duboisia Leaf

A dark greenish-brown powder with little odour and a slightly bitter taste.

The diagnostic characters are:

(*a*) The fragments of the *lamina in surface view*. The *upper epidermis* is composed of cells with straight or slightly sinuous walls which may show slight beading; the *cuticle* is strongly striated; *anisocytic* stomata may be present but they are extremely rare; the underlying palisade cells are fairly large and tightly packed. The cells of the *lower epidermis* are smaller than those of the upper epidermis and they are slightly more wavy-walled; the cuticle is less strongly striated; anisocytic stomata are very numerous. Fragments of the epidermis from over the veins are also fairly abundant; the cells are thin-walled, elongated and the cuticle is not striated; stomata only rarely occur in these regions.

(*b*) The *glandular trichomes*, which are fairly abundant; they are found scattered and attached to fragments of the epidermis. Each is composed of a short unicellular stalk and an ovoid head of three to five cells with granular, yellowish contents.

(*c*) The fragments of the *lamina in sectional view* showing the upper epidermis with strongly striated cuticle, a single layer of closely packed, wavy-walled palisade cells and the irregular cells of the spongy mesophyll several of which are filled with microsphenoidal crystals of calcium oxalate.

(*d*) The *idioblasts* composed of parenchymatous cells densely packed with *microsphenoidal crystals of calcium oxalate*. These occur in the spongy mesophyll and they are frequently broken so that the crystals are found scattered.

Duboisia leichardtii F. Moell. differs from *Duboisia myoporoides* in the following characters:
(*a*) the cuticle is not striated;
(*b*) fairly numerous stomata are present in the upper epidermis;
(*c*) the leaf is isobilateral with a palisade beneath both epidermises; that below the upper epidermis is occasionally two-layered.

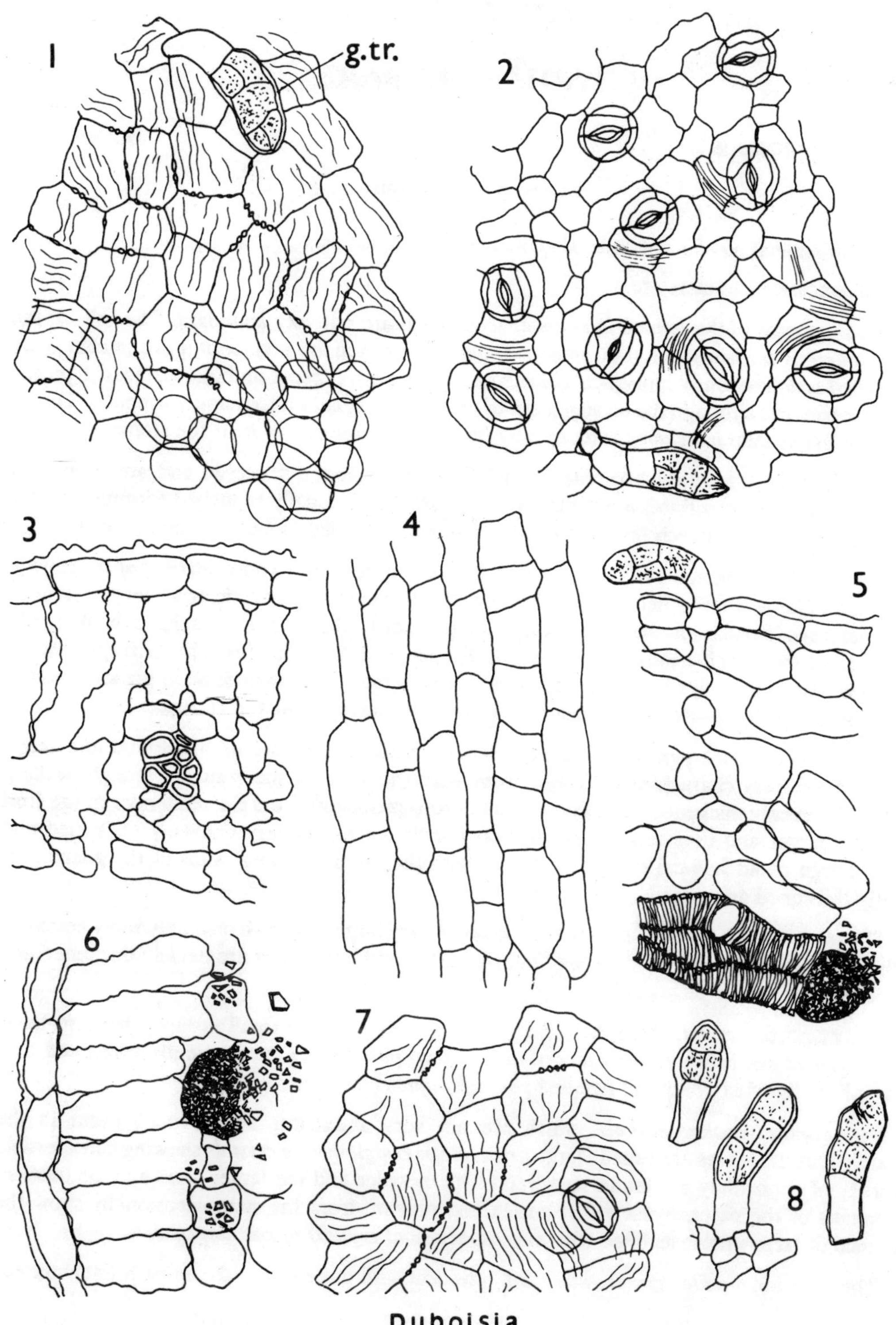

Duboisia

×330

1 Upper epidermis in surface view showing the striated cuticle, an attached glandular trichome (g.tr.) and part of the underlying palisade.

2 Lower epidermis in surface view showing numerous stomata and an attached glandular trichome.

3 Part of the lamina in sectional view showing the upper epidermis with striated cuticle, underlying palisade and part of a vein in the spongy mesophyll.

4 Epidermis over a vein in surface view.

5 Part of the lamina in sectional view showing the lower epidermis with an attached trichome, spongy mesophyll with part of a vein in longitudinal view and an idioblast containing microsphenoidal crystals of calcium oxalate.

6 Part of the lamina in sectional view showing the upper epidermis, palisade and cells of the spongy mesophyll containing microsphenoidal crystals of calcium oxalate.

7 Upper epidermis in surface view showing a stoma.

8 Glandular trichomes.

EGYPTIAN HENBANE

Hyoscyamus muticus L. Solanaceae

Egyptian Hyoscyamus

A pale brownish-buff powder with little odour and a slightly bitter taste.

The diagnostic characters are:

(*a*) The fragments of the *lamina in surface view*, which are not very abundant. The cells of the *upper epidermis* are large with thin, sinuous walls; those of the *lower epidermis* are smaller, very thin-walled and frequently indistinct. Numerous *stomata* are present on both surfaces; typically they are *anisocytic* although the arrangement of the subsidiary cells is frequently irregular. On the lower epidermis faint *cuticular striations* may be present, particularly near the stomata.

(*b*) The abundant *glandular trichomes*, which are usually found scattered and are frequently broken; they have uniseriate, multicellular stalks which are usually branched forming two (or occasionally four) arms each terminating in a one- or two-celled globular to ovoid head.

(*c*) The abundant fragments of the *calyx* and *stem in surface view*. The *epidermis of the calyx* is composed of large, thin-walled polygonal cells with occasional anomocytic or anisocytic stomata and numerous circular *cicatrices* marking the positions where trichomes have broken off; radiating out from each cicatrix are numerous distinct cuticular striations. The *stem epidermis* is similar to that of the calyx but the cells are more elongated; fewer cicatrices are present and the cuticle is frequently striated in all regions and not only surrounding the cicatrices.

(*d*) The *sclereids of the pericarp*, which are fairly abundant; they are usually found in a single layer and are very characteristic. Those from near the apex of the fruit are straight-walled, moderately evenly thickened and have very numerous pits; those from the remainder of the fruit are much larger and they have markedly wavy walls which are very unevenly thickened and pitted. Large ovoid *stomata* occur at intervals with the outer anticlinal walls of the guard cells slightly thickened and pitted.

(*e*) The *sclereids of the testa* composed of a layer of very large cells with distinctly wavy anticlinal walls; the outer walls are not thickened but the radial and inner walls are heavily thickened and striated; a few simple pits occur.

(*f*) The numerous *vessels* from the stem, which usually occur in small groups; they are fairly large, lignified and reticulately thickened or bordered pitted; they are frequently associated with thin-walled, lignified *fibres* and lignified *parenchymatous cells*.

(*g*) The *calcium oxalate crystals*, which are not very abundant. Those which occur in the mesophyll of the leaves are usually large *prismatic or conglomerate crystals* showing considerable diversity of form; they are found scattered in the powder and the larger ones may be broken. Fragments of the parenchyma of the cortex and phloem from the stem occasionally show the presence of large idioblasts filled with *microsphenoidal crystals of calcium oxalate*.

(*h*) The occasional *pollen grains*, which are spherical with three pores; the exine is finely pitted.

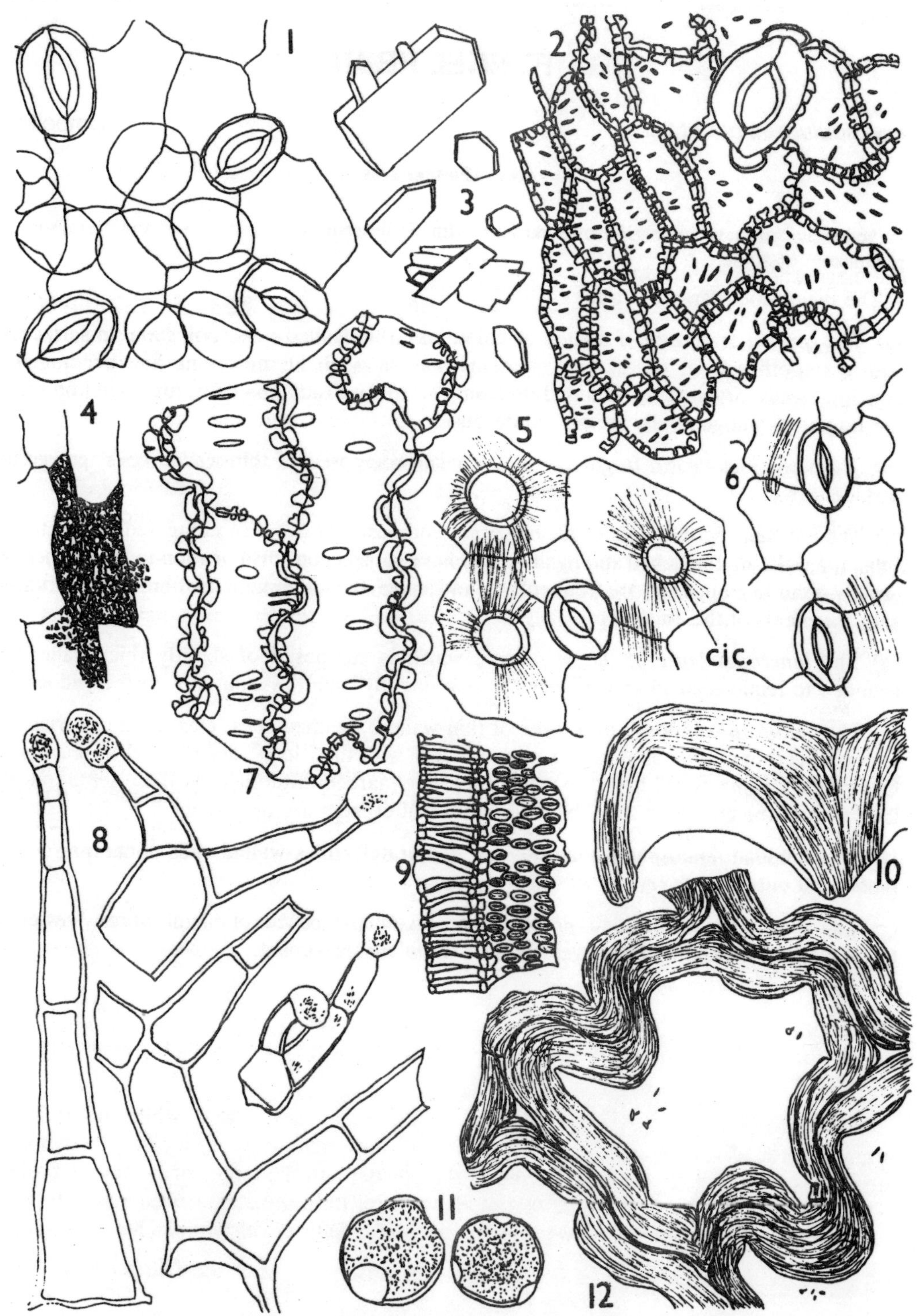

Egyptian Henbane

×330

1 Upper epidermis of the leaf in surface view showing stomata and part of the underlying palisade.
2 Sclereids of the pericarp from near the apex of the fruit.
3 Calcium oxalate crystals.
4 Parenchyma of the stem showing idioblasts containing microsphenoidal crystals of calcium oxalate.
5 Epidermis of the calyx in surface view showing cicatrices (cic.) and a stoma.
6 Lower epidermis of the leaf in surface view showing stomata and cuticular striations.
7 Sclereids of the pericarp.
8 Parts of glandular trichomes.
9 Part of a group of reticulately thickened and bordered pitted vessels from the stem.
10 Sclereids of the testa in sectional view.
11 Pollen grains.
12 Sclereids of the testa in surface view.

FENNEL FRUIT

Foeniculum vulgare Mill. Umbelliferae

Fennel

A yellowish-brown to greenish-brown powder with a pleasant, aromatic odour and taste somewhat reminiscent of Anise.

The diagnostic characters are:

(*a*) The *epicarp* composed of a layer of colourless, thin-walled cells, polygonal in surface view with a smooth cuticle; occasional fragments may show slight thickening and beading of the anticlinal walls. *Stomata*, surrounded by from two to four radiating cells, are found on some of the fragments but generally are not numerous.

(*b*) The numerous brown fragments of the *vittae* composed of thin-walled cells, polygonal in surface view.

(*c*) The *reticulate parenchyma of the mesocarp* composed of ovoid or elongated, subrectangular cells; the walls are thickened and lignified and have conspicuous oval or rounded pits. These cells usually occur in groups and are frequently found associated either with the fibro-vascular tissue or with fragments of the endocarp.

(*d*) The *innermost layer of the mesocarp*, which is composed of slightly thick-walled cells, rounded to rectangular in surface view; it is frequently found associated with the endocarp.

(*e*) The *endocarp* composed of a layer of thin-walled, lignified cells, elongated in surface view and arranged in groups of about six or more cells with their long axes parallel to one another. Occasional fragments are found in which there are marked differences in the orientation of the long axes of the groups of cells, but usually the differences are only slight.

(*f*) The abundant *endosperm* composed of moderately thick-walled cells containing *aleurone grains* and *microrosette crystals of calcium oxalate*.

(*g*) The fragments of lignified *fibro-vascular tissue* composed of small fibres, vessels and tracheids, and occasional larger vessels with reticulate thickening.

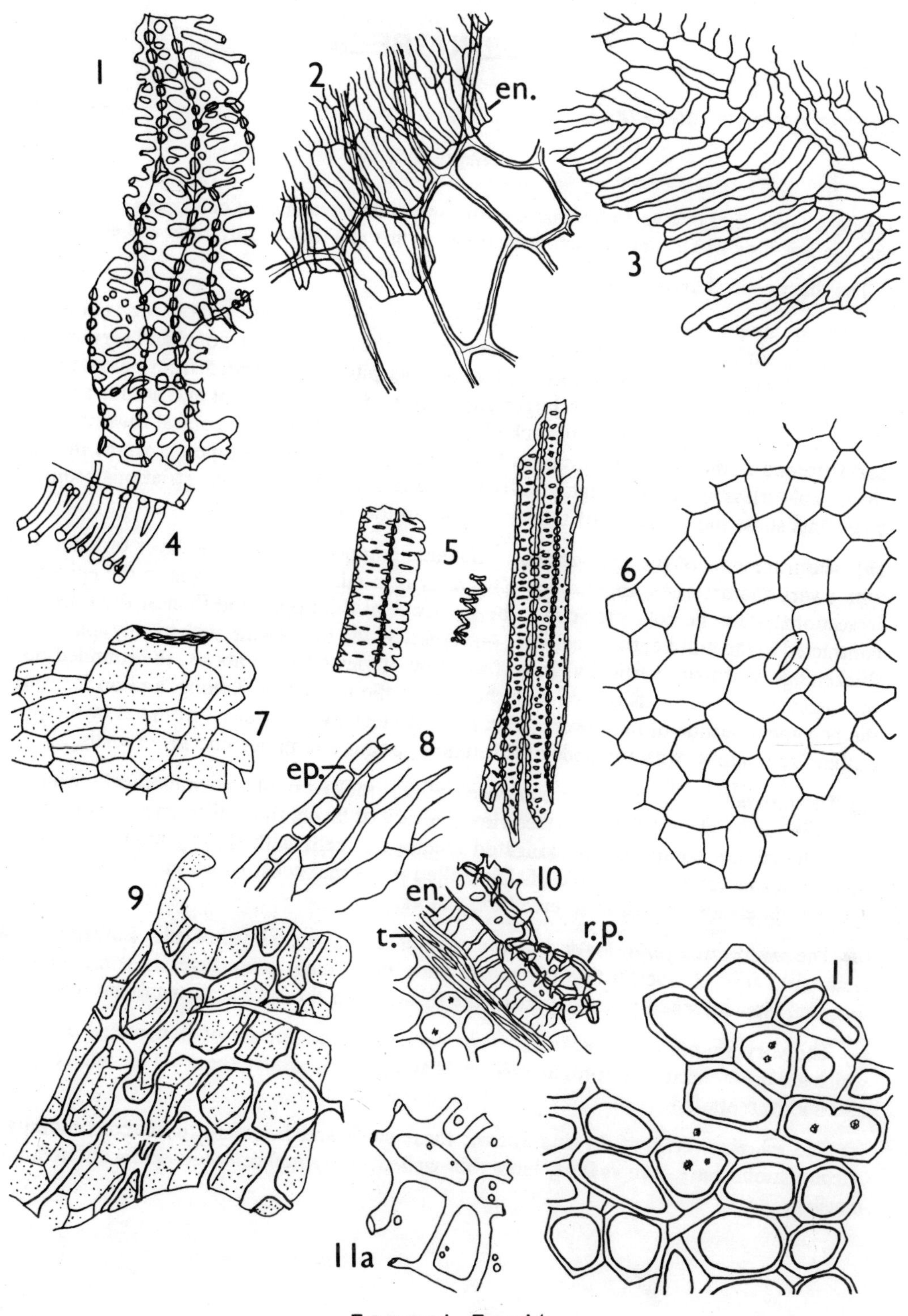

Fennel Fruit

×330

1 Reticulate parenchyma of the mesocarp.
2 Endocarp (en.) with overlying cells of the innermost layer of the mesocarp, in surface view.
3 Endocarp in surface view.
4 Fragment of a reticulately thickened vessel.
5 Elements from the fibro-vascular tissue.
6 Epicarp in surface view showing a stoma.
7 Fragment of a vitta.
8 Epicarp (ep.) and parenchyma of the mesocarp in sectional view.
9 Fragment of a vitta with overlying thick-walled cells of the innermost layer of the mesocarp, in surface view.
10 Part of the pericarp and seed in sectional view showing the reticulate parenchyma (r.p.), endocarp (en.), testa (t.) and endosperm.
11 Endosperm containing microrosette crystals of calcium oxalate.
11a Thicker-walled cells of the endosperm.

FOENUGREEK

Trigonella foenum-graecum L. Leguminosae

Fenugreek Seeds

A pale yellowish-buff powder with a characteristic, spicy odour reminiscent of Slippery Elm, and a strong, characteristic taste which is mealy and mucilaginous at first and then slightly bitter and unpleasant.

The diagnostic characters are:

(*a*) The fragments of the *epidermis of the testa* composed of cells containing yellowish-brown pigment. In surface view, when viewed from above, the cells are polygonal and regular with thick walls and a small lumen from which radiate distinct pits; when viewed from below the cells are similar in outline but the lumen is larger and filled with dense pigment and no pits are visible. In sectional view the cells are closely packed, longitudinally elongated, conical towards the outside and flattened at the base; the lumen is fairly wide at the base and tapers towards the apex; the thick, colourless walls are highly refractive and show longitudinal striations; some of the fragments show the presence of a thick cuticle on the outside.

(*b*) The fragments of the *hypodermis of the testa* composed of a single layer of colourless cells with a very characteristic appearance. This layer is usually found adherent to the epidermis, and in sectional view the cells are seen to be narrower at the upper end than at the lower end and contracted in the middle; these cells are thickened on the radial walls with evenly spaced, rod-like thickenings which run vertically. In surface view, if viewed from above, the rounded outline of the upper wall of the cells is seen with the tops of the rods of thickening, and on focusing down the polygonal outline of the lower wall comes into view; when viewed from below the polygonal outline is apparent, with the rods of thickening joining the upper and lower walls.

(*c*) The *parenchyma of the testa* composed of several layers of thin-walled cells which appear similar in sectional view but in surface view the various layers show differences in structure; some of the layers are composed of elongated rectangular cells with slightly thickened and beaded walls; other layers are composed of thin-walled polygonal cells, which may be very irregular in size or may enclose irregular intercellular spaces.

(*d*) The *outermost layer of the endosperm* composed of a single layer of cells, polygonal in surface view with very characteristic collenchymatous thickening. This layer is sometimes seen in sectional view attached to fragments of the testa, when the cells appear tabular and regular.

(*e*) The very abundant *parenchyma of the cotyledons*, composed of thin-walled cells, some of which are differentiated to form an epidermis and palisade while others are rounded or polygonal and undifferentiated.

(*f*) The *mucilage cells of the endosperm*; these swell and fragment in aqueous mounts but in *Alcohol* mounts are seen as fairly large thin-walled, polygonal cells containing striated masses of mucilage.

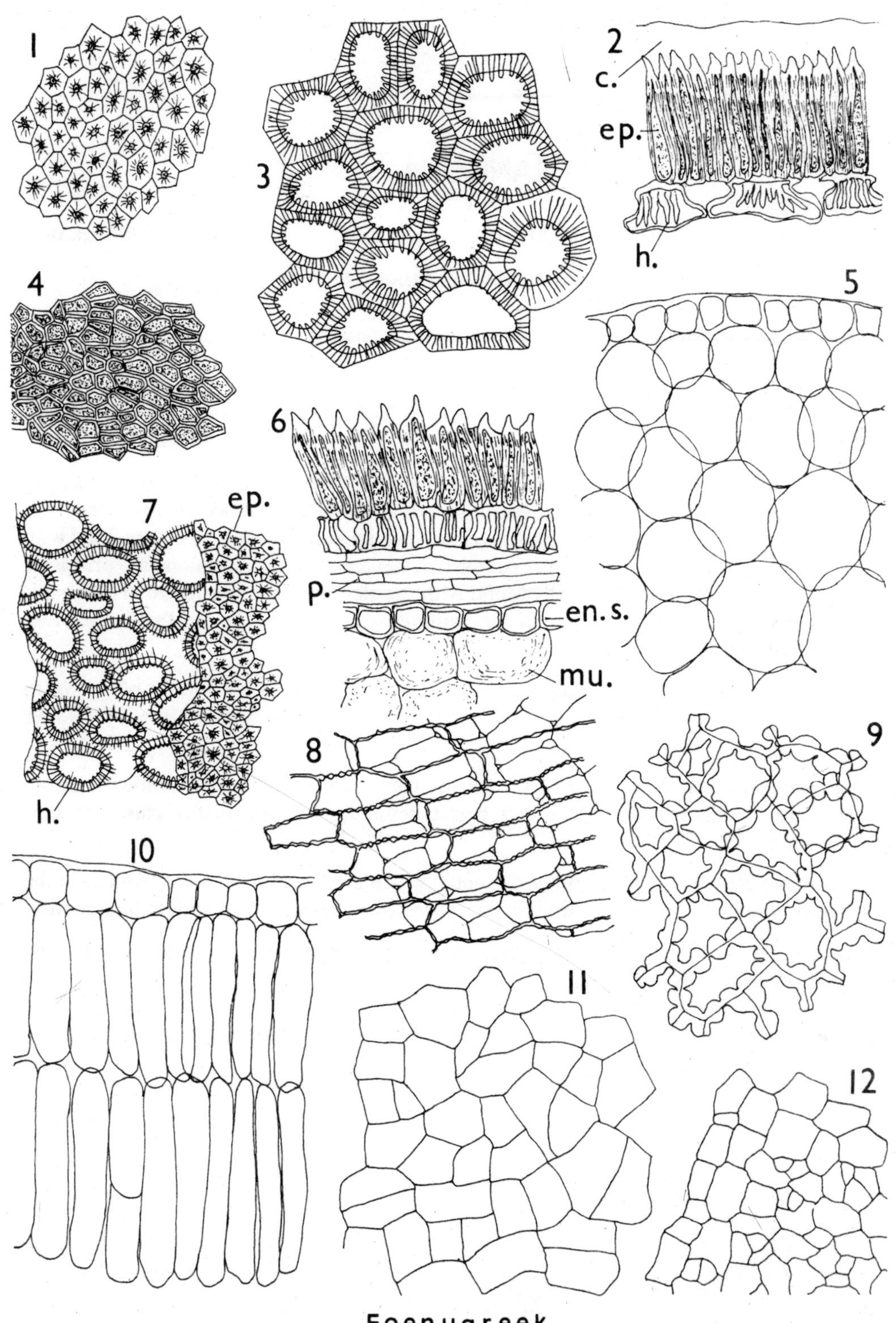

Foenugreek

×330

1 Epidermis of the testa in surface view, from above.
2 Cuticle (c.), epidermis (ep.) and hypodermis (h.) of the testa in sectional view.
3 Hypodermis of the testa in surface view, from below.
4 Epidermis of the testa in surface view, from below.
5 Epidermis and parenchymatous cells of the cotyledons in sectional view.
6 Part of the seed in sectional view showing the epidermis, hypodermis and parenchymatous layers (p.) of the testa and the outermost layer (en.s.) and the mucilage cells (mu.) of the endosperm.
7 Epidermis (ep.) and hypodermis (h.) of the testa in surface view, from above.
8 Layers of the parenchyma of the testa in surface view.
9 Outermost layer of the endosperm in surface view.
10 Epidermis and palisade of the cotyledons in sectional view.
11 Undifferentiated parenchyma of the cotyledons.
12 A single layer of the parenchyma of the testa in surface view.

FRANGULA

Rhamnus frangula L. (*Frangula alnus* Mill.) Rhamnaceae

Frangula Bark, Alder Buckthorn Bark

A yellowish-brown powder with a characteristic odour and an intensely bitter and nauseous taste.

The diagnostic characters are:

(*a*) The numerous groups of *fibres*, each surrounded by a calcium oxalate prism sheath; individual fibres are thick-walled, lignified, with a narrow lumen and few, inconspicuous pits.

(*b*) The *sieve tissue* consisting of thin-walled sieve tubes with well defined sieve plates on the oblique end walls, and thicker-walled phloem parenchyma. The parenchymatous cells are sometimes unevenly thickened and show characteristic beading on the walls; they are filled with yellow-brown contents and frequently also contain cluster crystals or, occasionally, prisms of calcium oxalate. *Medullary rays* are usually found with the sieve tissue either in radial longitudinal section or, less frequently, in tangential longitudinal section; the cells are thin-walled and filled with yellow-brown contents.

(*c*) The abundant fragments of *cork* composed of cells with slightly thickened walls, polygonal in surface view; the fragments appear bright orange-red when mounted in *Solution of Chloral Hydrate*.

(*d*) The *parenchyma* and *collenchyma* of the cortex composed of cells with yellowish-brown contents; the parenchymatous cells contain starch granules and, very occasionally, cluster crystals of calcium oxalate.

(*e*) The *prisms* and *cluster crystals of calcium oxalate*, which are found scattered as well as in the parenchymatous tissues; some of the cluster crystals are rather irregular and appear fragmented.

(*f*) The small, spherical *starch granules*, which are rarely found scattered but are present in some of the parenchymatous cells.

This powder is very similar to that of Cascara, page 46. It is distinguished from Cascara by the absence of sclereids and the red colour of the cork.

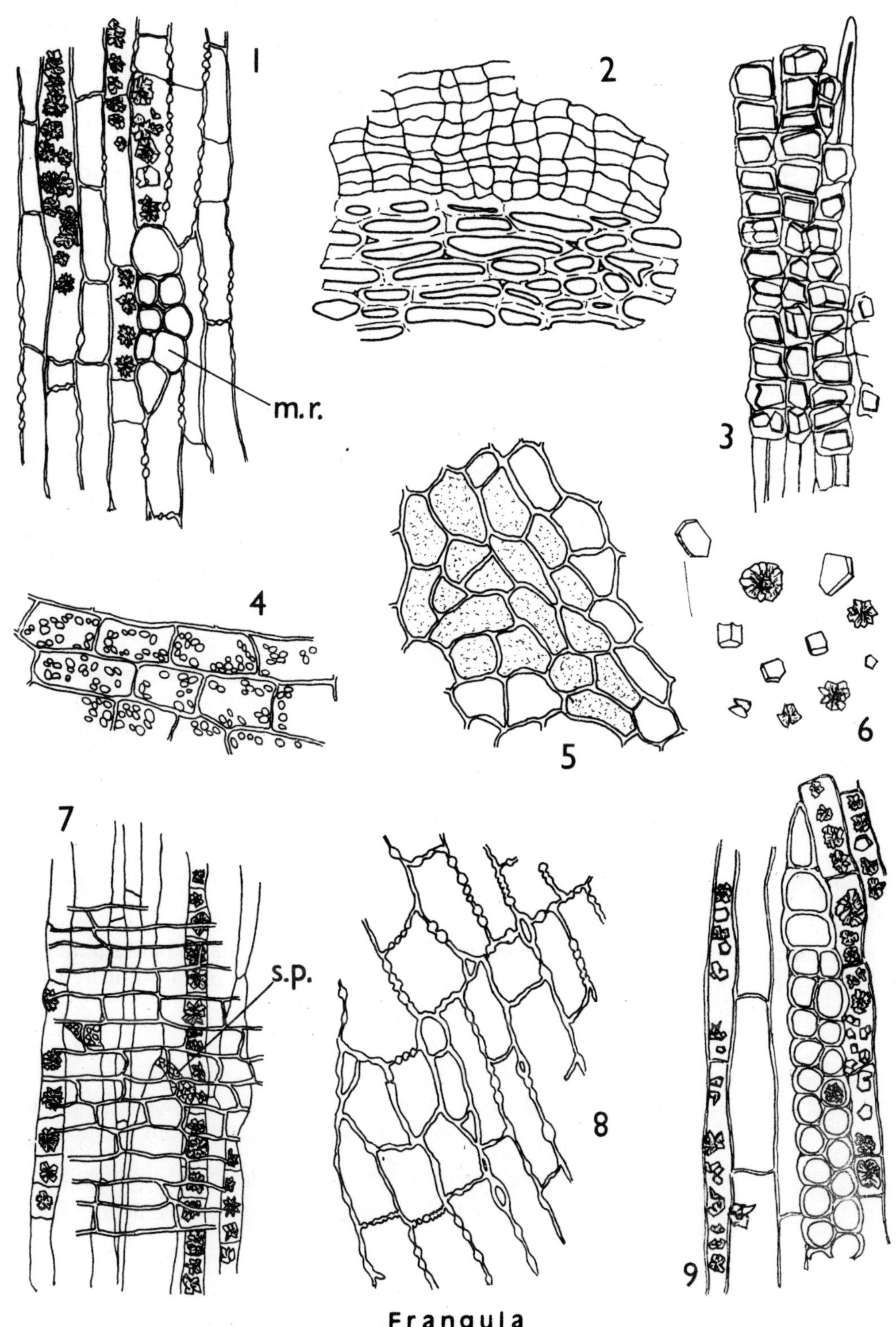

Frangula

×330

1 Phloem parenchyma containing cluster crystals of calcium oxalate and a medullary ray (m.r.) in tangential longitudinal section.
2 Cork and collenchyma in sectional view.
3 Part of a group of fibres with calcium oxalate prism sheath.
4 Parenchyma containing starch granules.
5 Cork in surface view.
6 Crystals of calcium oxalate.
7 Part of the phloem in radial longitudinal section showing sieve tubes with sieve plates (s.p.), phloem parenchyma containing cluster crystals of calcium oxalate and a medullary ray.
8 Phloem parenchymatous cells in tangential longitudinal section showing beaded walls.
9 Part of the phloem in tangential longitudinal section showing a medullary ray and phloem parenchyma containing crystals of calcium oxalate.

GALLS

Pathological outgrowths on
Quercus infectoria Olivier

Fagaceae

Aleppo Galls, Blue Galls, Oak Galls

A greyish-buff powder with a slight odour and a taste which is sweet at first, then astringent.

The diagnostic characters are:

(*a*) The abundant *sclereids*, which show great variation in size and are sometimes very large. The smaller cells are approximately isodiametric and have heavily thickened and striated walls with numerous pits; the lumen is usually filled with dense brown material. Some of the larger sclereids are much elongated and developed as *fibrous sclereids* with the ends sometimes markedly tapered; the walls are moderately and somewhat unevenly thickened, being thinner at the tapered ends; numerous pits are present and these are frequently branched; the lumen may be filled with dense brown material. The very large sclereids vary in shape but are usually more or less ovoid to rectangular; the walls are relatively thin giving a very large lumen which is filled with brown contents; fairly numerous pits are present. The smaller sclereids may be found in groups but the larger ones are usually found singly.

(*b*) The fairly abundant *parenchyma*, most of which is composed of rounded to polygonal cells with moderately thickened and pitted walls and distinct intercellular spaces; many of the fragments show collenchymatous thickening. Occasional groups of larger, more elongated parenchymatous cells also occur but these are usually found fragmented; these cells have thin, evenly thickened walls with few pits. All the parenchymatous cells frequently contain prisms or cluster crystals of calcium oxalate.

(*c*) The fairly abundant *crystals of calcium oxalate*, which are found scattered as well as in the parenchymatous tissue. The majority are in the form of rather irregular *cluster crystals*, varying considerably in size and sometimes quite large. *Prisms* also occur, some of which have a cluster crystal apparently adherent to one of the faces.

(*d*) The abundant angular fragments of *tannin*, which are only seen in a mount in which they are not soluble (e.g. *n-Hexanol*). The fragments occur in the parenchyma but are usually found scattered; they are rather thin and almost transparent.

(*e*) The *starch granules*, which are not very abundant; they are mostly simple but are frequently found massed together in groups; a small number of compound granules occur with two or three components. Individual granules are fairly large, ovoid to spherical or indistinctly polyhedral with a well marked radiate or slit-shaped hilum; some of the granules show faint striations.

(*f*) The very occasional groups of small, lignified *vessels* with spiral or annular thickening.

(*g*) The scattered brown *globular masses (lignin bodies)* which give a positive reaction for lignin.

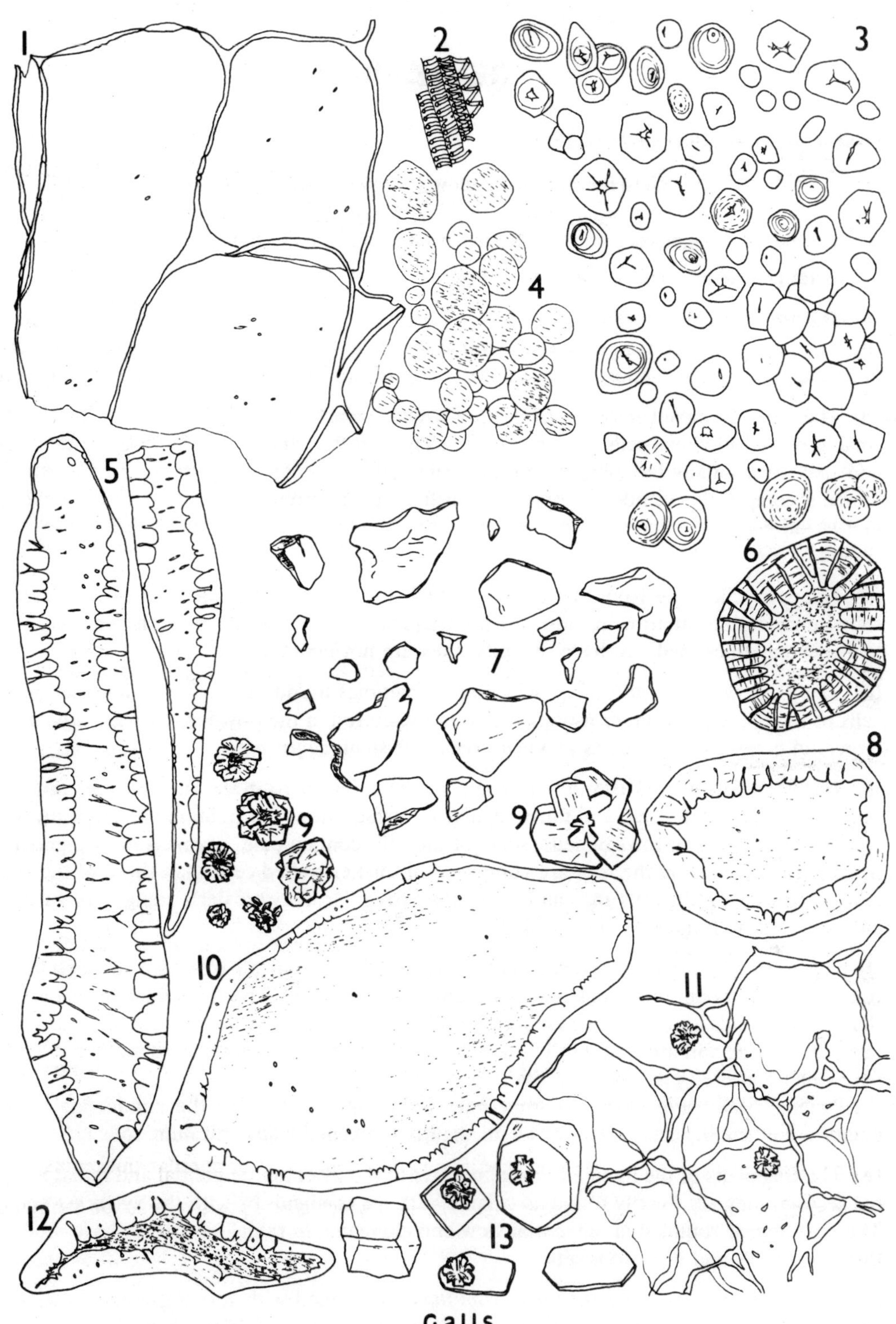

Galls

×330

1 Large-celled parenchyma showing pits.
2 Part of a group of vessels.
3 Starch granules.
4 Lignin bodies.
5 Fibrous sclereids.
6 A thick-walled sclereid with numerous pits and granular contents.
7 Fragments of tannin in a Hexanol mount.
8 A thinner-walled sclereid with fewer pits.
9 Cluster crystals of calcium oxalate.
10 A large thin-walled sclereid.
11 Smaller-celled parenchyma showing collenchymatous thickening, with cluster crystals of calcium oxalate in some of the cells.
12 A smaller fibrous sclereid with granular contents.
13 Prisms of calcium oxalate with associated cluster crystals.

GELSEMIUM

Gelsemium sempervirens (L.) Ait.*f.* Loganiaceae

Gelsemium Root, Yellow Jasmine Root, Yellow Root

A pale yellowish-fawn powder with a slight, mealy odour and a bitter taste.

The diagnostic characters are:

(*a*) The *starch granules*, which are not very abundant; they are small and usually simple but a small number of compound granules are found with two, three or occasionally more components; individual granules are spherical or somewhat polyhedral and a point hilum is sometimes visible.

(*b*) The fairly abundant *sclereids* from the rhizome, which occur singly or, more frequently, in small groups. Individual cells vary in size and shape but they are usually fairly small and irregular and may occasionally be considerably elongated; the walls are very thick and sometimes the lumen is completely occluded; simple or branched pits are present and the walls show numerous fine striations. The sclereids are sometimes found associated with thin-walled cortical parenchyma.

(*c*) The pericyclic *fibres* from the rhizome, which are very long and are found fragmented; they show considerable variation in width and are frequently swollen at the ends; the walls are strongly but unevenly thickened and have few pits; they are not lignified.

(*d*) The *prisms of calcium oxalate*, which are sometimes found in the thin-walled medullary ray cells of the phloem but more usually are found scattered in the powder; they are *tabular*, fairly large and occasionally occur as *twinned crystals* or small *aggregates*.

(*e*) The fragments of *cork* from the rhizome and root. Those from the rhizome are composed of thin-walled cells, polygonal and fairly regular in surface view; in sectional view they are seen to consist of a number of rows of cells; some of the cells contain pale, orange-yellow pigment. The fragments of cork from the root are composed of thicker-walled cells than those of the rhizome and in surface view the cells are smaller and more irregular; they are dark orange-brown in colour and some of the fragments give a slight reaction for lignin.

(*f*) The *tracheids, tracheidal-vessels* and *vessels* of the xylem, all of which are lignified. The tracheids have moderately thickened walls and numerous pits. The tracheidal vessels are larger than the tracheids and have a single perforation at each end; they also have numerous pits. The vessels are large and are frequently found fragmented; they are thin-walled and have scattered, very small bordered pits; they are not very abundant.

Lignified *xylem parenchyma* is sometimes found associated with the conducting elements, composed of small, rectangular cells with slightly thickened walls and numerous pits.

(*g*) The fragments of the lignified *medullary rays* of the xylem in tangential and radial longitudinal section; they are usually found associated with the tracheids or with the xylem parenchyma. The cells appear rounded in tangential view and elongated in radial view; they have moderately thickened walls and numerous pits.

(*h*) The small amount of *parenchyma from the cortex*, filled with starch granules; the cells are usually thin-walled and may be found associated with groups of sclereids or with fragments of cork.

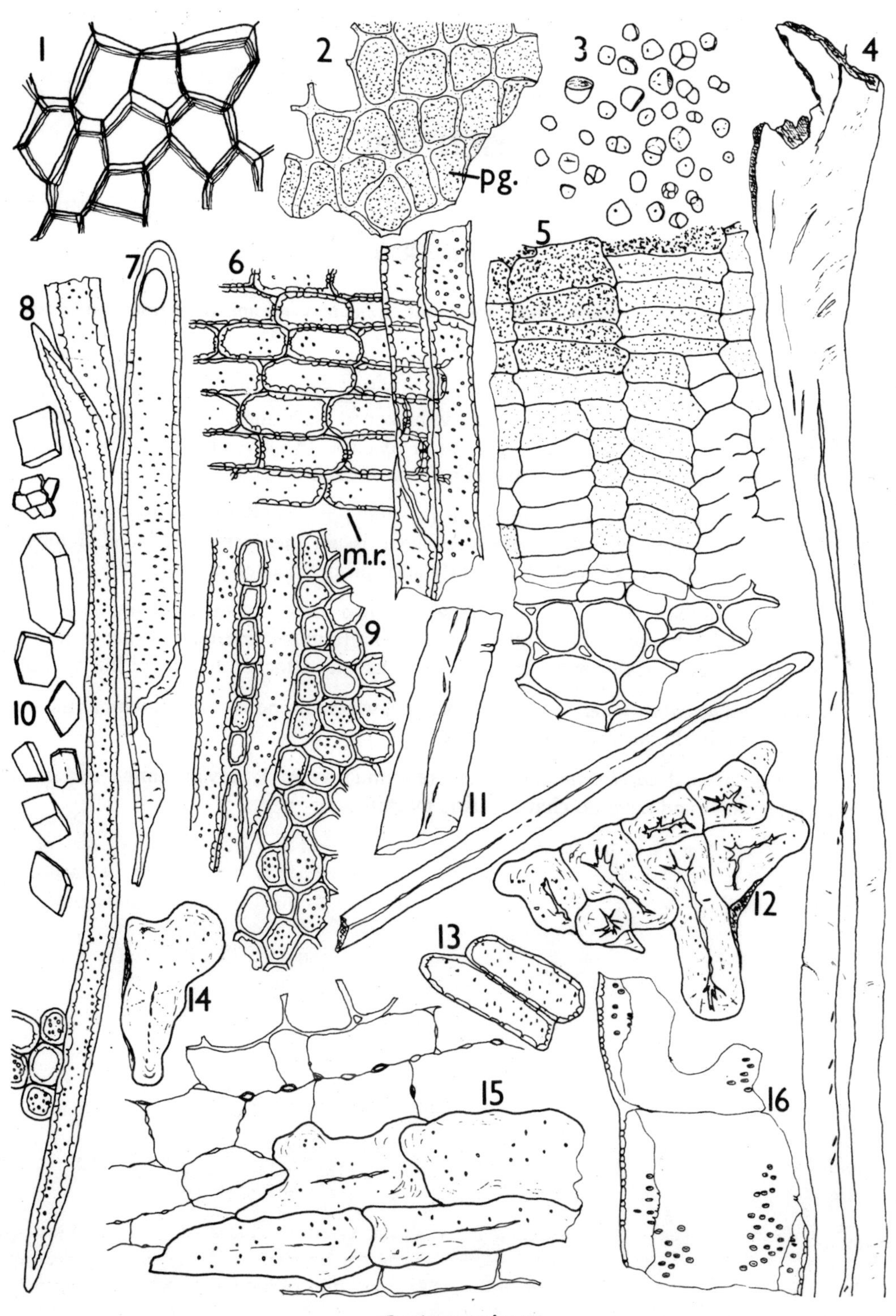

Gelsemium

×330

1 Cork from the rhizome in surface view.
2 Cork from the root in surface view, containing pigment (pg.).
3 Starch granules.
4 Part of a pericyclic fibre showing a swollen end.
5 Cork from the rhizome in sectional view with associated parenchyma of the cortex.
6 Part of the xylem in radial longitudinal section showing a medullary ray (m.r.), underlying tracheids and xylem parenchyma.
7 Part of a tracheidal vessel.
8 Tracheids.
9 Part of the xylem in tangential longitudinal section showing medullary rays (m.r.) and tracheids.
10 Calcium oxalate crystals.
11 Fragments of pericyclic fibres.
12 A group of sclereids.
13 Xylem parenchyma.
14 A single sclereid.
15 Part of a group of sclereids with associated parenchyma of the cortex.
16 Part of a bordered pitted vessel.

GENTIAN

Gentiana lutea L. Gentianaceae

Gentian Root

A tawny-brown powder with a characteristic, somewhat aromatic odour and an intensely bitter taste.

The diagnostic characters are:

(*a*) The abundant *parenchyma* composed of cells varying from rounded to elongated polygonal or rectangular in outline; they have moderately thickened walls and contain globules of fixed oil and abundant small, acicular crystals of calcium oxalate; the crystals of calcium oxalate are usually aggregated in one region near the periphery of each cell.

(*b*) The *vessels*, which may occur singly or in small groups; they are associated with the parenchyma or, occasionally, with thin-walled sieve tissue; they are fairly large, lignified and reticulately thickened. A few smaller, annularly and spirally thickened vessels are also present.

(*c*) The fairly abundant fragments of yellowish-brown *cork*; in surface view the cells are markedly elongated, thin-walled and filled with brown granular material; fragments in sectional view show from three to six or more layers of cells, usually attached to part of the phelloderm.

(*d*) The scattered *acicular crystals of calcium oxalate*, which are not very abundant as most of the crystals are found in the parenchymatous cells.

(*e*) The very occasional *starch granules*, which are found scattered; they are simple and spherical, usually rather small and have no characteristic markings.

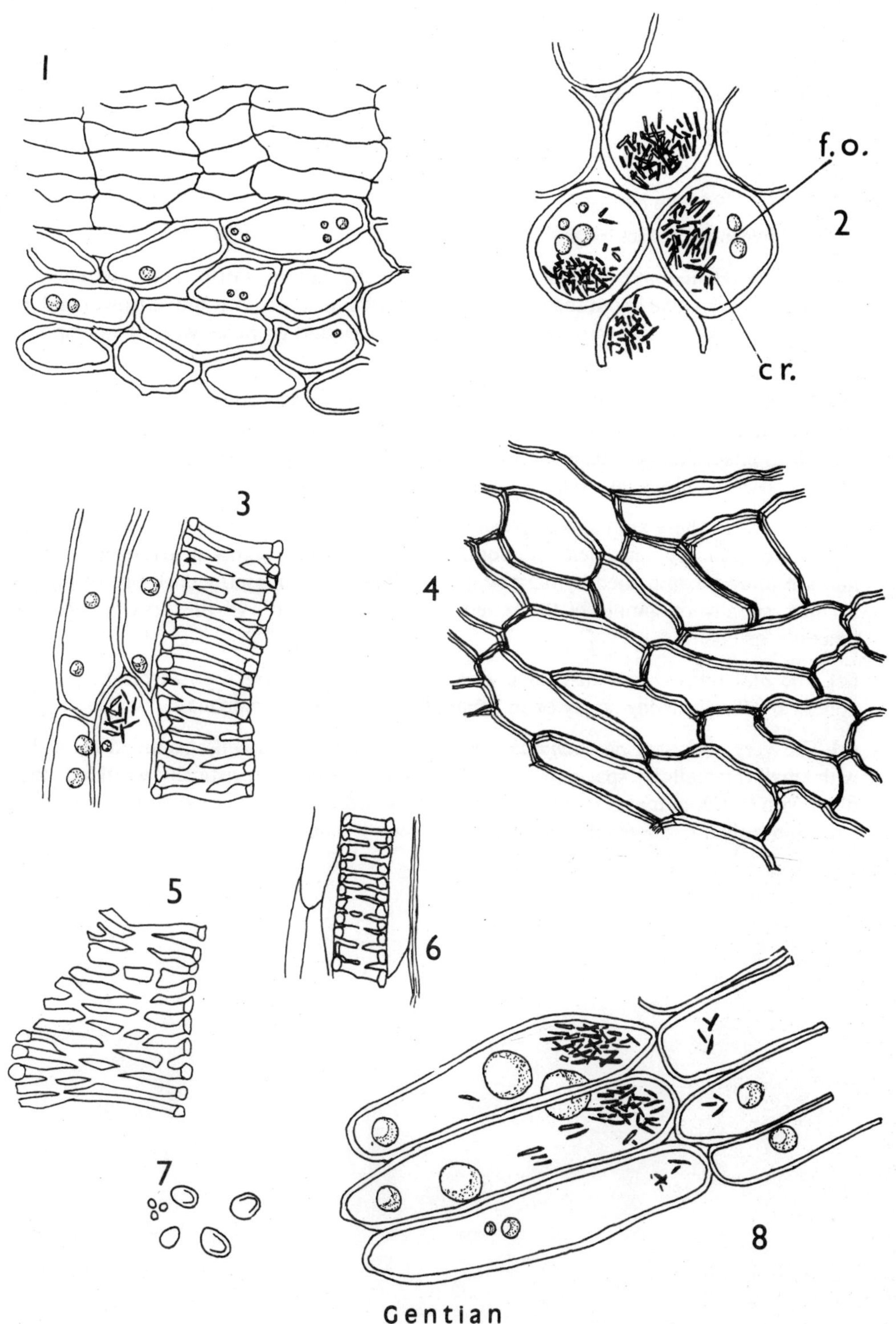

Gentian

×330

1 Cork and phelloderm in sectional view.
2 Rounded parenchymatous cells containing globules of fixed oil (f.o.) and acicular crystals of calcium oxalate (cr.).
3 A reticulately thickened vessel associated with parenchymatous cells containing calcium oxalate and fixed oil.
4 Cork in surface view.
5 Fragment of a reticulately thickened vessel.
6 A small reticulately thickened vessel associated with sieve tissue.
7 Starch granules.
8 Elongated parenchymatous cells containing globules of fixed oil and calcium oxalate crystals.

GINGER

Zingiber officinale Roscoe — Zingiberaceae

Ginger Rhizome, Jamaica Ginger

A pale yellow to cream powder with a pleasant, aromatic odour and a characteristic and pungent taste.

The diagnostic characters are:

(*a*) The abundant *starch granules*, which are mostly simple, fairly large, flattened, oblong to subrectangular to oval in outline with a small point hilum situated at the narrower end; infrequent granules show very faint transverse striations. Compound granules with two components occur very rarely.

(*b*) The *fibres*, which usually occur in groups and may also be found associated with the vessels; they are fairly large and one wall is frequently dentate; the walls are thin and marked with numerous pits which vary from circular to slit-shaped in outline; very thin transverse septa occur at intervals. The fibres give only a faint reaction for lignin.

(*c*) The *vessels*: these are fairly large and usually occur in small groups associated with the fibres; they are reticulately thickened, frequently showing distinct, regularly arranged rectangular pits, and are often accompanied by narrow, thin-walled cells containing dark brown pigment; a few smaller, spirally or annularly thickened vessels also occur. All the vessels give only a faint reaction for lignin.

(*d*) The *oleo-resin cells* which, in uncleared preparations, are seen as bright yellow ovoid to spherical cells occurring singly or in small groups in the parenchyma.

(*e*) The very abundant *parenchyma* composed of thin-walled cells, rounded to oval in outline with small intercellular spaces; many of the walls are characteristically wrinkled; the cells are filled with starch granules or oleo-resin. Very occasional groups of parenchyma are associated with thin-walled tissue composed of several rows of collapsed cells.

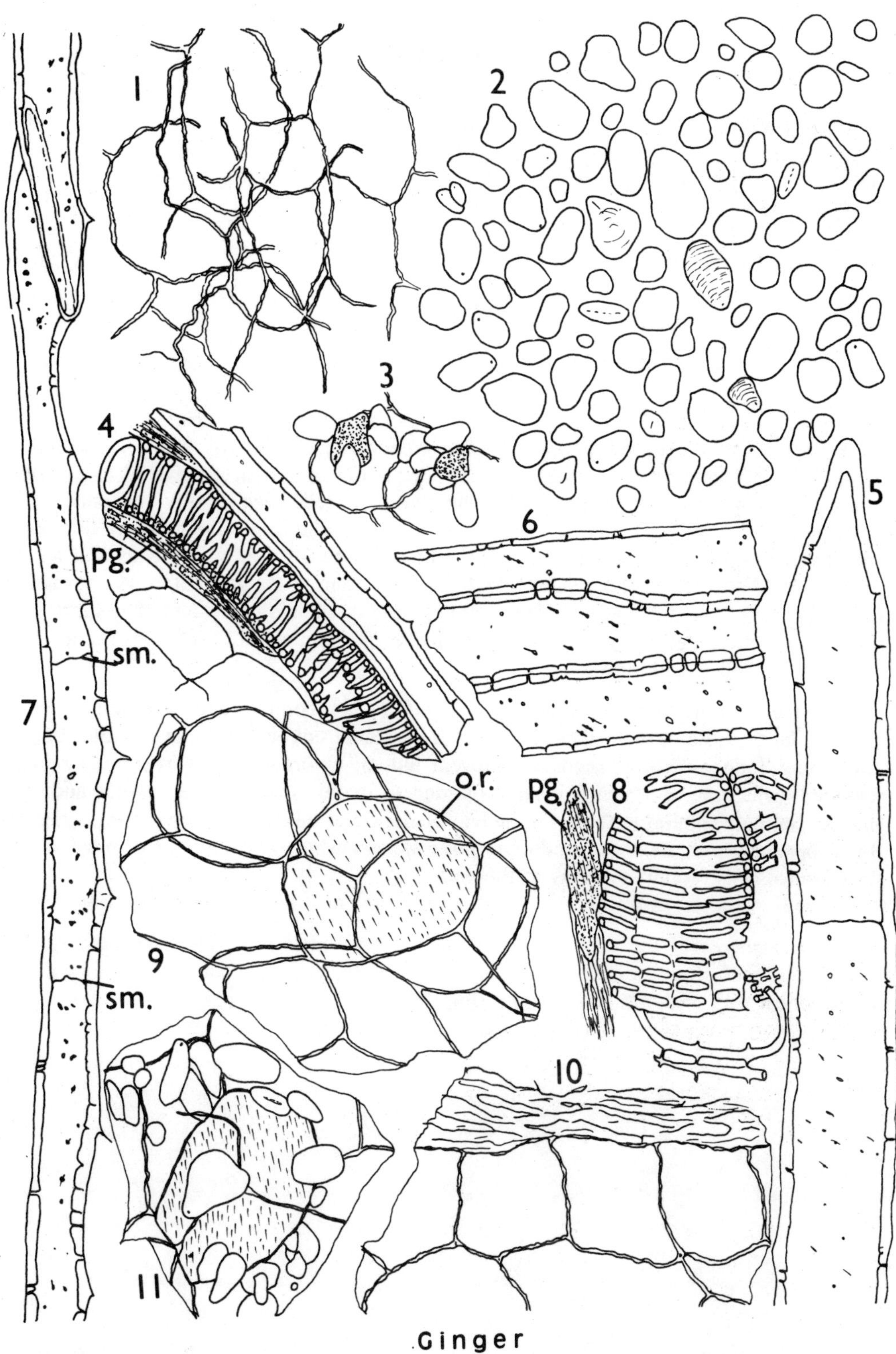

Ginger

×330

1 Parenchymatous cells showing wrinkled walls.
2 Starch granules.
3 Fragments of parenchyma with adherent oleo-resin and starch granules.
4 A small reticulately thickened vessel with associated pigment cells (pg.), fibres and parenchyma.
5 Part of a fibre.
6 Part of a group of fibres.
7 Fibres with dentate walls, showing septa (sm.).
8 Part of a larger reticulately thickened vessel with associated pigment cell (pg.).
9 Parenchyma and an oleo-resin cell (o.r.).
10 Parenchyma with associated collapsed tissue.
11 Parenchyma with adherent starch granules and an oleo-resin cell.

GRASS

Powdered Grass of commerce usually consists of one of several different grasses and although they all have a basically similar structure, the detailed histological characters vary with the species. Common Rye Grass has been selected as an example to indicate the types of structure which usually occur.

Lolium perenne L. Gramineae

Common Rye Grass

A greyish-green powder with a faint, characteristic grassy odour and a very slightly bitter taste.

The diagnostic characters are:

(*a*) Fragments of the *epidermises of the leaf blades in surface view*, which are composed of parallel, longitudinal files of elongated cells, frequently of two sizes referred to as '*long*' and '*short' cells*. On the *upper epidermis* over the ridges the cells have slightly thickened walls, and short, unicellular conical *trichomes* are present; between the ridges the cells are thinner-walled and stomata occur. The *stomata* are large with dumb-bell-shaped guard cells and a crescent-shaped subsidiary cell on either side; they frequently occur in longitudinal rows alternating with the 'long' cells. On the *lower epidermis* the walls are slightly wavy and the 'short' cells are sometimes represented by two smaller, '*twinned' cells*; stomata and trichomes occur, similar to those on the upper epidermis.

(*b*) Fragments of the *epidermis of the glume in surface view* composed of longitudinally elongated cells similar to those of the leaf blade but with markedly sinuous and unevenly thickened walls; alternating 'long' and 'short' cells are present but the 'short' cells are frequently replaced by 'twinned' cells, one of which is small, rounded to ovoid, and the other larger and crescent-shaped. Stomata, similar to those on the leaf blade, occur on the lower epidermis. Fragments of the upper epidermis show the underlying *hypodermis* which is composed of much-elongated, thick-walled cells, usually tapering at the ends.

The cells at the tip of the glume are pointed at the ends to form projecting teeth.

(*c*) The fragments of the *anthers*, consisting of very thin-walled, finely striated cells of the *epidermis in surface view* and the *fibrous layer* with characteristic, beaded walls. The *pollen grains* are spherical with a smooth exine and a single pore.

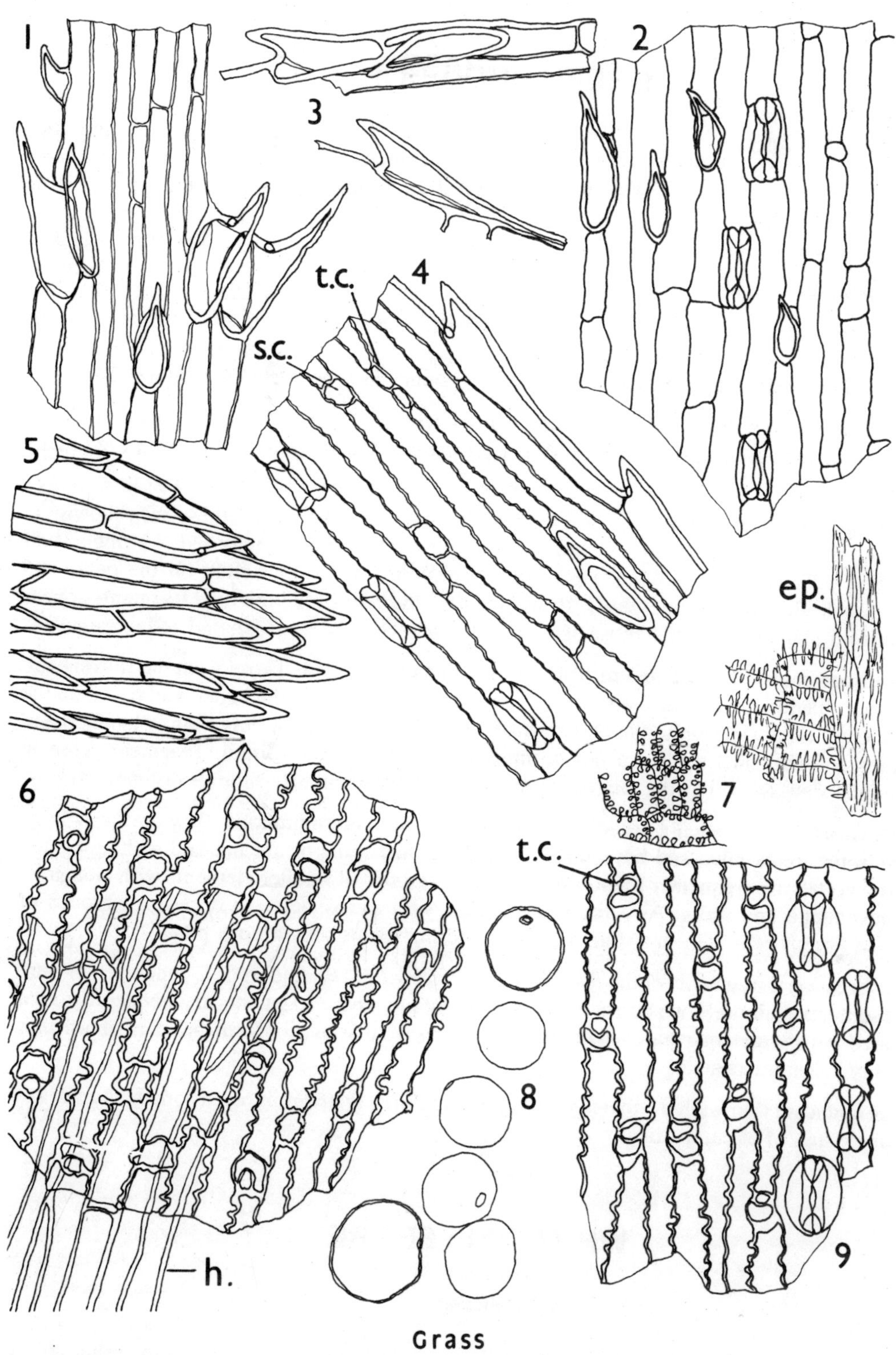

Grass

×330

1 Upper epidermis of the leaf blade over a ridge, in surface view, with trichomes.
2 Upper epidermis of the leaf blade between the ridges, in surface view, showing stomata, 'long' and 'short' cells and trichomes.
3 Fragments of the epidermis of the leaf blade over the ridges.
4 Lower epidermis of the leaf blade including the margin, in surface view, showing stomata, 'short' cells (s.c.) and 'twinned' cells (t.c.).
5 Tip of the glume with pointed projections.
6 Upper epidermis of the glume in surface view with part of the underlying hypodermis (h.).
7 Epidermis (ep.) and fibrous layer of the anther in surface view.
8 Pollen grains.
9 Lower epidermis of the glume in surface view showing stomata and 'twinned' cells (t.c.).

GREEN HELLEBORE

Veratrum viride Aiton — Liliaceae

American Veratrum, Veratrum

A greyish-fawn powder with little odour and a bitter and acrid taste; it is strongly sternutatory.

The diagnostic characters are:

(*a*) The abundant *starch granules*, which are mainly compound with two, three, four or occasionally more components; individual granules are fairly small, spherical and sometimes show a radiate or slit-shaped hilum. Some of the granules may be partially gelatinised.

(*b*) The *acicular crystals of calcium oxalate*, which are fairly large and occur in bundles almost filling some of the parenchymatous cells. A few crystals are found scattered but these are usually fragmented.

(*c*) The fragments of the *tegumentary tissue* from the rhizome and the root; these are yellowish in colour and the cells often contain patches of brown pigment; they are composed of a single layer of lignified cells which in sectional view are conspicuously more thickened on the outer and anticlinal walls than on the inner walls. In surface view the cells of the rhizome fragments appear rounded to oval in outline whilst those of the root fragments are more elongated and rectangular.

(*d*) The fragments of the *endodermis* from the rhizome and the root. Those from the rhizome are composed of lignified cells which are axially elongated and markedly thickened and pitted on the outer and anticlinal walls only; the endodermal cells from the root are only slightly lignified and the outer and anticlinal walls are not so markedly thickened and pitted. Fragments seen in longitudinal view show that the tangential walls have a conspicuously sinuous outline.

(*e*) The *vessels*, which usually occur in groups and are not very numerous; they are fairly large and the walls are lignified and have spiral or annular thickening or are marked with elongated pits. The vessels are frequently found associated with groups of smaller elements with elongated pits and oblique end walls. Also found associated with the vessels are occasional groups of elongated fibrous cells with thin, lignified walls and numerous conspicuous pits.

(*f*) The occasional fragments of the *leaf bases* in surface view; the epidermis is composed of thin-walled subrectangular cells which are pale yellow in colour. These fragments are frequently found associated with underlying parenchymatous cells, many of which contain bundles of acicular crystals of calcium oxalate.

(*g*) The abundant thin-walled *parenchyma* containing starch granules or, occasionally, bundles of acicular crystals of calcium oxalate.

WHITE HELLEBORE

Hellebore

Powdered White Hellebore, obtained from *Veratrum album* L., can be distinguished from powdered Green Hellebore by the length of the calcium oxalate crystals; in Green Hellebore they measure up to about 100 μm, whereas in White Hellebore they rarely exceed about 60 μm.

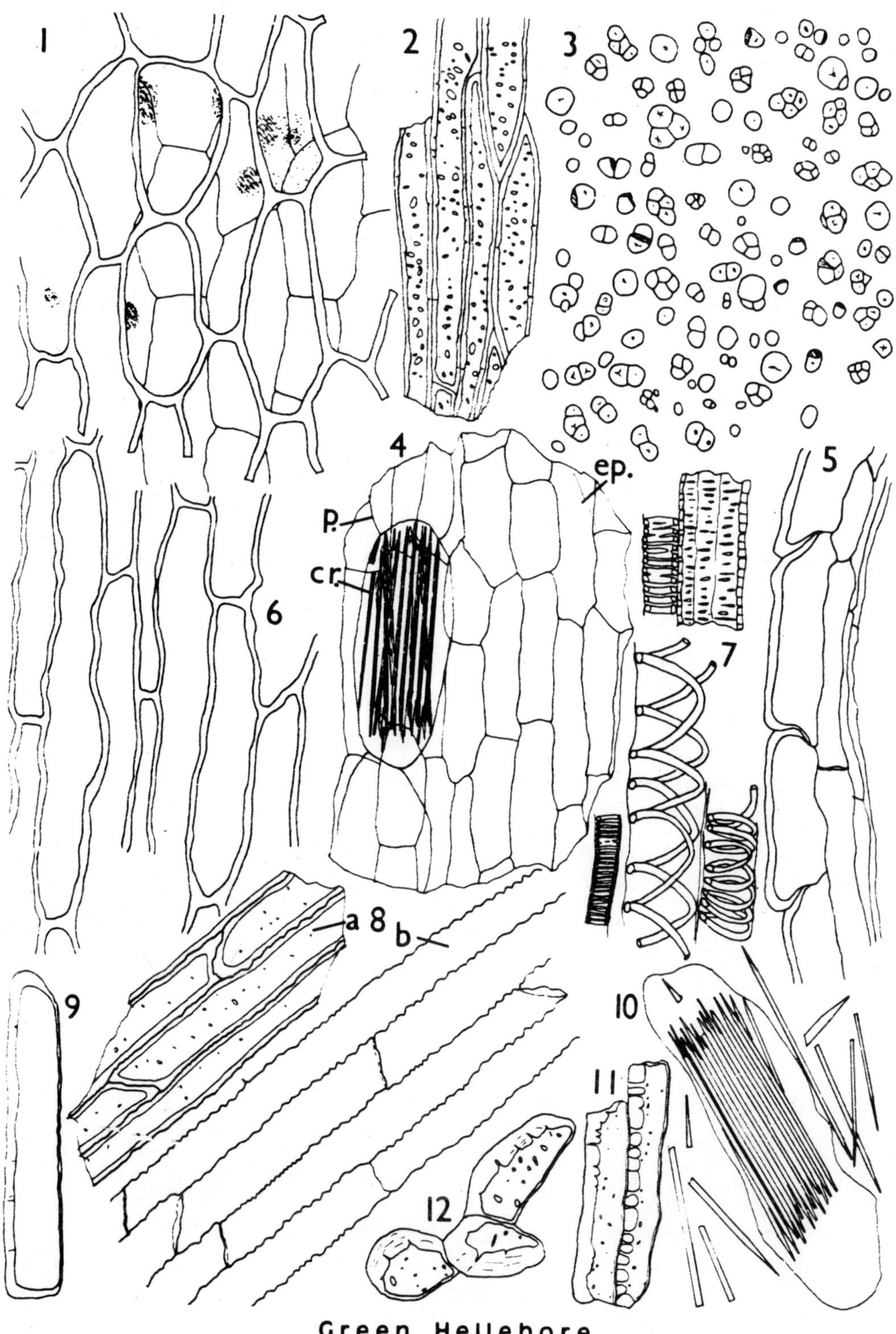

Green Hellebore

×330

1 Tegumentary tissue from the rhizome in surface view with underlying parenchyma.
2 Fibrous cells.
3 Starch granules.
4 Epidermis (ep.) of the leaf bases in surface view with underlying parenchyma (p.) containing acicular crystals of calcium oxalate (cr.).
5 Outer layers of the rhizome in sectional view.
6 Tegumentary tissue from the root in surface view.
7 Part of a group of vessels.
8 Endodermis of the root in tangential longitudinal view, (a) showing the thickening of the outer anticlinal walls and (b) showing the sinuous outline of the inner anticlinal walls.
9 Endodermal cell of the root in longitudinal view.
10 Acicular crystals of calcium oxalate, some contained in a parenchymatous cell.
11 Endodermal cells of the rhizome in longitudinal view.
12 Endodermal cells of the rhizome in transverse sectional view.

HEMLOCK FRUIT

Conium maculatum L. Umbelliferae

A greenish-brown powder with no odour or taste but, when treated with *Solution of Potassium Hydroxide*, develops a characteristic mouse-like odour.

The diagnostic characters are:

(*a*) The *epicarp*, composed of a layer of cells, polygonal in surface view, with a striated *cuticle* and slightly thickened walls; in sectional view some of the cells are seen to be somewhat papillose; *stomata* are very infrequent. Several of the cells contain sphaerocrystalline masses of *diosmin*, which also occur scattered.

(*b*) The *coniine layer*, which is very characteristic; it is composed of a layer of large, yellowish-brown cells, elongated in surface view and arranged with the long axes parallel to one another; this layer forms the *endocarp*. The cell walls sometimes have small, scattered pits and are strongly lignified and much thickened, particularly at the ends.

(*c*) The *innermost layer of the mesocarp*, which, like the coniine layer, is composed of fairly large, regularly arranged elongated cells although fragments from the ends of the fruit show a more random arrangement; the walls are lignified and evenly thickened. This layer is usually found associated with the coniine layer.

(*d*) The *fibres* and *vessels* of the vascular strands which usually occur in groups; the fibres have thick, lignified walls and occasional pits; the vessels are small, lignified, spirally or annularly thickened or, occasionally, have slit-shaped pits. Fragments of lignified and *pitted parenchyma* are also found scattered or associated with the vascular tissue.

(*e*) The *testa*, composed of a single layer of brown pigmented cells, polygonal in surface view; the anticlinal walls are thin but may show distinct beaded thickenings.

(*f*) The *endosperm*, composed of fairly large, thick-walled cells containing *aleurone grains* and *microrosette crystals of calcium oxalate*.

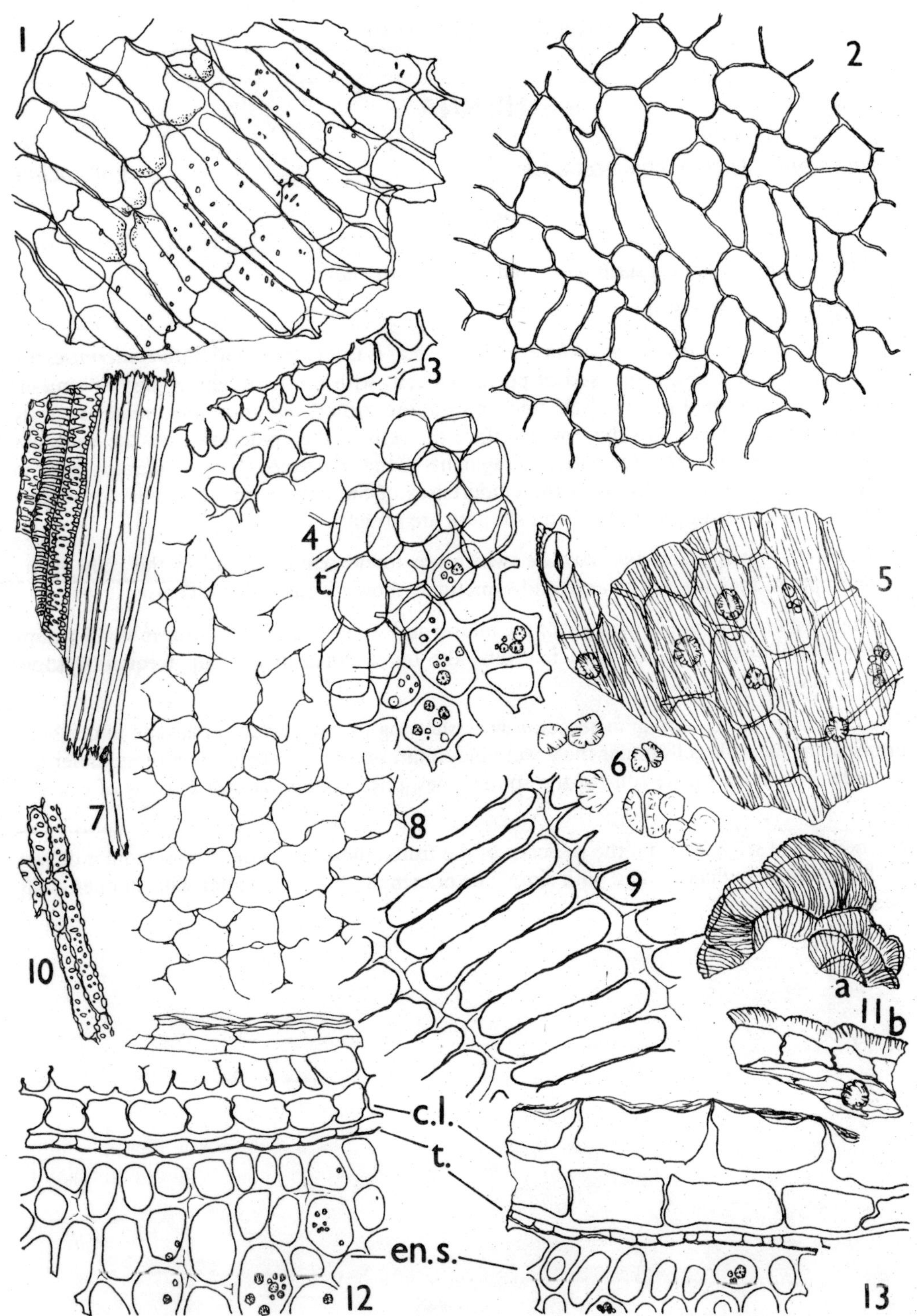

Hemlock Fruit

×330

1 Inner layers of the pericarp in surface view showing the thick-walled, pitted cells of the coniine layer and overlying thinner-walled cells of the adjacent layer of the mesocarp.
2 Innermost layer of the mesocarp from an end part of the fruit, in surface view.
3 Part of the coniine layer in sectional view showing the thickened end walls of the cells.
4 Testa (t.) in surface view with part of the underlying endosperm containing microrosette crystals of calcium oxalate.
5 Epicarp in surface view showing striated cuticle, a stoma and sphaerocrystalline masses of diosmin.
6 Sphaerocrystalline masses of diosmin.
7 Part of a group of fibres and vessels.
8 Testa in surface view.
9 Coniine layer in surface view.
10 Pitted parenchyma.
11 Epicarp in oblique surface view (a) and sectional view (b).
12 Pericarp and seed in sectional view showing part of the mesocarp, the coniine layer (c.l.), and the testa (t.) and endosperm (en.s.).
13 Part of the pericarp and seed in sectional view, similar to 12 but showing the coniine layer and adjacent layer of the mesocarp in longitudinal view.

HENNA

Lawsonia inermis L. (*Lawsonia alba* Lam.) Lythraceae

Henna Leaf

A yellowish-green powder with a slight odour and a faintly bitter taste.

The diagnostic characters are:

(*a*) The fragments of the *lamina in surface view*. The leaf is isobilateral and both *epidermises* are similar in appearance being composed of polygonal cells with thin, straight or slightly sinuous walls which may occasionally show slight thickening at the corners; *anomocytic stomata* are fairly numerous on both surfaces. On the lower surface the cells of the epidermis over the veins are more elongated and have a striated cuticle. Fragments of the *epidermis of the petiole* also occur in which the cells are similar to those of the epidermises of the lamina but the walls are slightly beaded; the *cuticle* is strongly striated and stomata are absent.

(*b*) The *cluster crystals of calcium oxalate*, which are found scattered and in the cells of the spongy mesophyll; they are fairly large and sometimes show a dense brown centre.

(*c*) The lignified *fibres* from the pericyle of the midrib and larger veins; they occur in small groups and are moderately thick-walled with few pits; the outer fibres in a group frequently show distinctly dentate walls.

(*d*) The fragments of the *lamina in sectional view* showing the two-layered palisade under both epidermises; the palisade cells under the lower epidermis are slightly shorter than those under the upper epidermis. Many of the cells of the spongy mesophyll contain cluster crystals of calcium oxalate.

(*e*) The occasional *sclereids* from the pericarp of the fruits; these occur in groups and are of two types—large and very thick-walled with simple or branched pits—or smaller with thinner walls and numerous simple pits.

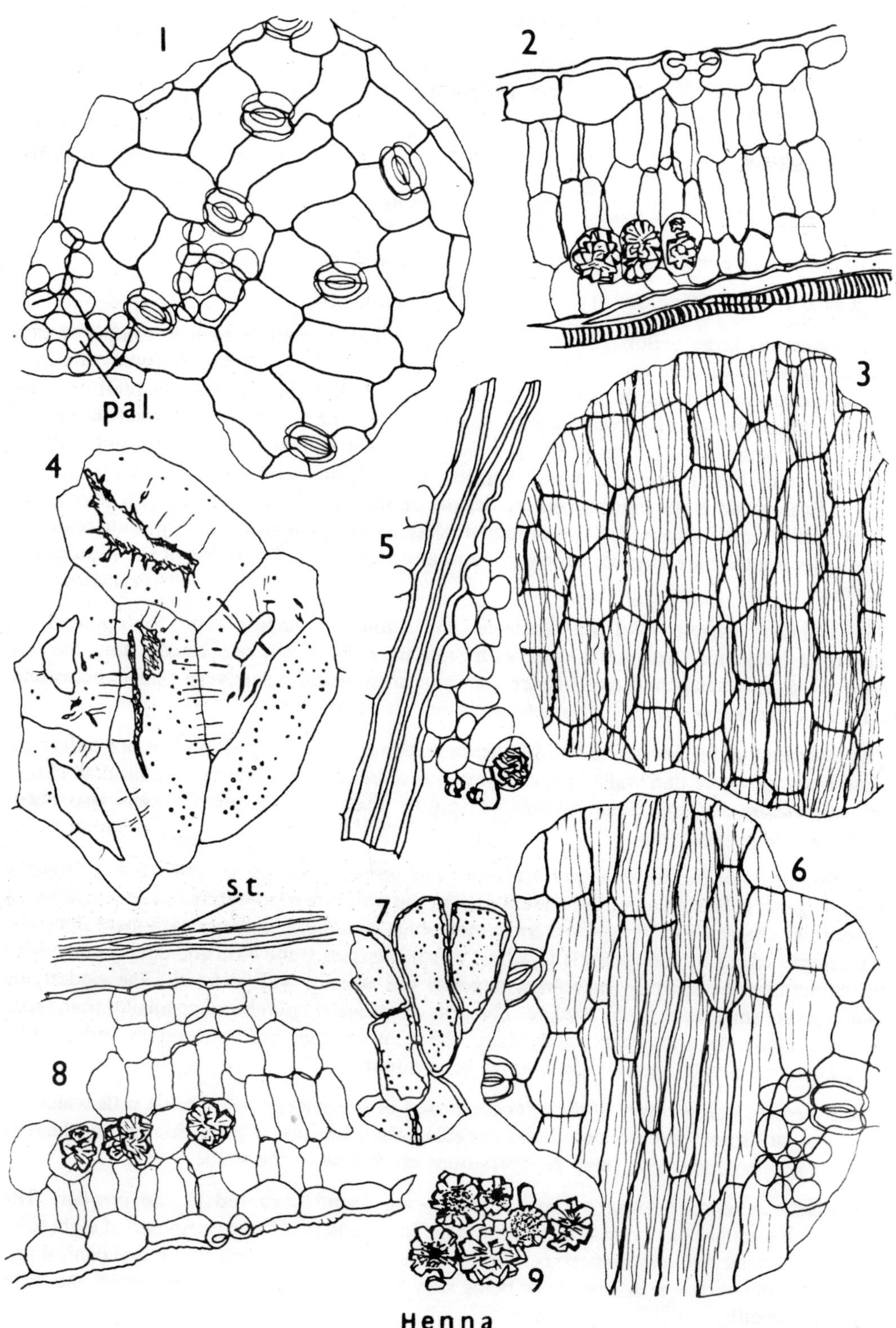

Henna

×330

1 Epidermis of the lamina in surface view with anomocytic stomata and part of the underlying palisade (pal.).

2 Part of the lamina in sectional view showing the upper epidermis, underlying two-layered palisade and spongy mesophyll cells containing cluster crystals of calcium oxalate.

3 Epidermis of the petiole in surface view showing cuticular striations.

4 Large, thick-walled sclereids from the pericarp.

5 Pericycle fibres and adjacent mesophyll cells

6 Lower epidermis of the lamina in surface view showing anomocytic stomata, underlying palisade cells and the region over a vein with cuticular striations.

7 Smaller, thinner-walled sclereids from the pericarp.

8 Part of the lamina in sectional view showing the lower epidermis, palisade, spongy mesophyll with cluster crystals of calcium oxalate, part of a fibre and crushed sieve tissue (s.t.).

9 Cluster crystals of calcium oxalate.

HOPS

Humulus lupulus L. Cannabaceae

Humulus, Lupulus

A pale brown powder with a characteristic, aromatic odour and a bitter, soapy taste.

The diagnostic characters are:

(*a*) The numerous large yellow *glands* which are very characteristic; each is composed of a number of thin-walled cells arranged in a single, hemispherical layer with a common cuticle which, on the concave surface, is raised to form a dome although this is often collapsed; the cells secrete a yellowish-brown oleo-resin into the space between the walls and the raised cuticle and this gives the characteristic colour to the glands. When seen in side view the cup shape of the glands is apparent, but in surface view they appear almost circular with the cells rather irregularly arranged. Each gland is attached to the epidermis of the stipule or bracteole, on which they occur, by a short stalk composed of two or four small cells. The glands are usually found scattered in the powder but they are also occasionally found attached to small portions of the stipules and bracteoles.

(*b*) The abundant fragments of the *bracteoles* and *stipules in surface view*: the epidermis is composed of irregularly polygonal cells with sinuous walls which are usually thin but are occasionally slightly thickened and beaded; *anomocytic stomata* occur very rarely; occasional irregular *cicatrices* occur where trichomes have been attached.

(*c*) The fragments of the *bracteoles* and *stipules in sectional view*; the mesophyll is not differentiated and is composed of thin-walled parenchymatous cells several of which contain small *cluster crystals of calcium oxalate*. Small groups of spirally thickened, lignified vessels also occur embedded in the parenchyma.

(*d*) The fragments of the *leaves in surface view*. The *upper epidermis* is composed of straight-walled, polygonal cells with a faintly striated *cuticle*; the walls are moderately thickened; stomata are absent but characteristic *cystolithic trichomes* occur containing calcium carbonate deposits; these trichomes are short and abruptly tapering, much enlarged at the base and deeply embedded in the epidermis; the calcium carbonate deposits are usually well defined. The underlying palisade cells are small and closely packed. The cells of the *lower epidermis* are smaller than those of the upper epidermis and are distinctly wavy; the walls are thin and occasionally very slightly beaded; numerous small, anomocytic stomata are present.

(*e*) The *sclerenchymatous layer of the testa* composed of fairly large pale brown cells which, in surface view, are somewhat elongated and irregular; the walls are slightly sinuous and heavily thickened with very numerous small pits; striations are visible in the walls.

(*f*) The *glandular* and *covering trichomes*, which are found scattered in the powder. The glandular trichomes have a two-celled biseriate stalk and a spherical head composed of eight thin-walled cells; they are not very numerous. The covering trichomes are unicellular and conical and show considerable variation in size, some being very long and frequently fragmented; the walls are thin and smooth.

(*g*) The very occasional fragments of the *pericarp*, seen in surface view to be composed of polygonal cells filled with very pale bluish-purple pigment; the walls are moderately thickened but rather indistinct.

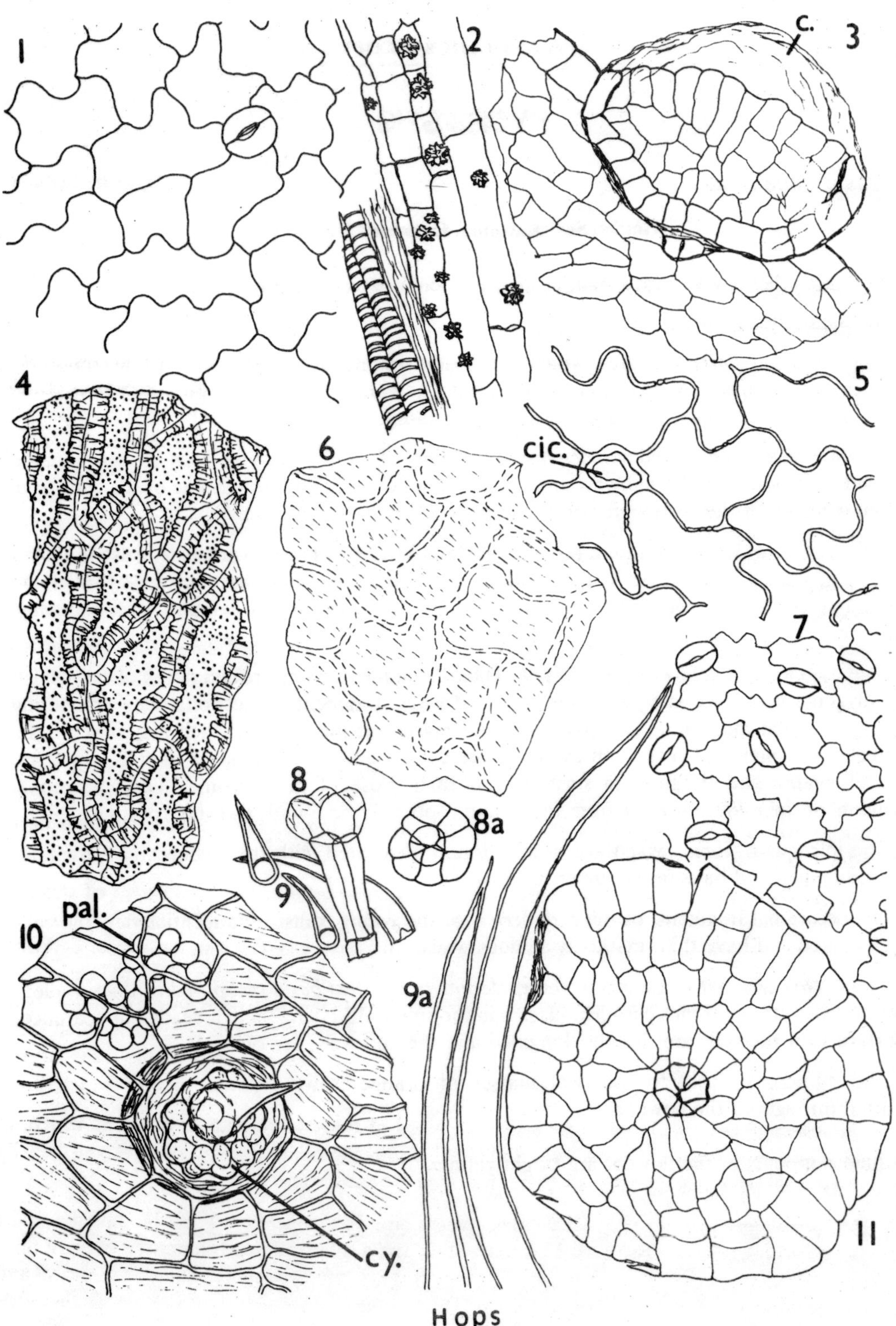

Hops

×330

1 Epidermis of a bracteole or stipule in surface view showing a stoma.

2 Part of the inner tissues from a bracteole or stipule showing parenchymatous cells containing cluster crystals of calcium oxalate and a group of vascular tissue.

3 A gland in side view, attached to part of the epidermis of a bracteole and showing the raised cuticle (c.).

4 Part of the sclerenchymatous layer of the testa in surface view.

5 Epidermis of a bracteole or stipule in surface view showing a cicatrix (cic.) and slight thickening and beading of the walls.

6 Part of the pericarp in surface view.

7 Lower epidermis of a leaf in surface view showing numerous stomata.

8 Glandular trichome in side view.

8a Glandular trichome viewed from above.

9 Small covering trichomes.

9a Large covering trichomes.

10 Upper epidermis of the leaf in surface view showing the underlying palisade cells (pal.), striated cuticle and a cystolithic trichome (cy.) with calcium carbonate deposits.

11 A gland in surface view.

HYDRASTIS

Hydrastis canadensis L. Ranunculaceae

Golden Seal Rhizome, Hydrastis Rhizome

A dull yellow-ochre powder with a faint, unpleasant odour and a persistently bitter taste.

The diagnostic characters are:

(*a*) The abundant *starch granules*, which are mostly simple and rather small; a few compound granules occur with two, three or four components. Individual granules are spherical to ovoid and occasionally show a small, rounded or slit-shaped hilum.

(*b*) The abundant thin-walled *parenchyma* containing starch granules; the cells are polygonal to rounded in transverse sectional view and elongated in longitudinal view. Some of the cells from the outer region of the cortex are somewhat collenchymatously thickened.

(*c*) The *vessels*, which are found in groups; they are fairly small and each element usually has a single conspicuous, circular perforation in each of the oblique end walls; they are lignified and have numerous small, slit-shaped pits. A very few larger vessels are found with reticulate thickening.

(*d*) The fragments of yellowish-brown *cork*. Those from the rhizome are composed of cells which are polygonal in surface view with thin, lignified walls; fragments in sectional view frequently show an irregular mass of dense brown granular matter on the outside which may obscure the cork cells. Fragments of cork from the roots are composed of a single layer of cells which are more elongated and irregular in surface view than those of the rhizome. Very occasional fragments of the *piliferous layer* from the young roots may be found, showing root hairs.

(*e*) The infrequent *fibres*, which are usually found associated with the vessels; they are thin-walled, lignified and have fairly numerous pits.

(*f*) The occasional fragments of the *endodermis* of the young roots; in tangential view the cells are elongated and have thin, markedly sinuous walls.

(*g*) The very occasional fragments of the *epidermis of the stem bases* composed of thick-walled, lignified cells with numerous conspicuous pits in the side walls giving them a beaded appearance; in surface view the cells are slightly elongated and the end walls are oblique.

(*h*) The numerous ovoid to spherical masses of orange-brown *granular matter* which are scattered throughout the powder.

Aqueous mounts of the powder are bright yellow.

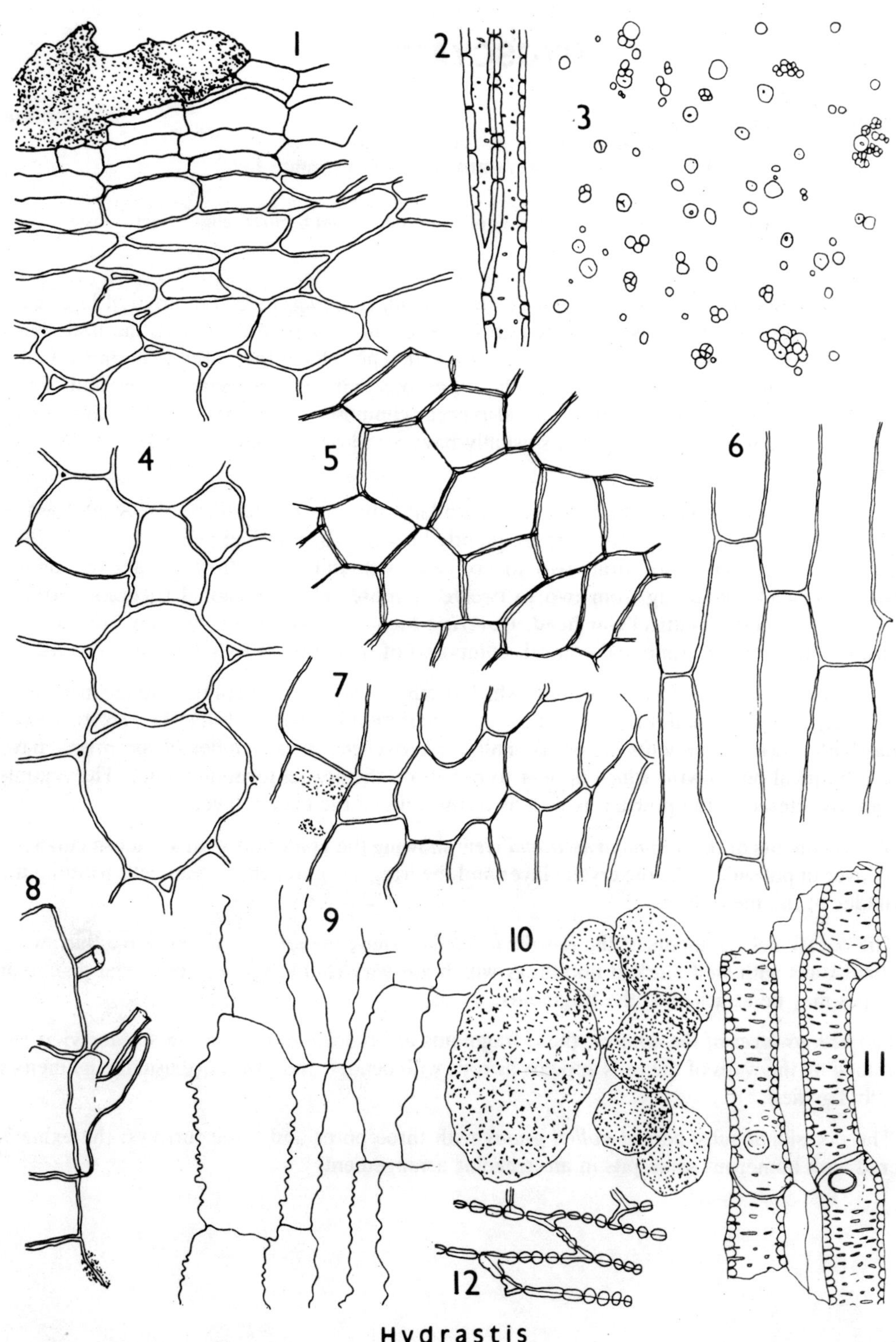

Hydrastis

×330

1 Outer tissues in sectional view showing dense granular matter in the cork.
2 Part of a group of fibres.
3 Starch granules.
4 Parenchyma in transverse section.
5 Cork from the rhizome in surface view.
6 Parenchyma in longitudinal section.
7 Cork from the root in surface view.
8 Piliferous layer in sectional view showing root hairs.
9 Endodermis of the young roots in tangential view.
10 Orange-brown granular masses.
11 Vessels and xylem parenchyma.
12 Epidermis of the stem base in surface view showing beaded walls.

HYOSCYAMUS

Hyoscyamus niger L. Solanaceae

Henbane Leaf, Hyoscyamus Herb, Hyoscyamus Leaf

A yellowish-green powder with a characteristic, unpleasant odour and a bitter, slightly acrid taste.

The diagnostic characters are:

(*a*) The fragments of the *lamina in surface view*. The *upper epidermis* is composed of large cells with thin, slightly sinuous walls; fairly numerous *anisocytic stomata* are present; the underlying palisade cells are moderately large and loosely packed. The cells of the *lower epidermis* are also large and have thin, markedly sinuous walls; numerous anisocytic stomata are present. Fragments of the epidermis from over the veins also occur composed of elongated cells with straight, slightly thickened walls; these fragments usually have attached trichomes or show the *cicatrices* left by them.

(*b*) The *glandular trichomes*, which are very abundant; they are found scattered or attached to fragments of the epidermis and they are frequently broken. They are very characteristic, with a uniseriate stalk composed of from two to six cells with thin, smooth walls and an ovoid, multicellular head containing from two to twelve or more cells; occasional trichomes have a unicellular stalk and a multicellular head. *Covering trichomes* also occur but they are not very numerous; they are uniseriate and conical, composed of from two to four thin-walled cells.

(*c*) The abundant *calcium oxalate crystals*, which occur in a layer of cells in the spongy mesophyll immediately below the palisade. They show great variation in form and may be *prisms, cluster crystals* with a few components or, occasionally, *microsphenoids*; a number of the prisms have dense cylindrical outgrowths which appear to penetrate the crystal forming a plug. The crystals are found scattered in the powder as well as in the cells of the crystal layer.

(*d*) The fragments of the *lamina in sectional view* showing the epidermis with a smooth cuticle, a single layer of palisade cells, the crystal layer and the irregular parenchymatous cells forming the remainder of the mesophyll.

(*e*) The occasional fragments of the *corolla in surface view*; the *epidermal cells* have thin, wavy anticlinal walls with well marked infoldings which are very characteristic; occasional glandular trichomes may be attached to the fragments.

(*f*) The *fibrous layer of the anthers*; these fragments are reddish-purple and in surface view the thickening on the walls of the cells appears as rods with beaded ends; they are usually lignified or partially lignified.

(*g*) The occasional subspherical *pollen grains* with three pores and three furrows; the exine is covered with numerous small pits in an irregular arrangement.

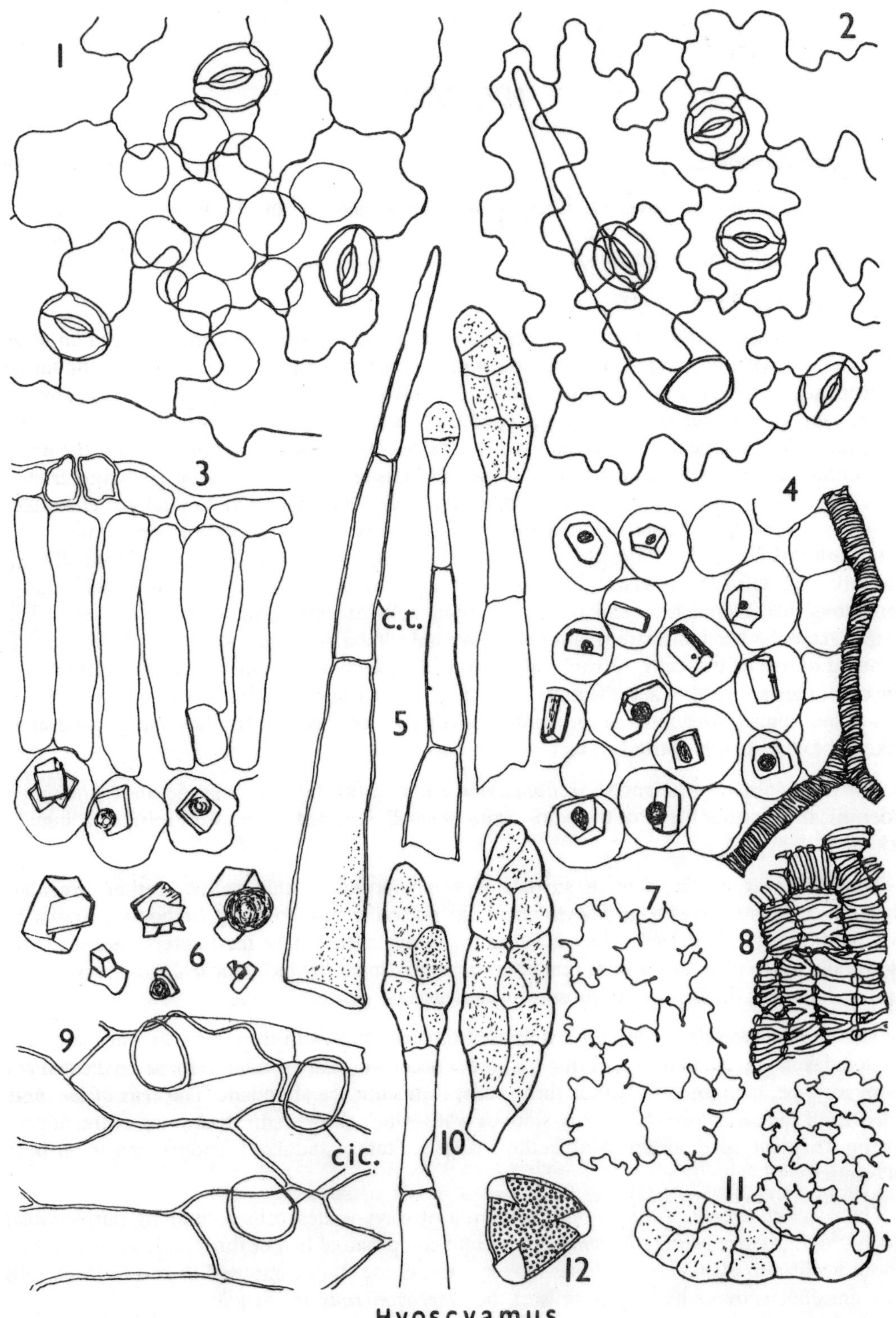

×330

1. Upper epidermis in surface view showing anisocytic stomata and part of the underlying palisade.
2. Lower epidermis in surface view showing anisocytic stomata and a covering trichome.
3. Part of the lamina in sectional view showing the upper epidermis, palisade and crystal layer.
4. Crystal layer in surface view, with part of a vein in longitudinal section.
5. A covering trichome (c.t.) and parts of two glandular trichomes.
6. Calcium oxalate crystals.
7. Epidermis of the corolla in surface view.
8. Fibrous layer of the anther in surface view.
9. Epidermis from over a vein in surface view showing part of an attached trichome and cicatrices (cic.).
10. Parts of two glandular trichomes.
11. Epidermis of the corolla in surface view with a glandular trichome.
12. Pollen grain.

HYSSOP

Hyssopus officinalis L. **Labiatae**

Occurs as the fresh or dried leaves, stems and occasional flowering tops; the leaves are greyish green and distinctly punctate on both surfaces; the flowers are a deep violet. It has a very strong, aromatic odour and an aromatic, camphoraceous and bitter taste.

The diagnostic characters are:

(*a*) The *epidermises of the leaves* in surface view, composed of cells with thin, sinuous to wavy walls; *diacytic stomata* occur abundantly on both surfaces. The palisade cells under the upper epidermis are fairly large and loosely packed. *Crystals of hesperidin* occur in both epidermises and are especially numerous in the upper epidermis; in *Chloral Hydrate* mounts of the fresh or dried material they appear as sphaerocrystalline masses of very fine, radiating crystals, but when the material has been stored in *Alcohol* they are seen as larger needle crystals radiating from a point; they slowly dissolve in *Solution of Potassium Hydroxide* giving a yellow colour. *Glandular trichomes* of both multicellular and capitate types are very numerous on both epidermises; the multicellular trichomes are large and each has a short, unicellular stalk and a head formed from eight radiating cells around which the common cuticle is raised to form a bladder; these occur in depressions in the epidermis and the surrounding cells are arranged to form a rosette. The capitate glandular trichomes are smaller and have unicellular stalks and spherical to ovoid heads composed of one or two cells. Occasional *covering trichomes* also occur, especially on the lower epidermis; they are conical and the majority are short and unicellular but in the regions over the veins a few longer trichomes occur composed of two or three cells; they have moderately thickened and distinctly warted walls.

(*b*) The leaf is dorsiventral and in *sectional view* shows a two-layered palisade under the upper epidermis; the vascular tissue of the veins contains small, lignified *vessels* with spiral and annular thickening.

(*c*) The *epidermis of the stem* in surface view composed of thin-walled, rather irregular, polygonal cells with occasional diacytic stomata; glandular and covering trichomes, similar to those on the leaf, are present. *Fibres* occur in the pericyle; they have moderately thickened and pitted walls which give only a faint reaction for lignin. Small lignified *tracheids* and *vessels* with spiral and annular thickening are present in the vascular tissue.

(*d*) The *outer epidermis of the calyx* composed of small cells with thin, sinuous walls and very occasional stomata. Numerous covering trichomes occur which are similar to those on the leaf but the longer type, composed of two or three cells, is much more abundant. The *cells of the inner epidermis* of the calyx lobes have very sinuous walls which show slight thickening at the angles; covering trichomes are absent. Multicellular and capitate glandular trichomes occur on both epidermises.

(*e*) The *outer epidermis of the corolla* composed of wavy-walled cells containing purple-violet pigment; uniseriate *covering trichomes* are present composed of two or three cells with very thin, smooth walls; also *glandular trichomes* having a uniseriate stalk composed of two or three cells and a unicellular, ovoid head. The cells of the *inner epidermis* are *papillose*.

(*f*) The *pollen grains* are spherical with six pores and furrows and a finely granular exine.

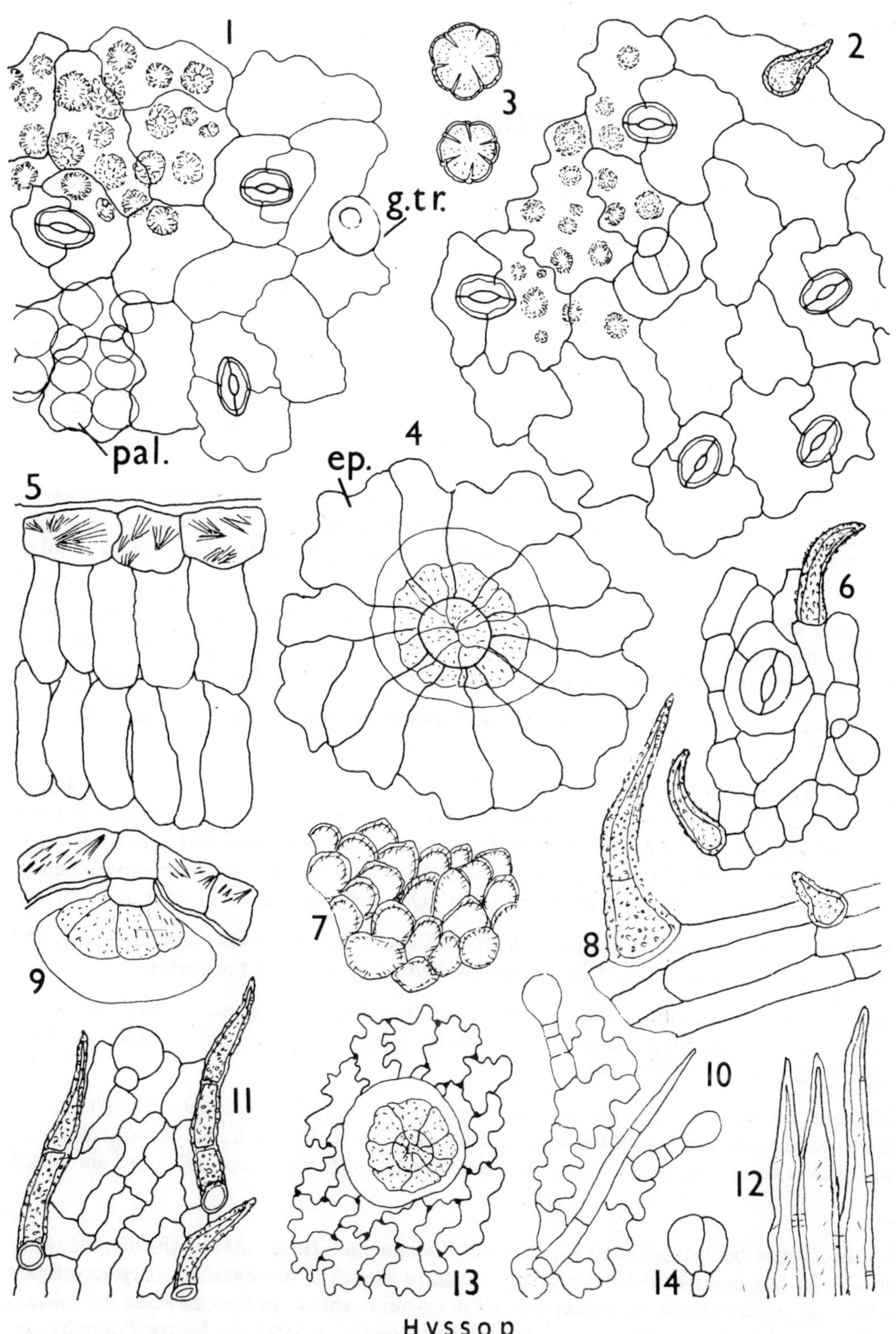

Hyssop

×330

1 Upper epidermis of the leaf in surface view showing stomata, radiating masses of hesperidin, a capitate glandular trichome (g.tr.) and part of the underlying palisade (pal.).
2 Lower epidermis of the leaf in surface view showing stomata, radiating masses of hesperidin, a capitate glandular trichome and a covering trichome.
3 Pollen grains.
4 A multicellular glandular trichome in surface view with surrounding cells of the lower epidermis (ep.) of the leaf.
5 Part of the lamina in sectional view showing the two-layered palisade and hesperidin crystals in
6 Epidermis of the stem in surface view showing a stoma, a capitate gland and covering trichomes.
7 Inner epidermis of the corolla with papillae.
8 Epidermis of the leaf over a vein, in surface view.
9 Lower epidermis of the lamina in sectional view with hesperidin crystals and a multicellular glandular trichome.
10 Outer epidermis of the corolla in surface view.
11 Outer epidermis of the calyx in surface view.
12 Part of a group of pericyclic fibres from the stem.
13 Inner epidermis of a calyx lobe in surface view.
14 A capitate gland in side view.

INDIAN PODOPHYLLUM

Podophyllum emodi Wall. *ex* Hook. *f. et* Thoms (*Podophyllum hexandrum* Royle) — Berberidaceae

Indian Podophyllum Rhizome

A light brown powder with a slight odour and a bitter taste.

The diagnostic characters are:

(*a*) The abundant *starch granules*, which are mostly compound with two, three or possibly up to twenty or more components but larger aggregations are usually broken; individual granules are rather small; a circular to crescent-shaped hilum is sometimes visible.

(*b*) The *vessels*, which occur singly or, more usually, in small groups accompanied by thin-walled xylem parenchyma; they are lignified, reticulately thickened or sometimes marked with irregularly arranged, slit-shaped pits surrounded by inconspicuous borders; a few vessels with spiral or annular thickening also occur.

(*c*) The fairly abundant *sclereids*, which occur in groups and are frequently fragmented; individual cells are elongated rectangular in outline and have moderately thickened, pitted walls. The groups of sclereids are often found associated with thin-walled parenchyma of the pith.

(*d*) The brown fragments of *cork* from the rhizome composed of thin-walled, lignified cells which are polygonal and somewhat elongated in surface view.

(*e*) The abundant brown fragments of the *outer layer of the rootlets*; this is composed of cells which, in surface view, are elongated rectangular in outline with evenly thickened walls and few pits; in sectional view the cells are seen to be thickened on the outer and side walls only. Frequently associated with this outer layer is the underlying layer, the *exodermis* composed of cells similar in size and shape to those of the outer layer but with thin, very sinuous walls.

(*f*) The *cluster crystals of calcium oxalate*, which are not very abundant; they are fairly large and are found scattered or, occasionally, in the thin-walled parenchyma of the cortex.

(*g*) The occasional fragments of the *endodermis* of the rootlets composed of cells which, in tangential view, are somewhat similar to those of the exodermis but are more regular in shape and the walls are less markedly sinuous.

(*h*) The abundant *parenchyma* containing starch granules and, very occasionally, cluster crystals of calcium oxalate; the majority of the cells are thin-walled and elongated, but occasional groups of rounded cells occur. The parenchymatous cells from the pith often have thickened and pitted walls.

This powder may be distinguished from that of Podophyllum (page 184) by the abundance of sclereids and fragments of the outer layers of the rootlets, the presence of a well developed cork and the smaller size of the cluster crystals of calcium oxalate. In Podophyllum the calcium oxalate cluster crystals measure up to 100 μm in diameter, whereas in Indian Podophyllum they rarely exceed 60 μm in diameter.

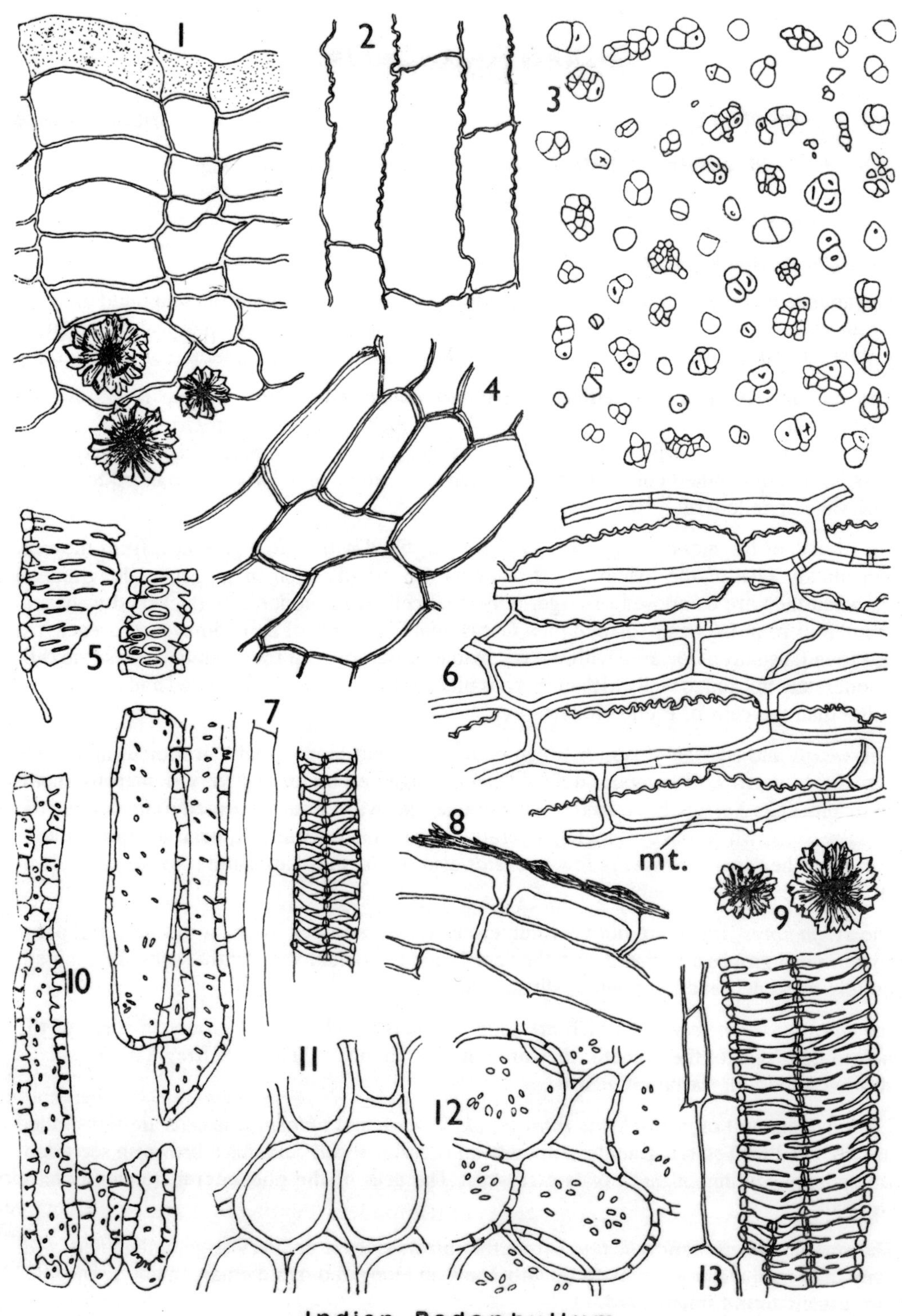

Indian Podophyllum

×330

1 Part of the cork and cortex from the rhizome in sectional view with cluster crystals of calcium oxalate.
2 Endodermis from the root in tangential view.
3 Starch granules.
4 Cork in surface view.
5 Fragments of pitted vessels.
6 Outer layer of the rootlets (mt.) in surface view with underlying exodermis.
7 Part of a group of sclereids with associated parenchyma and spirally thickened vessels.
8 Outer layers of the rootlets in sectional view.
9 Cluster crystals of calcium oxalate.
10 Part of a group of sclereids.
11 Thick-walled parenchyma.
12 Pitted parenchyma from the pith.
13 Part of a group of reticulately thickened vessels and xylem parenchyma.

INDIAN RAUWOLFIA

Rauwolfia serpentina Benth. Apocynaceae

Chootachand, Indian Snake Root, Sarpagandha, Rauwolfia

A pale brownish-yellow powder with a slight odour and a bitter taste.

The diagnostic characters are:

(*a*) The abundant *starch granules*, which are mostly simple but a number of compound granules also occur with two, three or four components; individual granules are spherical to irregular, often quite large, and usually have a well marked hilum in the form of a simple or radiate split.

(*b*) The abundant fragments of reddish-brown *cork* composed of three or four layers of thin-walled cells which, in surface view, are polygonal and more or less isodiametric; some of these fragments are strongly lignified while others do not give a reaction for lignin. Occasional fragments of the unlignified cork cells may be seen in sectional view, usually attached to part of the thin-walled phelloderm.

(*c*) The abundant fragments of *lignified parenchyma*, filled with starch granules, from the very wide medullary rays of the xylem; the fragments are usually seen in tangential longitudinal section when they are composed of large, polygonal cells with moderately thickened walls and very numerous rounded to slit-shaped pits. Occasional fragments of lignified xylem parenchyma are also found, usually associated with the tracheidal-vessels or with the medullary rays; the cells have moderately thickened walls with numerous pits but they are more elongated and rectangular in outline than the cells of the medullary rays.

(*d*) The *vessels* and *tracheidal-vessels* which occur singly but more usually are found in groups; they are fairly narrow with moderately thickened, lignified walls and very numerous small, bordered pits. The vessels have somewhat oblique end walls and are usually larger than the tracheidal-vessels, which have a single perforation in the lateral walls at, or at a short distance from, each of the tapering ends. A few *tracheids* also occur; these are similar to the tracheidal-vessels but have no perforations.

(*e*) The *xylem fibres*, which are not very numerous; they are rather irregular in shape and occur singly or in small groups associated with the vessels and tracheidal-vessels; the walls are lignified, moderately thickened and have small, slit-shaped pits.

(*f*) The *calcium oxalate crystals* which are found scattered and in small groups in some of the parenchymatous cells of the phloem; they are not very abundant. They are irregularly prismatic and show considerable variation in size.

(*g*) The small amount of *parenchyma from the phelloderm* and *phloem*; the cells are thin-walled and usually filled with starch granules although an occasional cell contains a brownish secretion, and others may contain calcium oxalate crystals. The cells of the phelloderm frequently have sinuous walls.

(*h*) The very occasional *pericyclic fibres* from the rhizome; these are very large, unlignified, with unevenly thickened walls and they frequently show an elongated ovoid enlargement at one end; they are usually found fragmented.

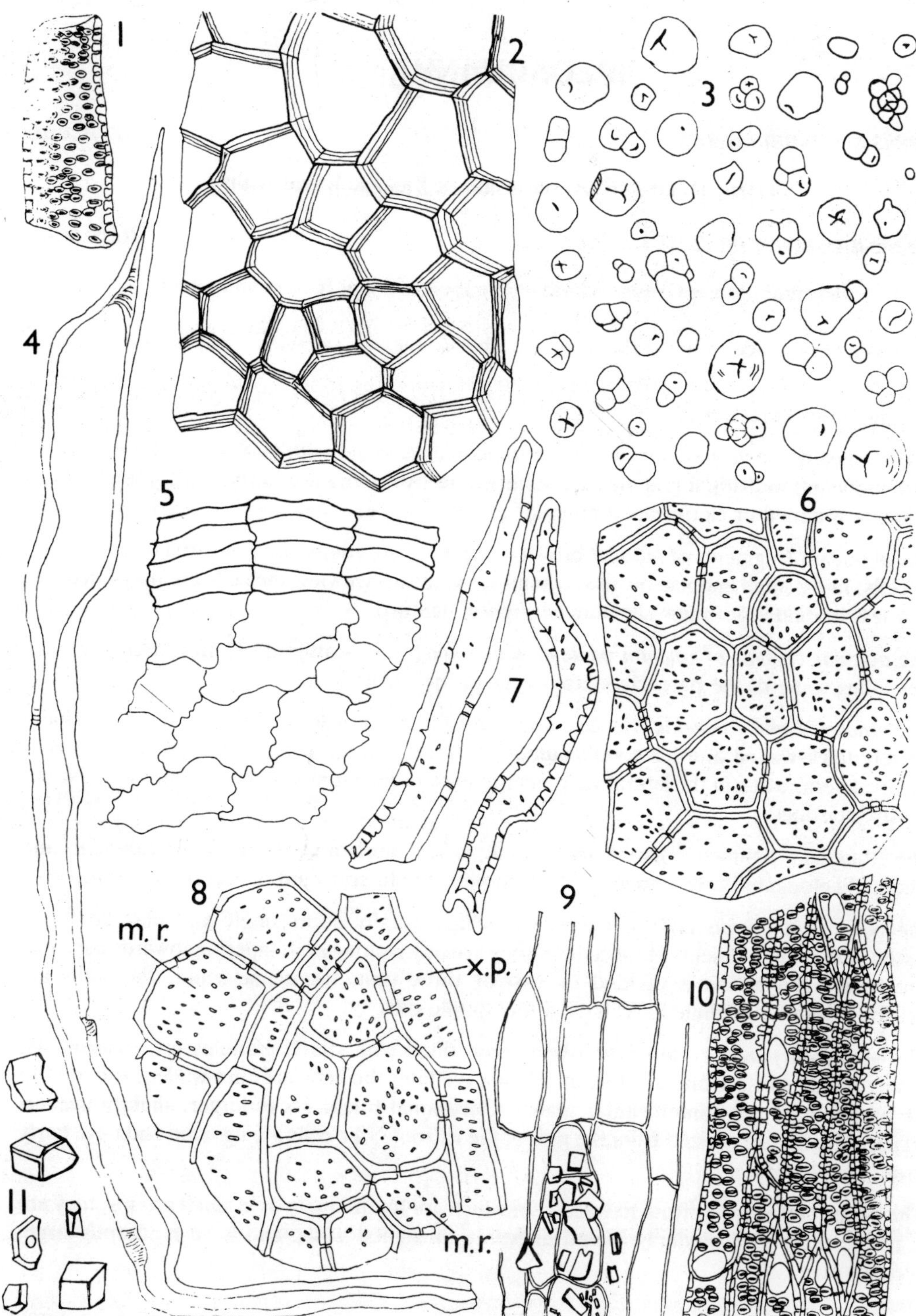

Indian Rauwolfia

×330

1 Fragment of a bordered pitted vessel.
2 Cork in surface view.
3 Starch granules.
4 Part of a pericyclic fibre from the rhizome.
5 Cork and phelloderm in sectional view.
6 Fragment of a medullary ray from the xylem in tangential longitudinal section.
7 Xylem fibres.
8 Xylem parenchyma (x.p.) and part of two medullary rays (m.r.), in tangential longitudinal section.
9 Phloem tissue in tangential longitudinal section with crystals of calcium oxalate.
10 Part of a group of tracheids and tracheidal vessels.
11 Calcium oxalate crystals.

IPECACUANHA

Cephaelis acuminata Karsten — Rubiaceae

Cartagena, Costa Rica, Nicaragua or Panama Ipecacuanha

Cephaelis ipecacuanha (Brot.) A. Rich. — Rubiaceae

Brazilian, Matto Grosso, Minas or Rio Ipecacuanha; Ipecacuanha Root

A light greyish-fawn powder with a slight odour and a bitter taste; it is sternutatory and irritant to mucous membranes.

The diagnostic characters are:

(*a*) The abundant *starch granules*, which are mostly compound with two, three, four or up to eight components; individual granules are spherical to ovoid and are fairly small; they occasionally show a rounded or cleft-shaped hilum.

(*b*) The abundant fragments of reddish-brown *cork*; these are composed of several layers of thin-walled cells, fairly small and narrow in sectional view; in surface view the cells are polygonal and more or less isodiametric; the walls may be slightly lignified.

(*c*) The *acicular crystals of calcium oxalate*, which are found scattered or, more frequently, in bundles filling some of the parenchymatous cells of the phelloderm.

(*d*) The *tracheids and tracheidal-vessels*, which are found in groups; they are small, lignified, moderately thick-walled and have very numerous small, bordered pits. The tracheidal-vessels have an oval perforation in the lateral walls near to each of the bluntly pointed ends, but these are frequently indistinct.

(*e*) The abundant lignified *parenchyma of the xylem* composed of small, rectangular and longitudinally elongated cells, moderately thick-walled with scattered bordered or simple pits.

(*f*) The occasional *fibrous cells of the xylem*, which usually occur singly and may be found associated with other elements of the xylem; they are much elongated, tapering towards each end and frequently the lumen is divided by two or three thin, transverse septa; the walls are moderately thickened, lignified and have a few simple pits.

(*g*) The abundant *parenchyma of the phelloderm*, filled with starch granules or, occasionally, containing bundles of acicular crystals of calcium oxalate; the cells are thin-walled, rounded to oval in outline with small intercellular spaces. Occasional fragments of larger, slightly thicker-walled parenchyma are present from the pith of the rhizome; the cells are lignified and have fairly numerous simple pits.

(*h*) The occasional *sclereids* from the rhizome, which are found singly or in small groups; they are large, rectangular, with moderately and unevenly thickened walls, and have numerous large, conspicuous pits.

Cephaelis ipecacuanha can be distinguished from *Cephaelis acuminata* by the size of the starch granules; in *C. ipecacuanha* they rarely exceed 15 μm in diameter, whereas in *C. acuminata* they frequently attain a diameter of 22 μm.

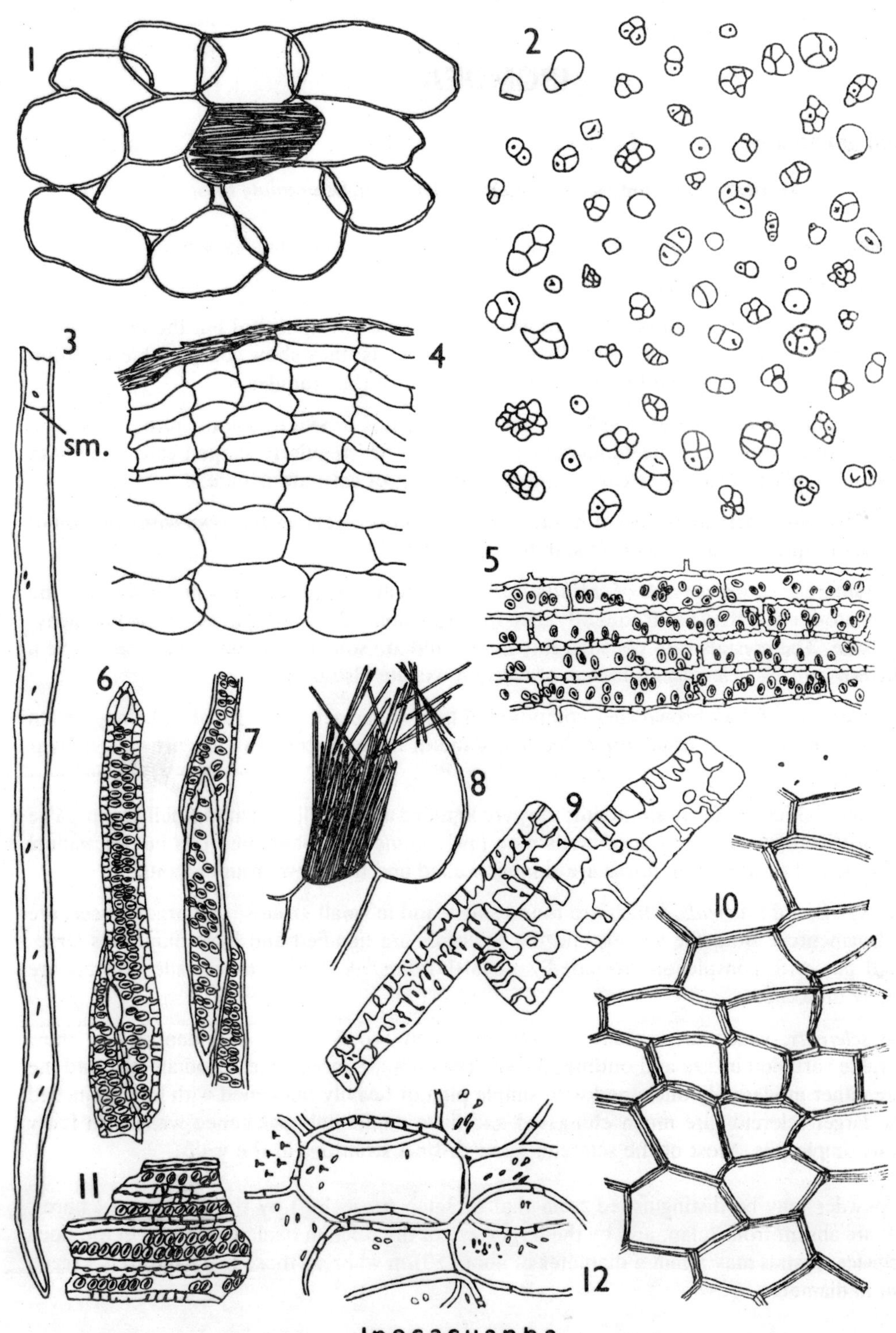

Ipecacuanha

×330

1 Parenchymatous cells of the phelloderm showing a bundle of acicular crystals of calcium oxalate in one of the cells.
2 Starch granules.
3 Part of a fibrous cell showing septa (sm.).
4 Part of the cork and phelloderm in sectional view.
5 Lignified xylem parenchyma in longitudinal section.
6 Tracheidal vessels.
7 Part of a group of tracheids.
8 Parenchyma with acicular crystals of calcium oxalate.
9 Sclereids from the rhizome.
10 Cork in surface view.
11 Fragment of xylem elements.
12 Parenchyma of the pith of the rhizome.

IPOMOEA

Ipomoea orizabensis (Pellet.) Ledanois Convolvulaceae

Mexican Scammony Root, Orizaba Jalap Root, Scammony Root

A light brown powder with a slight, characteristic odour and a bitter and nauseous taste.

The diagnostic characters are:

(*a*) The abundant *starch granules*, a few of which are simple and spherical but the majority are compound with two to four or occasionally more components; they show considerable variation in size. A rounded or slit-shaped hilum is visible in most of the granules.

(*b*) The abundant *thin-walled parenchyma*, much of which is brown in colour, rather indistinct and composed of *resin cells*; the remainder is composed of irregularly shaped cells filled with starch granules or cluster crystals (or occasionally prisms) of calcium oxalate.

(*c*) The numerous spherical masses of *resin*, which stain a deep yellowish-brown with *Solution of Iodine*; they frequently have adherent starch granules.

(*d*) The numerous *cluster crystals of calcium oxalate* which are found scattered and in some of the parenchymatous cells; they are frequently seen in longitudinal files in fragments of the parenchymatous tissue. The crystals vary considerably in size and are sometimes quite large; they have a dense brown centre. A few small *prisms* of calcium oxalate also occur.

(*e*) The fragments of dark brown *cork* composed of thin-walled cells, polygonal and elongated in surface view; the walls are usually lignified and some of the cells contain dark brown, granular pigment.

(*f*) The *fibres*, which are fairly abundant; they are lignified and usually occur in small groups. The majority have moderately thickened walls with fairly numerous slit-shaped pits but occasional groups are found in which the fibres are thinner-walled and have few, rounded pits.

(*g*) The *vessels* and *tracheids*, which are found singly and in small groups; the larger vessels are usually fragmented. Both the vessels and the tracheids are lignified and have numerous large, elongated pits with conspicuous rounded or oval borders. A few of the smaller vessels are reticulately thickened.

(*h*) The *sclereids*, which are usually found singly and are not very abundant. They show considerable variation in size and outline; the smaller ones are more or less isodiametric and the walls are either moderately thickened with simple pits, or heavily thickened with few, branched pits; the larger sclereids are much elongated and have moderately thickened walls with fairly numerous simple pits. Most of the sclereids show distinct striations in the walls.

This powder may be distinguished from that of Jalap (page 140) by the presence of fibres, which are absent from Jalap, and by the larger size of the calcium oxalate crystals; in Ipomoea the cluster crystals may attain a diameter of about 50 μm whereas those in Jalap rarely exceed 30 μm in diameter.

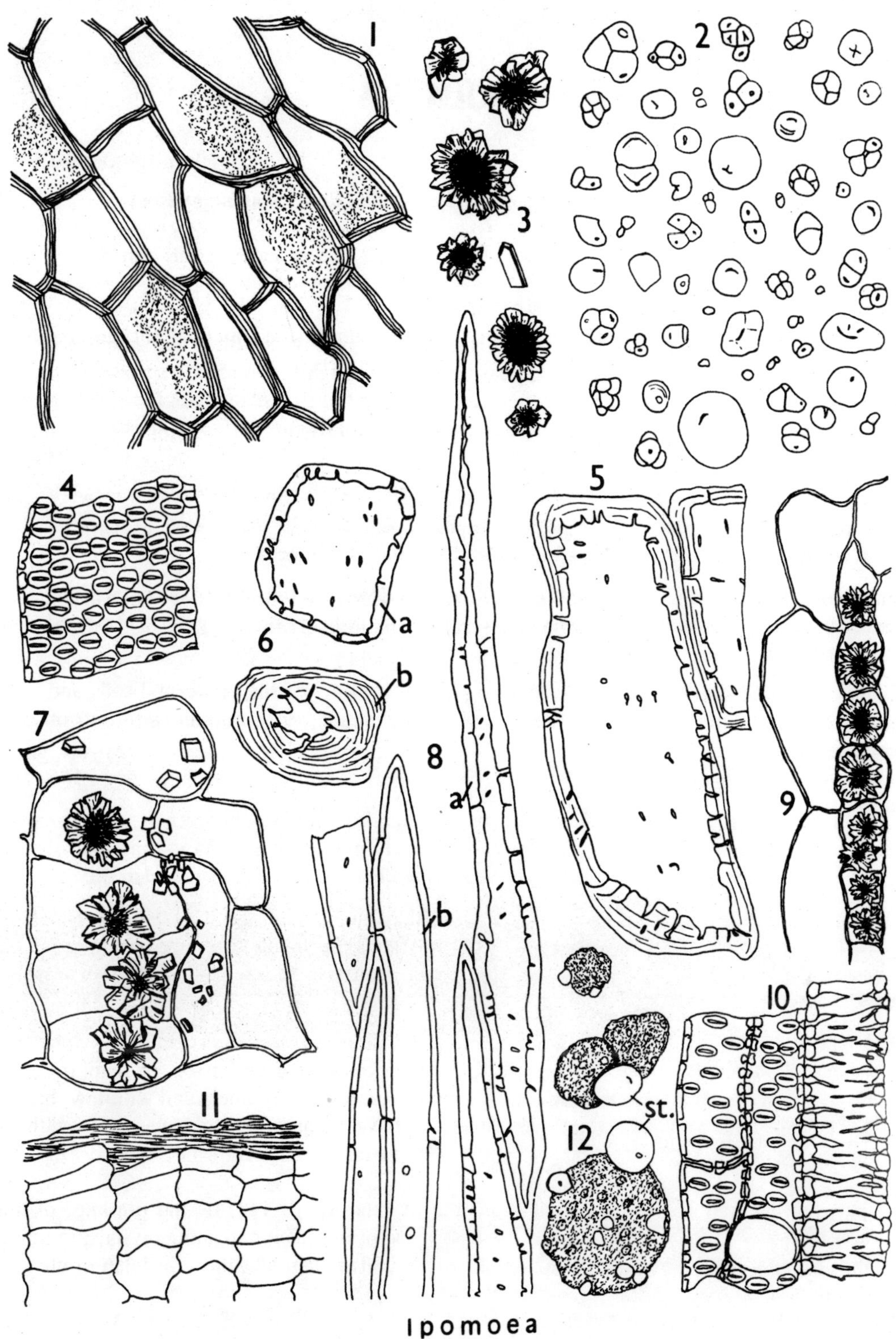

Ipomoea

×330

1 Cork in surface view.
2 Starch granules.
3 Calcium oxalate crystals.
4 Fragment of a large bordered pitted vessel.
5 Large elongated sclereids.
6 Smaller sclereids (a) with moderately thickened walls and simple pits and (b) with heavily thickened walls and branched pits.
7 Parenchymatous cells containing prisms and cluster crystals of calcium oxalate.
8 Parts of groups of fibres showing (a) the thicker-walled type with fairly numerous pits and (b) the thinner-walled type with few pits.
9 Parenchyma with part of a file of calcium oxalate cluster crystals, in longitudinal section.
10 Part of a group of vessels and xylem parenchyma.
11 Cork in sectional view.
12 Masses of resin with adherent starch granules (st.).

ISPAGHULA

Plantago ovata Forssk. Plantaginaceae

Spogel Seeds, Isafgul

A pale, pinkish-fawn powder with a slight odour and a very mucilaginous taste.

The diagnostic characters are:

(*a*) The *epidermis of the testa* composed of large cells with transparent walls, filled with *mucilage*; the cells swell rapidly in aqueous mounts and appear polygonal to slightly rounded in surface view when viewed from above, whilst from below they appear elongated to rectangular; the swelling takes place mainly in a radial direction, as is seen in the occasional fragments found in side view. The mucilage stains with *Solution of Ruthenium Red*.

(*b*) The fragments of the *endosperm* composed of thick-walled cells with numerous large, very conspicuous pits. These fragments are frequently found attached to the *inner layer of the testa* composed of rather indistinct, thin-walled cells containing brown pigment.

(*c*) The fragments of the *embryo* composed of small, thin-walled cells; the cells of the cotyledons are polygonal to slightly rounded; fragments of the tips of the radicles show regularly arranged layers of uniform cells.

(*d*) The very occasional *starch granules*, which are present in some of the epidermal cells and may be found embedded in the mucilage; they are small and simple, or compound with four or more components.

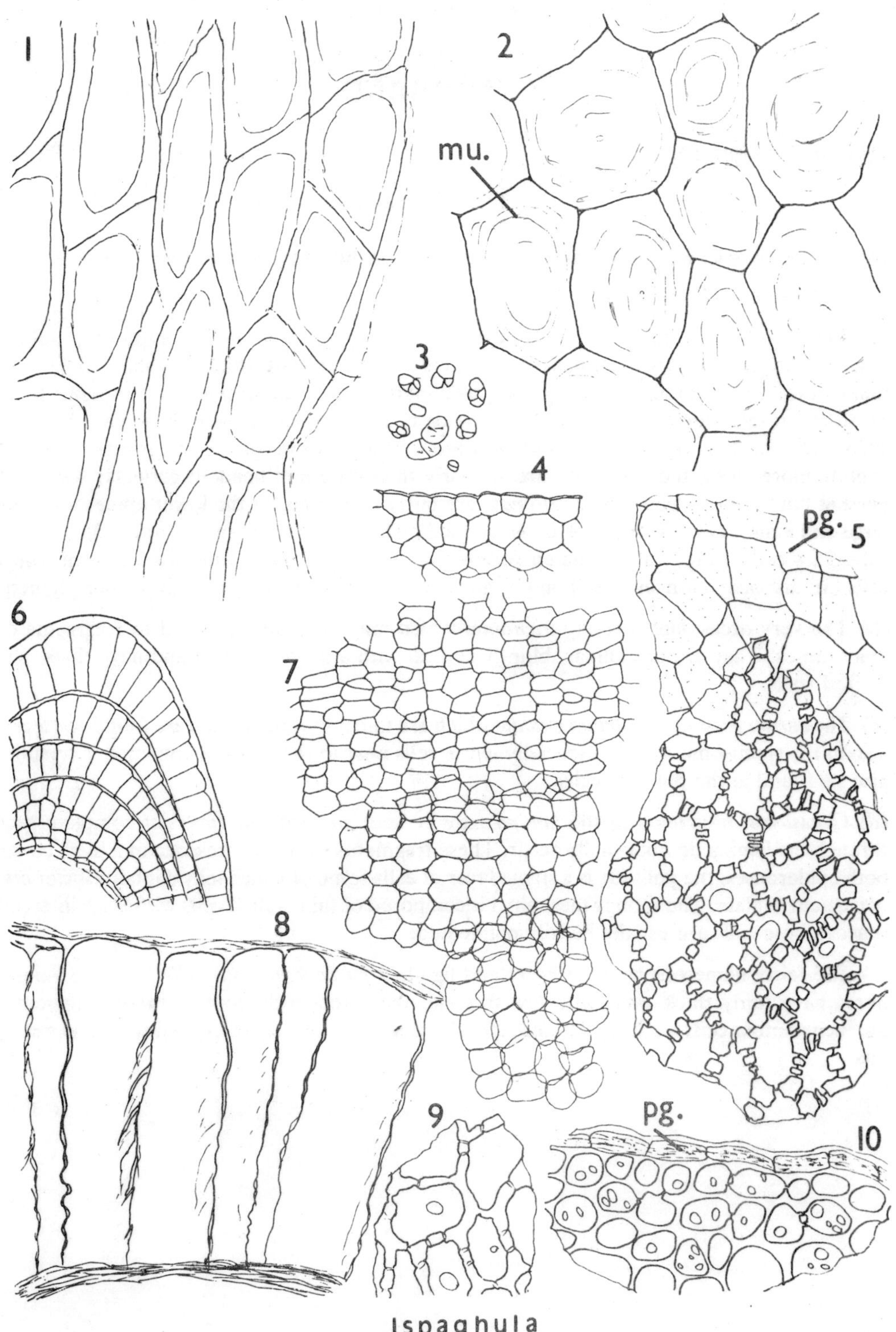

Ispaghula

×330

1 Epidermis of the testa in surface view, from below, in an aqueous mount.
2 Epidermal cells of the testa in surface view, from above, showing mucilage (mu.) in a Ruthenium Red mount.
3 Starch granules.
4 Part of a cotyledon in sectional view.
5 Part of the endosperm in surface view, with associated layer of the testa containing pigment (pg.).
6 Part of the radicle of the embryo.
7 Layers of the cotyledons in surface view.
8 Epidermis of the testa in side view showing the swollen cells containing mucilage.
9 Part of the endosperm in surface view.
10 Inner layer of the testa containing pigment (pg.) and part of the endosperm, in sectional view.

JABORANDI

Pilocarpus microphyllus Stapf. Rutaceae

Jaborandi Leaves

A mid-brown powder with a faint, aromatic odour and a slightly pungent taste which produces salivation.

The diagnostic characters are:

(*a*) The fragments of the *lamina in surface view*. The *upper epidermis* is composed of subrectangular to polygonal cells with straight, moderately thickened walls which may show slight beading; many of the cells contain brown pigment; well marked *cuticular striations* are present; there are no stomata; the underlying thin-walled palisade cells are small, irregularly arranged and rather indistinct. The cells of the *lower epidermis* are similar to those of the upper epidermis but are slightly more elongated; the walls are similarly thickened and beaded; cuticular striations are present but are less well marked. *Stomata* are fairly numerous on the lower epidermis; they are large and almost circular and each is surrounded by from four to six small, tangentially elongated subsidiary cells. Fragments of the epidermis from over the larger veins also occur in which the cells are distinctly elongated and only slightly striated; they usually contain brown pigment.

(*b*) The very occasional *covering trichomes* which may be found attached to fragments of the epidermises. They are unicellular, bluntly conical with a narrow lumen and have thick, slightly warted walls.

(*c*) The *cluster crystals of calcium oxalate* which are fairly abundant; they are found scattered and also in the spongy mesophyll, especially in the cells near to the veins; a few smaller crystals may also be found in the palisade cells.

(*d*) Occasional fragments of the *lamina* may be seen *in sectional view* but complete sections through the lamina do not usually occur. These fragments show the presence of a thick cuticle on both epidermises; the palisade is a single layer of cells some of which may contain cluster crystals of calcium oxalate. The spongy mesophyll is composed of thin-walled cells with large intercellular spaces; these cells are usually heavily pigmented.

(*e*) The fairly numerous lignified *fibres* and lignified *parenchymatous cells* from the veins. The fibres have fairly thick walls with few pits and they frequently contain brown pigment. The parenchymatous cells are irregular in shape; they have moderately thickened walls and numerous pits.

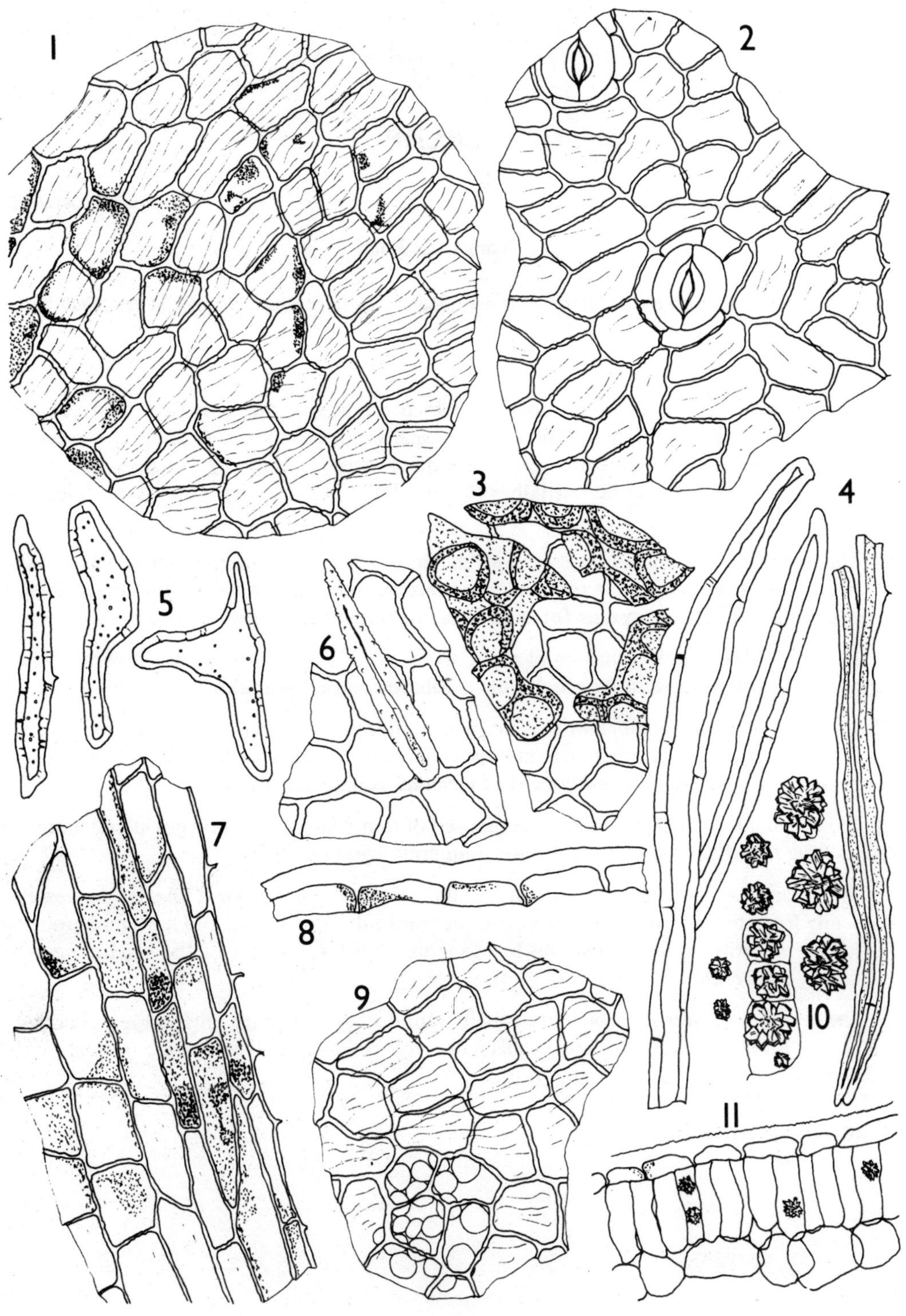

Jaborandi

×330

1 Upper epidermis in surface view showing the strongly striated cuticle and the pigment in some of the cells.
2 Lower epidermis in surface view showing stomata and the faintly striated cuticle.
3 Cells of the spongy mesophyll in surface view containing dense brown pigment, with part of the epidermis lying beneath.
4 Parts of fibres, some containing pigment.
5 Lignified parenchymatous cells from the veins.
6 Fragment of the upper epidermis in surface view with an attached trichome.
7 Part of the epidermis from over a vein in surface view showing faint striations and pigment in many of the cells.
8 Part of the upper epidermis in sectional view showing the thick cuticle and granules of pigment in the cells.
9 Upper epidermis in surface view showing cuticular striations and part of the underlying palisade.
10 Cluster crystals of calcium oxalate.
11 Part of the lamina in sectional view showing the upper epidermis with thick cuticle, palisade cells (some containing cluster crystals of calcium oxalate) and part of the spongy mesophyll.

JALAP

Ipomoea purga Hayne Convolvulaceae

Vera Cruz Jalap

A mid-brown powder with a characteristic, fruity odour and a taste which is sweet at first, then bitter and acrid.

The diagnostic characters are:

(*a*) The abundant *starch granules*, some of which are simple and spherical to ovoid but the majority are compound with two, three or occasionally more components; they vary considerably in size and individual granules are sometimes quite large; a linear or radiate hilum is usually visible. A few granules may be partially gelatinised and in these the hilum is conspicuous and enlarged.

(*b*) The abundant thin-walled *parenchyma*, much of which is brown in colour, rather indistinct and composed of *resin cells*; the remainder is composed of rounded to elongated cells filled with starch granules or cluster crystals (or occasionally prisms) of calcium oxalate.

(*c*) The numerous spherical masses of *resin*, which stain a deep yellow-brown with *Solution of Iodine*; they vary in size and frequently have adherent starch granules.

(*d*) The *cluster crystals of calcium oxalate*, which are fairly abundant; they are found scattered and in groups in some of the parenchymatous cells; they are fairly uniform in size and most show a dark brown centre. A very few *prisms* of calcium oxalate also occur.

(*e*) The fragments of dark brown *cork* composed of thin-walled cells, polygonal and more or less isodiametric in surface view; the cells are frequently lignified.

(*f*) The *vessels* and *tracheids*, which are found singly and in groups; the larger vessels are frequently fragmented. Both the vessels and the tracheids are lignified and have numerous large, slit-shaped pits with conspicuous oval to hexagonal borders. A few of the smaller vessels are reticulately thickened.

(*g*) The occasional *sclereids*, which are usually found singly; they are fairly large, rectangular to elongated with moderately thickened walls and conspicuous pits; striations are frequently visible in the walls.

Compare Ipomoea, page 134.

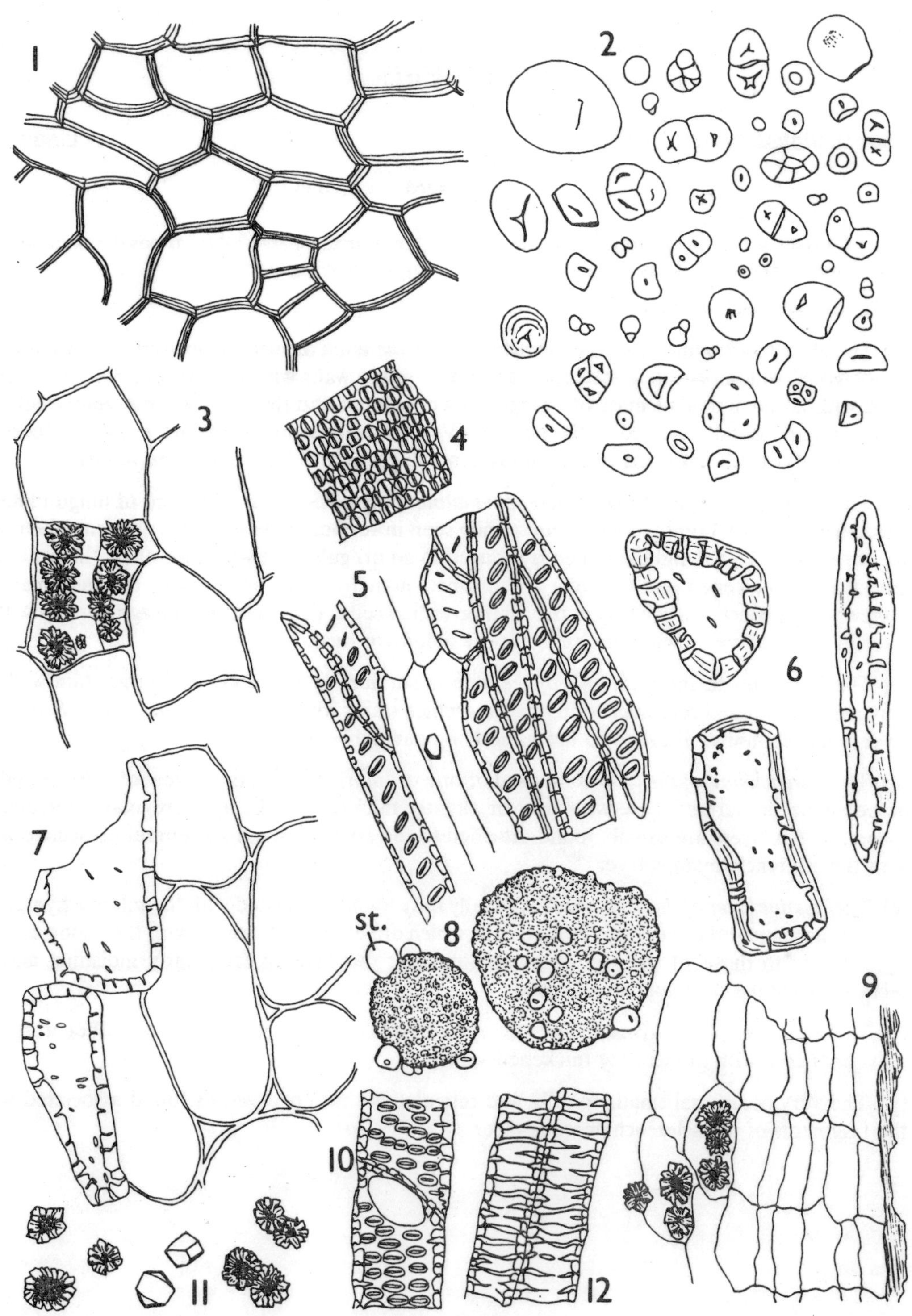

Jalap

×330

1 Cork in surface view.
2 Starch granules.
3 Parenchyma containing cluster crystals of calcium oxalate.
4 Fragment of a bordered pitted vessel.
5 Part of a group of tracheids with adjacent parenchyma.
6 Sclereids.
7 Part of a small group of sclereids with associated parenchyma.
8 Masses of resin with adherent starch granules (st.).
9 Cork and part of the phelloderm in sectional view.
10 Bordered pitted vessels.
11 Prisms and cluster crystals of calcium oxalate.
12 Reticulately thickened vessels.

LINSEED

Linum usitatissimum L. **Linaceae**

Flaxseed

Linseed usually occurs in the form of 'crushed linseed', a coarse, yellowish-brown powder with distinct darker brown fragments; it has a slight odour and an oily and mucilaginous taste.

The diagnostic characters are:

(*a*) The abundant fragments of the *pigment layer of the testa*; in surface view the cells are square to polygonal with moderately thickened and finely pitted walls which are colourless; each cell is filled with an homogenous mass of orange-brown pigment and these masses frequently fall out intact and are found scattered in the powder. Very occasional fragments are found in sectional view, usually attached to part of the endosperm; the cells are then seen to be tabular.

(*b*) The colourless or pale brown *sclerenchymatous layer of the testa* composed of longitudinally elongated cells with bluntly pointed ends when seen in surface view; in some fragments the walls are strongly thickened and the lumen is reduced to an irregular line whilst in others the walls are less strongly thickened and the lumen is distinct; numerous pits are present but they may be somewhat indistinct, particularly in the thinner-walled cells. Very occasional fragments show this layer in sectional view, when the cells appear oblong or oval.

(*c*) The fragments of the *epidermis of the testa* in surface view composed of large, thin-walled, polygonal to rounded cells filled with *mucilage* which stains with *Solution of Ruthenium Red*. This layer is usually found attached to the underlying parenchyma.

(*d*) The *parenchyma of the testa* composed of one or, more usually, two layers of cells, rounded or polygonal in surface view with thin or slightly thickened walls and irregular intercellular spaces. These layers are usually found attached to the epidermis and sometimes associated also with the sclerenchymatous layer.

(*e*) The *hyaline layer of the testa* which is usually only found associated with the sclerenchymatous layer; it is composed of very thin-walled cells which are elongated and lie with their long axes at right angles to those of the sclerenchymatous cells; this layer is frequently indistinct and in sectional view the cells appear collapsed.

(*f*) The abundant *parenchyma of the endosperm* and *cotyledons* composed of rather irregular polygonal cells with moderately thickened walls.

(*g*) The very occasional small, spirally and reticulately thickened *vessels* found associated with the fragments of the sclerenchymatous layer.

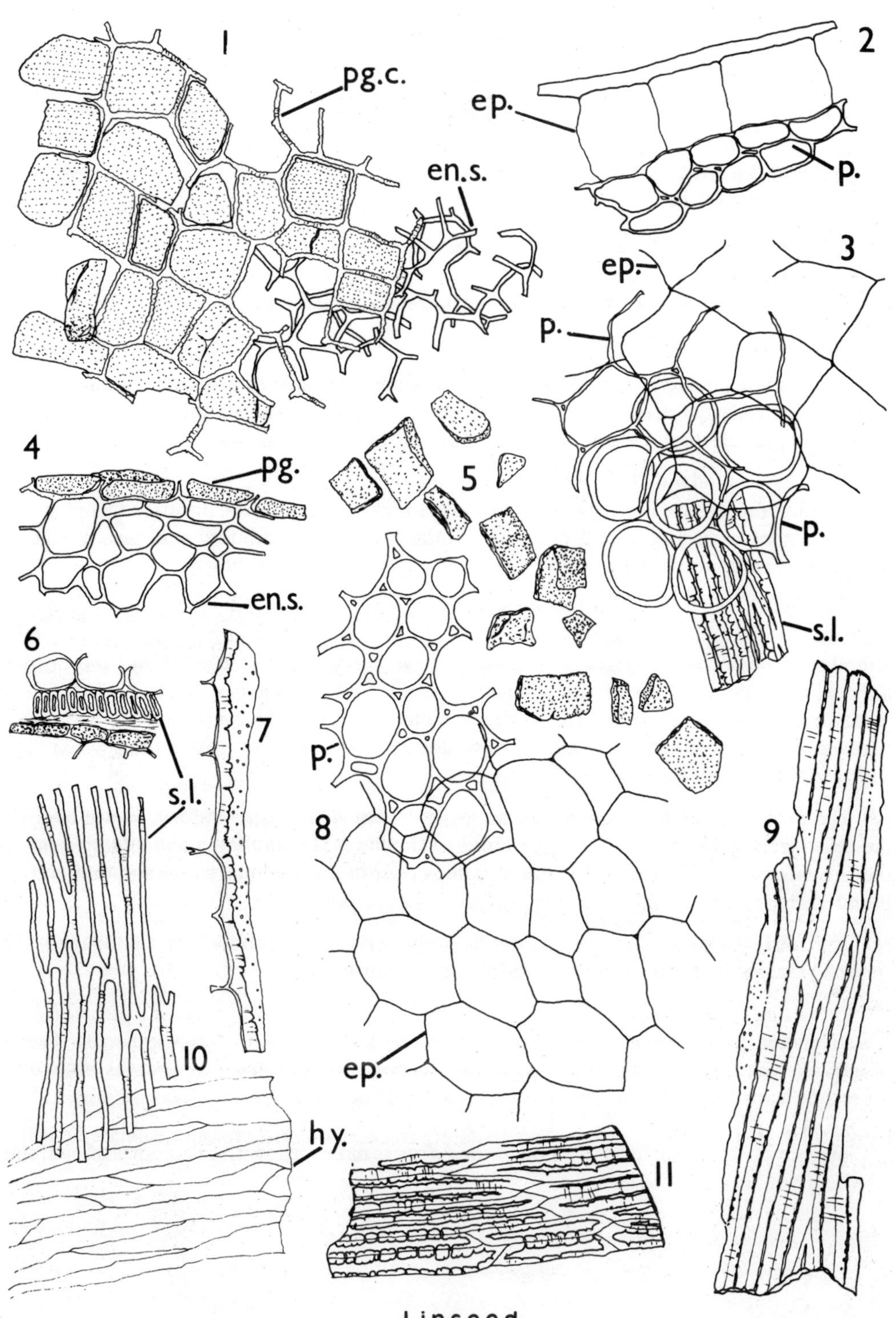

Linseed

×330

1 Pigment layer of the testa in surface view showing the cells containing pigment (pg.c.) and underlying endosperm cells (en.s.).
2 Epidermis (ep.) and two layers of parenchyma of the testa (p.) in sectional view.
3 Part of the testa in surface view showing the epidermis (ep.), two layers of parenchyma (p.) and sclerenchyma (s.l.).
4 Pigment layer of the testa (pg.) and endosperm (en.s.) in sectional view.
5 Isolated masses of pigment.
6 Part of the testa in sectional view showing the sclerenchymatous layer (s.l.), collapsed hyaline layer and pigment layer.
7 Part of a cell of the sclerenchymatous layer in longitudinal sectional view, showing the dentate outline corresponding to the adjacent parenchymatous cells.
8 Part of the testa in surface view showing the epidermis (ep.) and underlying parenchyma (p.).
9 Thick-walled cells of the sclerenchyma layer in surface view.
10 Thin-walled cells of the sclerenchyma layer (s.l.) in surface view, with associated hyaline layer (hy.).
11 Moderately thickened cells of the sclerenchyma layer in surface view.

LIQUORICE

Glycyrrhiza glabra L. and varieties of *Glycyrrhiza glabra* — Leguminosae

Liquorice Root

A pale, yellowish-brown powder with a faint, characteristic odour and a sweet taste.

The diagnostic characters are:

(*a*) The abundant *starch granules*, most of which are simple; they are rather small, spherical to ovoid and slightly flattened; a slit-shaped hilum is visible in some of the larger granules. A few compound granules are present with two, three or four components.

(*b*) The very abundant *fibres* which occur in groups surrounded by a calcium oxalate prism sheath. Individual fibres are very thick-walled with few, small pits; the different layers in the walls are sometimes clearly seen and only the middle lamella and primary wall give a reaction for lignin; frequently no lumen is visible.

(*c*) The *vessels*, which are found singly or in small groups; some of the individual vessels are very large and are frequently found fragmented. They are lignified and usually bordered pitted, although in some of the larger vessels the pits are very much elongated and the borders are difficult to discern. Many of the smaller, narrower vessels show a single perforation in the somewhat oblique end walls. The larger vessels are usually accompanied by lignified xylem parenchyma composed of moderately thin-walled cells, square to elongated rectangular in outline with variably pitted walls.

(*d*) The *prisms of calcium oxalate*, the majority of which are fairly uniform in size and occur in the cells forming the crystal sheath surrounding the fibres. In addition a few larger prisms occur; they are present in some of the parenchymatous cells of the medullary rays and pith and may be found in these cells or, more usually, scattered in the powder.

(*e*) The fairly abundant fragments of orange-brown *cork* composed of thin-walled cells; in surface view the cells are polygonal and fairly regular in outline.

(*f*) The abundant thin-walled *parenchyma from the cortex, medullary rays* and *pith*; the cells vary from rounded to rectangular in outline and are usually filled with starch granules. Occasional groups of sieve tissue, composed of very thin-walled cells with faint sieve areas, may be found associated with the medullary rays. A small amount of collenchyma is also present.

Liquorice powder prepared from the *peeled drug* is more yellowish in colour and contains very infrequent cork fragments.

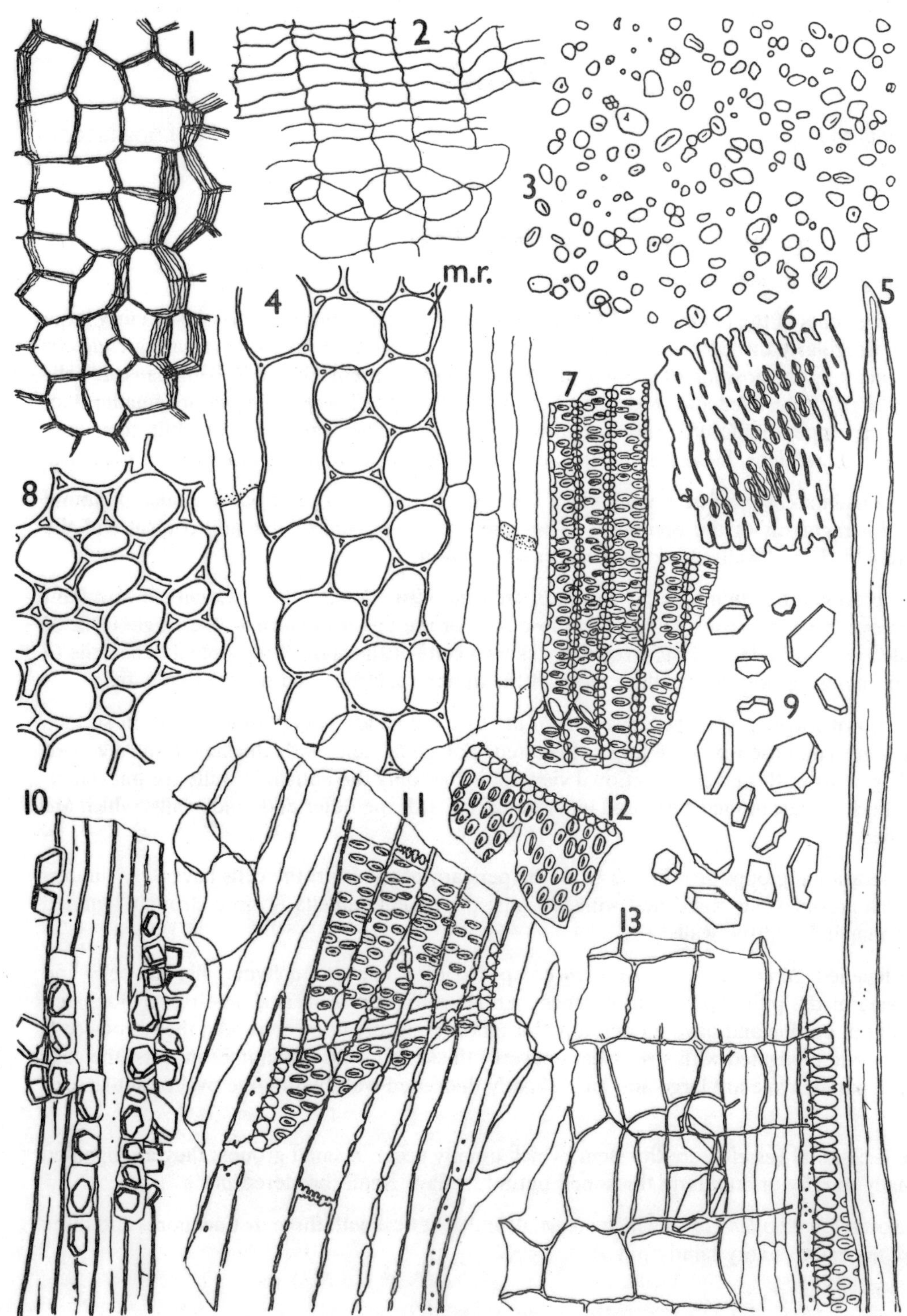

Liquorice

×330

1 Cork in surface view.
2 Part of the cork and cortex in sectional view.
3 Starch granules.
4 Part of a medullary ray (m.r.) in tangential longitudinal section with associated sieve tissue.
5 Part of a single fibre.
6 Fragment of a large vessel with elongated pits.
7 Part of a group of smaller vessels with bordered pits.
8 Collenchyma from the cortex.
9 Prisms of calcium oxalate.
10 Part of a group of fibres with incomplete calcium oxalate prism sheath.
11 Lignified xylem parenchyma with part of an underlying bordered pitted vessel and adjacent thin-walled parenchyma.
12 Fragment of a bordered pitted vessel.
13 Part of a medullary ray in radial longitudinal section with underlying thin-walled parenchyma and part of a bordered pitted vessel.

LOBELIA

Lobelia inflata L. Lobeliaceae

Lobelia Herb, Indian Tobacco

A dull yellowish-green powder with a faint odour and a pungent, acrid taste.

The diagnostic characters are:

(*a*) The fragments of the *lamina in surface view*. The *upper epidermis* is composed of fairly large cells with irregularly thickened, slightly sinuous walls; occasional cells show radiating *cuticular striations* marking the position of small *papillae*; stomata are absent; the underlying palisade cells are fairly large, thin-walled and loosely packed. The cells of the *lower epidermis* are smaller than those of the upper epidermis and are distinctly sinuous; the walls are thin but they may occasionally show slight thickening at the corners; numerous *anomocytic* stomata are present.

(*b*) The abundant *covering trichomes* which usually are found scattered but may also be found attached to fragments of the epidermis. They are very large, unicellular and conical and the moderately thickened walls show faint scattered striations.

(*c*) The occasional fragments of the *lamina in sectional view* showing the thick cuticle with faint striations overlying the large, slightly papillose cells of the upper epidermis, the single layer of thin-walled palisade cells and the irregularly shaped cells of the spongy mesophyll. The cells of the lower epidermis are smaller than those of the upper epidermis and have a thin cuticle.

(*d*) The brown fragments of the *epidermis of the testa* which are very characteristic. In surface view they are composed of very large elongated, polygonal cells with thickened and lignified walls. Fragments of this layer in sectional view show that only the anticlinal walls are thickened, with the thickest part in the centre and tapering off towards the outer and inner walls, which are not lignified.

(*e*) The occasional groups of *sclereids* from the pericarp of the fruit; the cells have very sinuous walls which are unevenly thickened with few pits; the middle lamella is more strongly lignified than the remainder of the walls.

(*f*) The lignified *parenchyma of the stem* composed of xylem parenchyma, fibrous cells and parenchyma of the pith. The xylem parenchymatous cells vary from isodiametric to elongated rectangular in outline and have moderately thickened walls and numerous pits; the fibrous cells are narrow and elongated with somewhat unevenly thickened walls and numerous pits; the cells of the pith parenchyma are large and have slightly thickened walls with large oval or slit-shaped pits.

(*g*) The occasional *vessels* from the stem, which usually occur in small groups; they are lignified and usually spirally or annularly thickened but a few have small, bordered pits.

(*h*) The occasional *pollen grains* which are small and spherical with three distinct pores and three furrows; the exine is very faintly pitted.

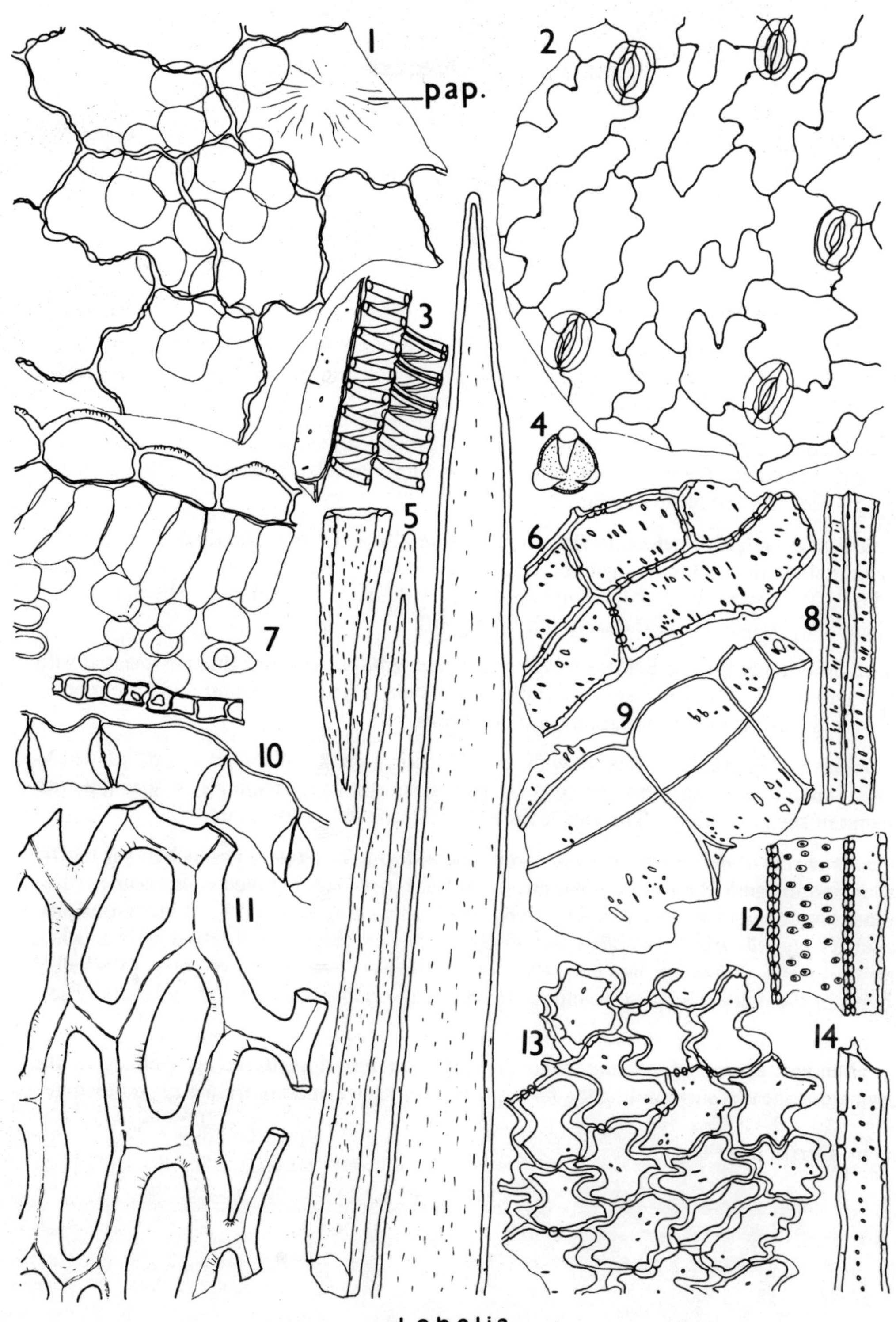

Lobelia

×330

1 Upper epidermis in surface view showing a papilla (pap.) and underlying palisade cells.
2 Lower epidermis in surface view with anomocytic stomata.
3 Spirally thickened vessels and a fragment of xylem parenchyma from the stem.
4 Pollen grain.
5 Parts of covering trichomes.
6 Xylem parenchyma from the stem.
7 Part of the lamina in sectional view.
8 Fibrous cells from the stem.
9 Parenchyma of the pith.
10 Epidermis of the testa in sectional view.
11 Epidermis of the testa in surface view.
12 Part of a bordered pitted vessel and adjacent fibrous cell from the stem.
13 Sclereids from the pericarp in surface view.
14 Part of a fibrous cell from the stem.

LONCHOCARPUS

Lonchocarpus spp. Leguminosae

Barbasco, Cube Root

A cream to fawn powder with little odour and a taste which at first is slight then becomes acrid and produces an unpleasant, numbing sensation in the mouth and throat.

The diagnostic characters are:

(*a*) The very abundant *starch granules*; they are simple or compound with up to four or more components. Individual granules are frequently quite large and are spherical or polyhedral with a distinct, rather small, radiate hilum.

(*b*) The abundant *fibres*, which are usually found in groups surrounded by a calcium oxalate prism sheath. Individual fibres are long and narrow with variably thickened walls which are partially lignified; pits are fairly numerous.

(*c*) The very large *vessels*, which occur singly or, occasionally, in small groups and are sometimes found fragmented; the walls are lignified and have numerous fairly large, closely arranged bordered pits. The vessels are usually found associated with lignified xylem parenchymatous cells or with lignified parenchyma of the medullary rays.

(*d*) The occasional *sclereids*, which are found singly or in groups of two or three associated with unlignified parenchyma; they are isodiametric or slightly elongated rectangular and have moderately thickened walls with faint striations and numerous pits.

(*e*) The fragments of *cork*; in surface view the cells are polygonal, thin-walled and pale fawnish-brown in colour; in sectional view the cells occur in several layers, frequently associated with parenchyma of the phelloderm. The cork cells give a faint reaction for lignin.

(*f*) The *parenchyma of the xylem, medullary rays* and *phloem*. The xylem parenchyma is mostly thin-walled and unlignified but occasional groups of thicker-walled, lignified cells occur particularly in association with the vessels; they are longitudinally elongated and have numerous pits. The medullary ray cells are also mostly unlignified, but they are thicker-walled and lignified when adjacent to vessels, fibres or lignified xylem parenchyma. Fragments of very thin-walled parenchyma of the phloem are also found occasionally; the cells are elongated and more or less uniform.

(*g*) The abundant *prisms of calcium oxalate*, which are found scattered as well as in the parenchymatous sheaths surrounding the fibres; they vary in size and are frequently quite large.

Compare Derris, page 86.

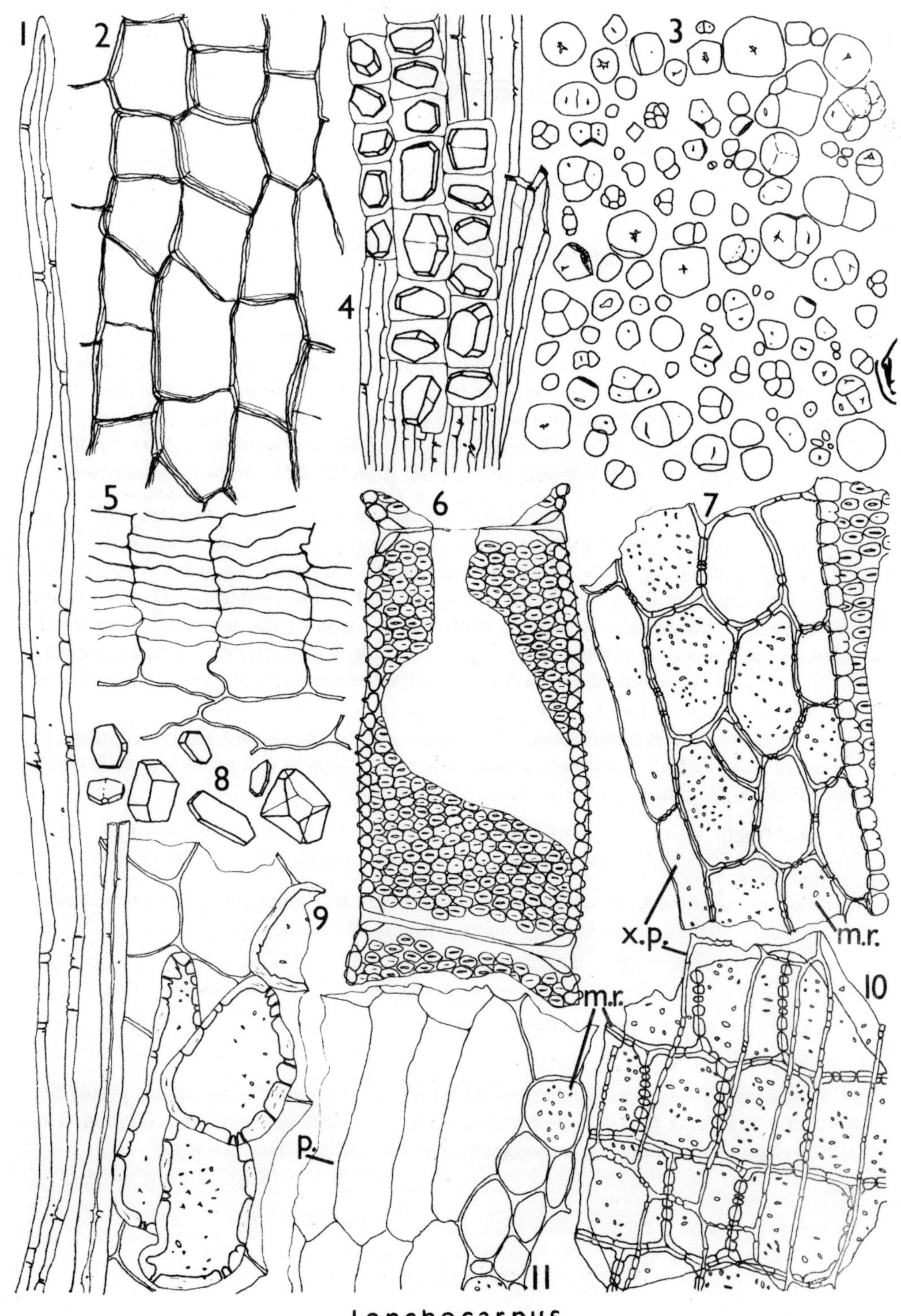

Lonchocarpus

×330

1 Part of a single fibre.
2 Cork in surface view.
3 Starch granules.
4 Part of a group of fibres with calcium oxalate prism sheath.
5 Part of the cork and phelloderm in sectional view.
6 A bordered pitted vessel.
7 Part of the xylem in tangential longitudinal section showing lignified xylem parenchyma (x.p.), lignified medullary ray cells (m.r.) and part of a bordered pitted vessel.
8 Prisms of calcium oxalate.
9 A group of sclereids with adjacent parenchyma and part of a fibre.
10 Lignified xylem paraenchyma (x.p.) and part of a medullary ray (m.r.) in radial longitudinal section.
11 Phloem parenchyma (p.) with part of a medullary ray (m.r.) in tangential longitudinal section.

LUCERNE

Medicago sativa L. subsp. *sativa* Leguminosae

Alfalfa

A mid greenish-brown powder with a slight odour and taste.

The diagnostic characters are:

(*a*) The fragments of the *leaf lamina in surface view*. The *upper epidermis* is composed of sinuous cells with thin walls which show occasional beading; the underlying palisade cells are small and loosely packed. The cells of the *lower epidermis* are larger and more sinuous in outline than those of the upper epidermis and the walls are distinctly and regularly beaded, although beading does not occur at the junctions of the cells; occasional fragments show a rounded *cicatrix* which is surrounded by radiating cells. *Anisocytic* and *anomocytic stomata* occur on both epidermises.

(*b*) The *covering trichomes*, which are very characteristic; they are fairly abundant and occur scattered or attached to portions of the lower epidermis. They are uniseriate, composed of two short basal cells and a very long, undulating, terminal cell which tapers towards the apex, and they are usually bent near the base so that they lie appressed to the epidermis. The two small basal cells have smooth, moderately thickened walls but the wall of the terminal cell is much thickened so that a lumen is only rarely visible, and the *cuticle* is coarsely warted and irregular. When these trichomes are detached they usually break off at the second basal cell so that only the long terminal cells are seen scattered in the powder.

Very occasional *glandular trichomes* may be found scattered or, more usually, attached to fragments of the calyx epidermis; they have a uniseriate stalk composed of up to four cells and a rounded, unicellular or bicellular head.

(*c*) The occasional fragments of *vascular tissue* from the veins with lignified, spirally or annularly thickened *vessels* and associated *calcium oxalate prism crystal sheath*.

(*d*) The fragments of *leaf lamina in sectional view*, which are not abundant; they show a two-layered palisade and a spongy mesophyll containing strands of vascular tissue.

(*e*) The fragments of *lignified parenchyma* from the stem composed of large, longitudinally elongated cells with moderately thickened walls and fairly numerous pits; these are sometimes found associated with groups of lignified vessels with spiral or annular thickening or, in the larger elements, with bordered pits.

(*f*) The *pollen grains* and fragments of the *petals*, which are very rare. The pollen grains are spherical with three indistinct pores, three furrows, a smooth exine and granular contents. The epidermis of the petals is papillose, with elongated *papillae* and a striated *cuticle*.

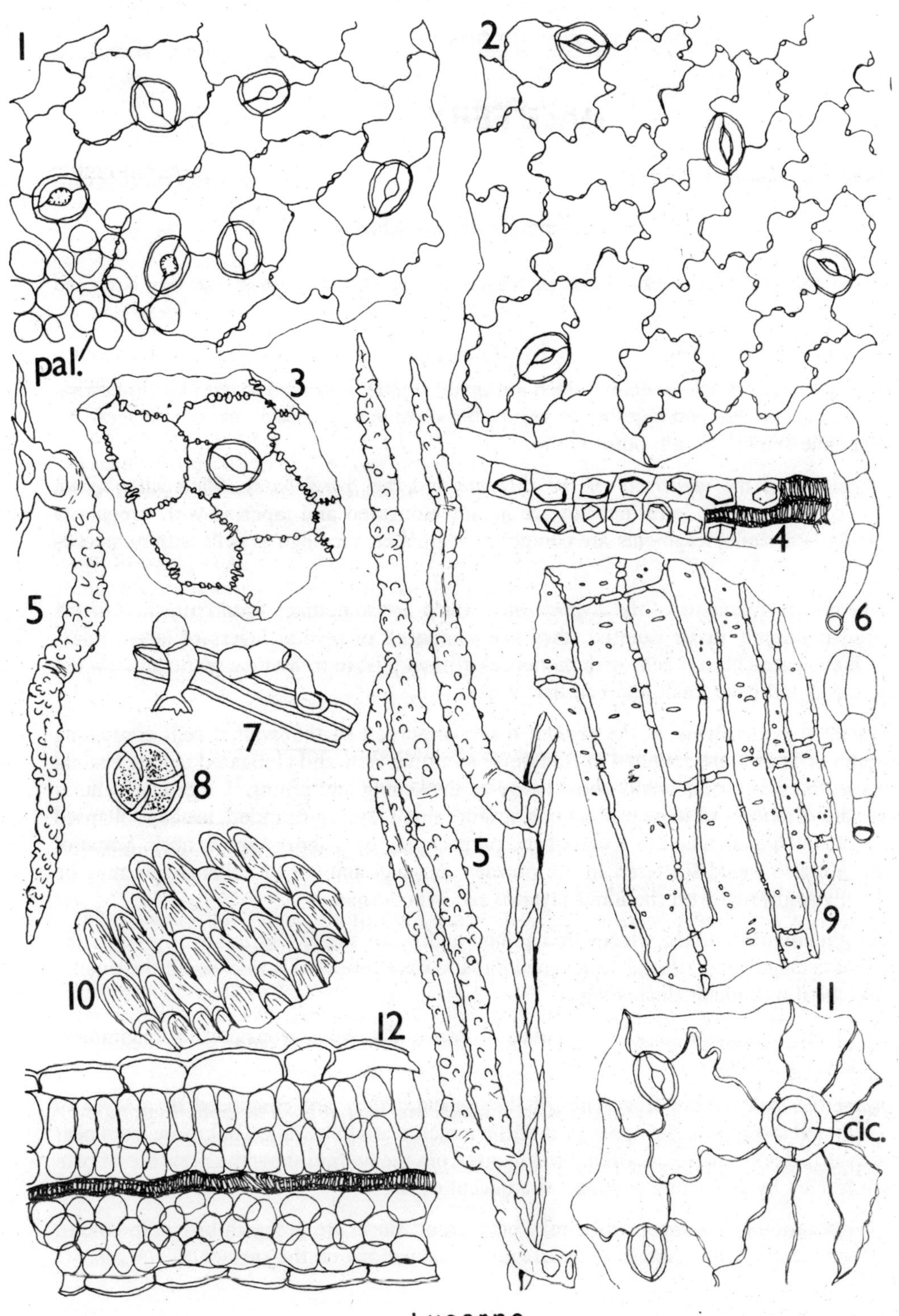

Lucerne

×330

1 Upper epidermis of the leaf in surface view showing anomocytic and anisocytic stomata and part of the underlying palisade (pal.).
2 Lower epidermis of the leaf in surface view showing stomata.
3 Outer epidermis of the calyx in surface view.
4 Part of a vascular strand showing vessels and part of the calcium oxalate prism crystal sheath.
5 Covering trichomes.
6 Glandular trichomes.
7 Glandular trichomes on a fragment of the calyx.
8 Pollen grain.
9 Pitted parenchyma from the stem, in longitudinal view.
10 Papillose epidermis of a petal.
11 Lower epidermis of the leaf in surface view showing a cicatrix (cic.).
12 Part of the leaf lamina in sectional view.

MALE FERN

Dryopteris filix-mas agg. Polypodiaceae

Aspidium, Filix-mas, Male Fern Rhizome

A mid-brown powder with paler specks; the odour is slight and the taste sweetish at first, then bitter and nauseous.

The diagnostic characters are:

(*a*) The fairly abundant *starch granules*, which are small, simple, spherical to ovoid or somewhat polyhedral; they occur clumped together in groups but compound granules are not present. An occasional granule shows a small, point hilum.

(*b*) The fragments of the *epidermis of the rhizome* and the *frond bases*, filled with brown pigment; the cells are rather indistinct but are mainly elongated and tapering with irregularly thickened walls; occasional fragments are composed of smaller, rectangular cells with numerous pits.

(*c*) The dark brown fragments of the *hypodermis*, which are sometimes found attached to the epidermis but frequently occur isolated; they are composed of several layers of large, thick-walled, much elongated fibrous cells with numerous distinct pits; in transverse sectional view the cells are rounded and have small intercellular spaces.

(*d*) The abundant *parenchyma of the ground tissue* composed of thin-walled cells containing starch granules. The cells are rounded in transverse sectional view and elongated in longitudinal sectional view; the walls occasionally show irregular thickening and pitting. Large intercellular spaces occur and into some of these project one or more small, oval or rounded, usually collapsed *glands* each of which is attached to a cell of the parenchyma by a short narrow neck. Some of these glands are also found scattered in the powder. A small amount of collenchyma may be present, usually associated with the inner layer of the hypodermis.

(*e*) The fairly numerous *vessels*, which are lignified and occur singly and in small groups; the larger vessels are mainly scalariformly thickened but a few are reticulately thickened; the smaller vessels show spiral or annular thickening.

(*f*) The fragments of the *endodermis* composed of thin-walled cells, elongated in longitudinal view with a sinuous outline.

(*g*) The numerous pale brown fragments of the *ramenta*; they are composed of a layer of elongated cells and those from the upper part of the ramenta are thin-walled but those from near the base are fairly thick-walled; occasional fragments from the margin show the presence of two-celled teeth formed by projecting portions of adjacent cells.

(*h*) The very occasional *sporangia* which may be present; these are greenish-brown in colour, reniform in outline and have characteristic irregular reticulations on the surface.

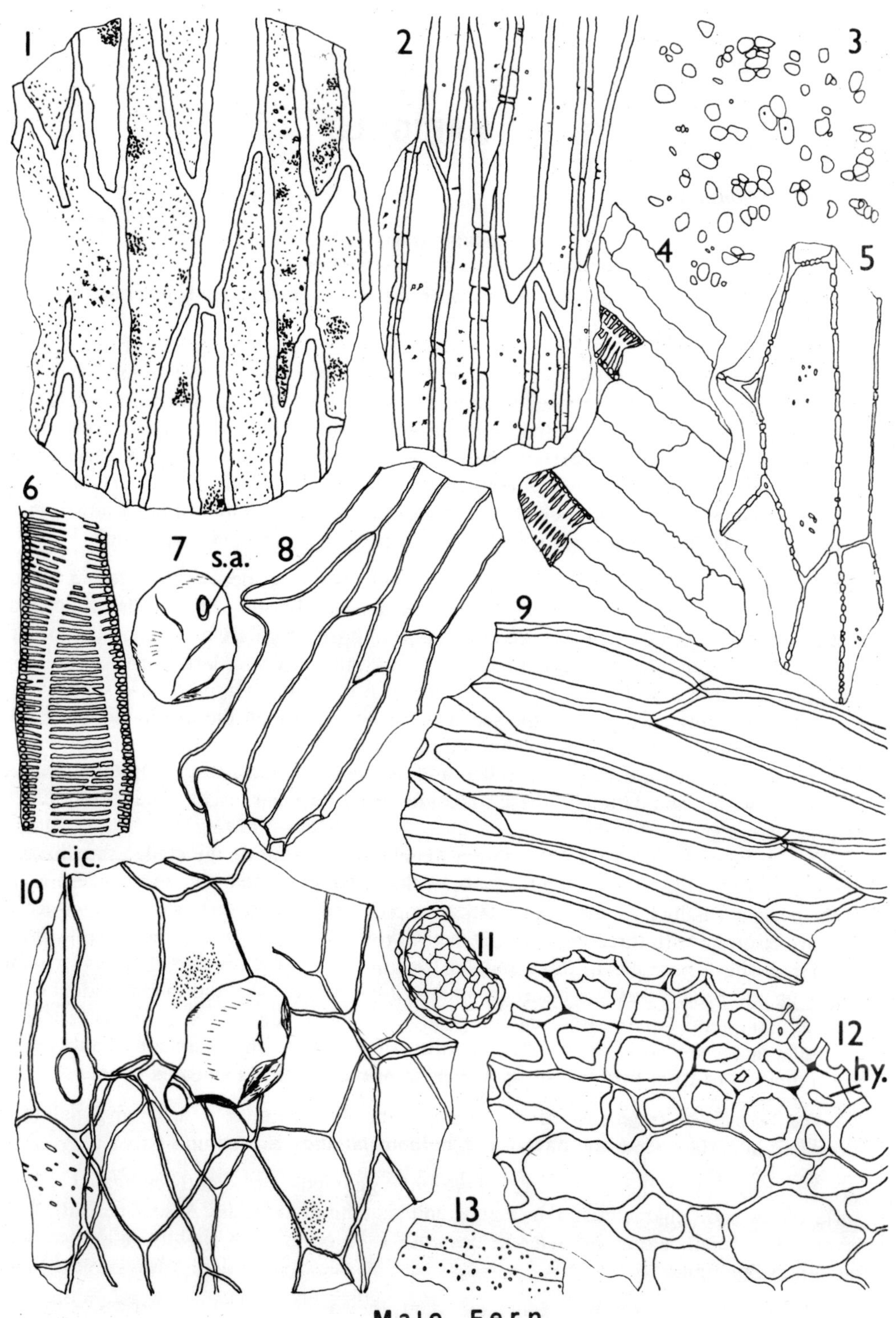

Male Fern

×330

1 Epidermis of the frond bases in surface view showing pigment in some of the cells.
2 Hypodermis in surface view.
3 Starch granules.
4 Endodermis in longitudinal view with part of adjacent vessels.
5 Pitted parenchyma of the ground tissue in longitudinal view.
6 Part of a scalariformly thickened vessel.
7 A detached gland showing the scar of attachment (s.a.).
8 Part of the upper part of a ramentum showing the two-celled marginal projections.
9 Thicker-walled cells from the basal region of a ramentum.
10 Parenchyma of the ground tissue in transverse sectional view showing an attached gland and the cicatrix (cic.) of another.
11 A spore.
12 Part of the hypodermis (hy.) and adjacent collenchyma in transverse sectional view.
13 Fragment of the epidermis in surface view showing pitted walls.

MARIGOLD

Calendula officinalis L. Compositae

Calendula, Marigold Florets

A yellowish-brown powder with a characteristic, aromatic odour and a slightly bitter and aromatic taste.

The diagnostic characters are:

(*a*) The very abundant fragments of the *corollas of the ligulate florets in surface view*. The *inner epidermis* is composed of elongated rectangular cells which are irregularly and finely sinuous in outline; the cuticle is faintly striated; in the apical region of the corolla the cells are smaller and less regularly arranged; at the extreme base there is a single layer of cells with marked thickening on the outer walls and these cells contain prisms and very small cluster crystals. The *outer epidermis* is similar to the inner epidermis except that a small number of fairly large, *anomocytic stomata* occur in the apical region; these are not present on the inner epidermis.

(*b*) The *covering* and *glandular trichomes*, which are very occasionally found attached to fragments of the epidermises on which they occur, but the majority are detached and found scattered. The covering trichomes are of two types; those which are more abundant occur on the involucral bracts and the basal region of the corollas; they are very large, biseriate, multicellular and conical with a rounded apex; the cells of which they are composed have slightly thickened walls. The covering trichomes of the second type occur only on the involucral bracts; they are uniseriate, conical and very long, composed of four or five cells with the apical cell much longer than the others; they are very thin-walled and all the cells, and particularly the apical cell, are frequently twisted and flattened; these trichomes usually appear bright reddish-purple in *Chloral Hydrate* mounts.

The glandular trichomes show variation mainly in the form of the stalks; they occur on the involucral bracts, the corollas and the walls of the ovaries. Those from the corollas and the walls of the ovaries usually have uniseriate stalks composed of from three to five cells but occasionally they are biseriate with three or four cells in each row; very occasionally there is no stalk and the gland is sessile. The stalks of the glandular trichomes from the involucral bracts frequently are very long and broad; they are biseriate, multicellular and conical and the individual cells at the base are frequently quite large and irregularly arranged. On all the glandular trichomes the glandular heads are ovoid, multicellular and usually biseriate; they vary considerably in size and are composed of from two or four up to twelve or more thin-walled cells.

(*c*) The occasional fragments of the *stigmas*; the epidermal cells are polygonal to slightly elongated in surface view and have short, bulbous *papillae*.

(*d*) The fragments of the *fibrous layer of the anthers* composed of slightly elongated cells which in surface view show characteristic thickening and beading of the walls. Associated with the fibrous layer a few small, elongated *sclerenchymatous cells* occur with slightly thickened walls and numerous large pits.

(*e*) The *pollen grains*, which are quite abundant; they are fairly large, spherical, with three very distinct pores; the exine is sharply spiny and also has very faint granulations.

(*f*) The occasional fragments of the *walls of the ovaries* composed of small cells, polygonal in surface view and containing brown pigment.

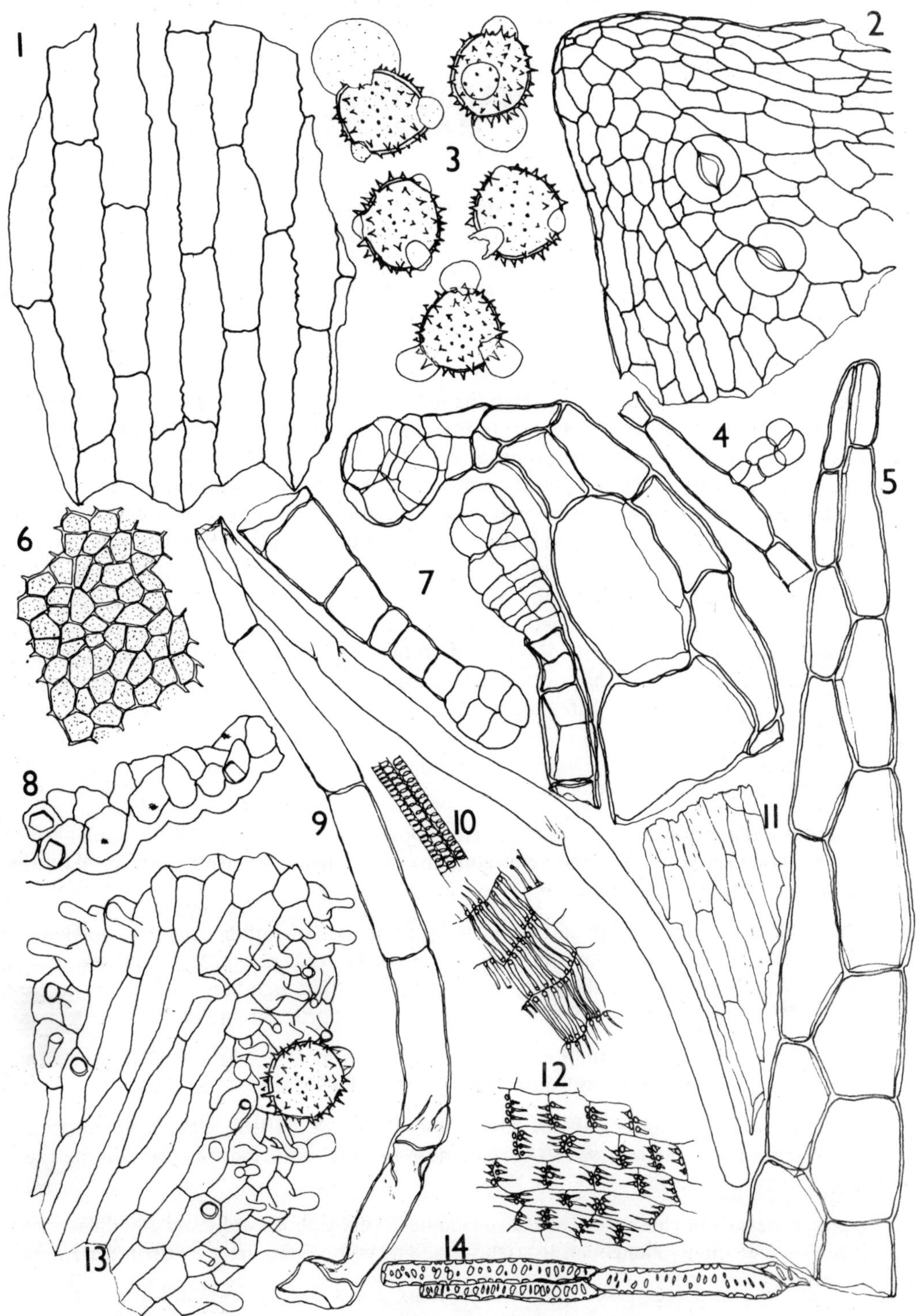

Marigold

×330

1 Epidermis of the corolla in surface view.
2 Outer epidermis at the apex of the corolla in surface view showing stomata.
3 Pollen grains.
4 A sessile glandular trichome attached to a fragment of the corolla.
5 A biseriate, multicellular covering trichome from the corolla.
6 Part of the ovary wall in surface view showing cells containing pigment.
7 Glandular trichomes.
8 Cells from the base of the corolla in surface view containing crystals.
9 A covering trichome from an involucral bract.
10 A fragment of vascular tissue.
11 Epidermis of the corolla from near the apex in surface view.
12 Fibrous layer of the anther in surface view.
13 Part of a stigma in surface view showing bulbous papillae with an adherent pollen grain.
14 Sclerenchymatous cells from the anther.

MARJORAM

Origanum vulgare L. Labiatae

Wild Marjoram, Oregano

Occurs as the fresh or dried leaves, stems and flowering heads; the flowers and the surrounding bracts are a deep pinkish-purple. It has a strong, aromatic, characteristic odour and a warm, aromatic and slightly bitter taste.

The diagnostic characters are:

(*a*) The *upper epidermis of the leaf*, which, in surface view, is composed of cells with sinuous to wavy walls sometimes showing occasional beading although in the regions over the veins the walls are distinctly thickened and beaded; *diacytic stomata* occur only rarely; the underlying palisade cells are small and closely packed. The cells of the *lower epidermis* are smaller than those of the upper epidermis and the thin walls are markedly sinuous; numerous diacytic stomata are present. *Glandular trichomes* are abundant on both surfaces and those which are more conspicuous are of the typical labiate type with a short, unicellular stalk and a radiate head composed of a number of indistinct cells around which the common cuticle is raised to form a bladder; the epidermal cells surrounding these glands are arranged to form a rosette. Capitate glandular trichomes are also widely distributed and the majority of these are composed of a unicellular stalk and a small ovoid to spherical unicellular head, but occasional glands occur in which the stalk is uniseriate and composed of two or, rarely, three cells. *Covering trichomes* also occur scattered on both epidermises, particularly over the veins; they are uniseriate with from two to six cells, conical and bluntly pointed and sometimes curved at the apex; the walls are slightly thickened and show scattered longitudinal striations.

(*b*) The leaf is dorsiventral and *in sectional view* shows a single-layered palisade under the upper epidermis; the vascular tissue of the veins contains small, lignified *vessels*, with spiral or annular thickening.

(*c*) The *epidermis of the stem* in surface view, is composed of rather irregular, polygonal cells with a strongly striated *cuticle*; occasional diacytic stomata occur and both glandular and covering trichomes, similar to those on the leaf, are also present. The lignified vascular tissue contains occasional *fibres*, *xylem parenchyma* and *vessels* showing bordered pits or annular thickening.

(*d*) The *bracts* are similar to the leaves but in addition have a single row of *teeth* along the margins; these are thin-walled and show faint longitudinal striations.

(*e*) The *outer epidermis of the calyx* is also similar to that of the leaf, although stomata are not abundant. The *inner epidermis* shows very numerous, long, covering trichomes in the region at the base of the calyx teeth.

(*f*) The cells of the *outer epidermis of the corolla* have very sinuous walls and glandular trichomes occur abundantly, also some covering trichomes. The cells of the *inner epidermis* are *papillose*.

(*g*) The *pollen grains* are small, spherical, with six pores and furrows and a smooth or finely pitted exine.

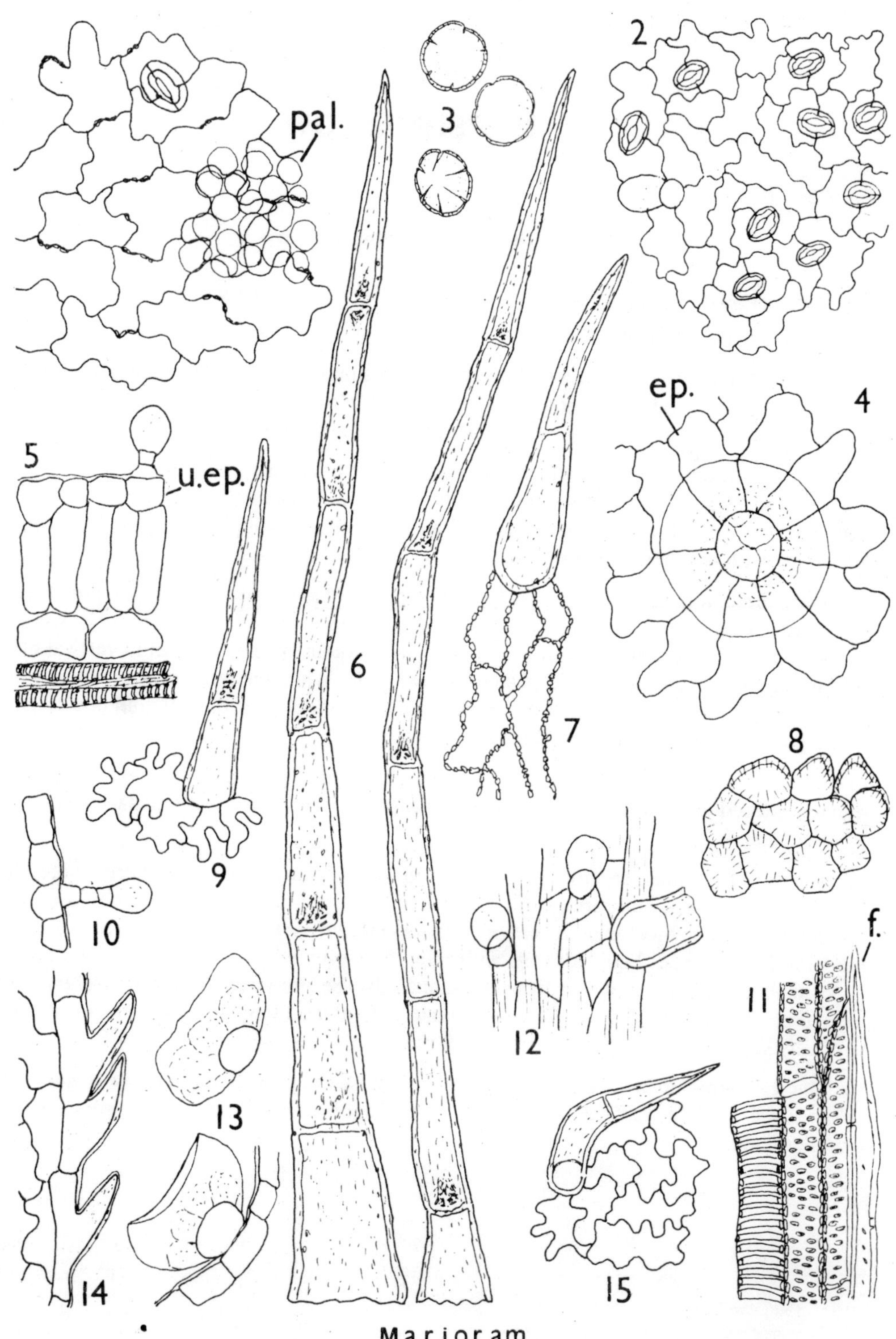

Marjoram

×330

1 Upper epidermis of the leaf in surface view with part of the underlying palisade (pal.).
2 Lower epidermis of the leaf in surface view showing diacytic stomata and a capitate gland.
3 Pollen grains.
4 A multicellular glandular trichome in surface view with surrounding cells of the upper epidermis (ep.) of the leaf.
5 Part of the lamina in sectional view showing a capitate gland in the upper epidermis (u.ep.).
6 Covering trichomes.
7 Upper epidermis of the leaf over a vein in surface view.
8 Inner epidermis of the corolla showing papillae.
9 Outer epidermis of the corolla in surface view.
10 Upper epidermis of the leaf in sectional view showing a capitate gland.
11 Part of the xylem of the stem showing a fibre (f.), xylem parenchyma, a bordered pitted vessel and an annularly thickened vessel.
12 Epidermis of the stem in surface view showing capitate glands and part of a covering trichome.
13 Multicellular glandular trichomes in side view.
14 Outer epidermis on the margin of a bract.
15 Outer epidermis of the calyx in surface view.

MARSHMALLOW

Althaea officinalis L. Malvaceae

Guimauve, Marshmallow Root

A pale buff powder with a faint, aromatic odour and a mucilaginous taste.

The diagnostic characters are:

(*a*) The abundant *starch granules*; they are mostly simple but a few are compound with two or three components; individual granules are small, spherical to ovoid or subreniform and rather irregular and frequently have a well marked circular or slit-shaped hilum.

(*b*) The very abundant *fibres*, which occur singly and in groups; individual fibres are very long, fairly thin-walled and usually unlignified although the middle lamella may occasionally be slightly lignified; they are rather irregular in outline and have few, small pits. They are frequently found associated with lignified xylem parenchyma.

(*c*) The abundant thick-walled *parenchyma* composed of axially elongated, polygonal cells with a few conspicuous pits on the side walls; some of the cells contain large cluster crystals of calcium oxalate and, in longitudinal section, these cells are frequently seen to occur in vertical files; other cells of the parenchyma are developed as *mucilage cells*, while the remainder are filled with starch granules. The mucilage cells are more rounded in outline than the surrounding cells and the mucilage stains with *Solution of Ruthenium Red*.

(*d*) The *cluster crystals of calcium oxalate* and the amorphous masses of *mucilage*, which are found scattered as well as in the parenchymatous cells. The masses of mucilage frequently have adherent starch granules.

(*e*) The *vessels*, which are found singly or in small groups; they are fairly large, lignified, bordered pitted or scalariformly thickened and have oblique end walls. They are sometimes accompanied by subrectangular *xylem parenchymatous cells* which are fairly large and have moderately thickened, lignified walls with numerous pits.

A small amount of lignified parenchyma may also be present from the *medullary rays of the stem base*; these cells are rounded to ovoid and more elongated than those of the xylem parenchyma and they have numerous small pits.

(*f*) The fragments of *cork*, which are present in most samples to a greater or lesser extent; the cells are polygonal in surface view and have thin, lignified walls; the outer layers are filled with granular contents.

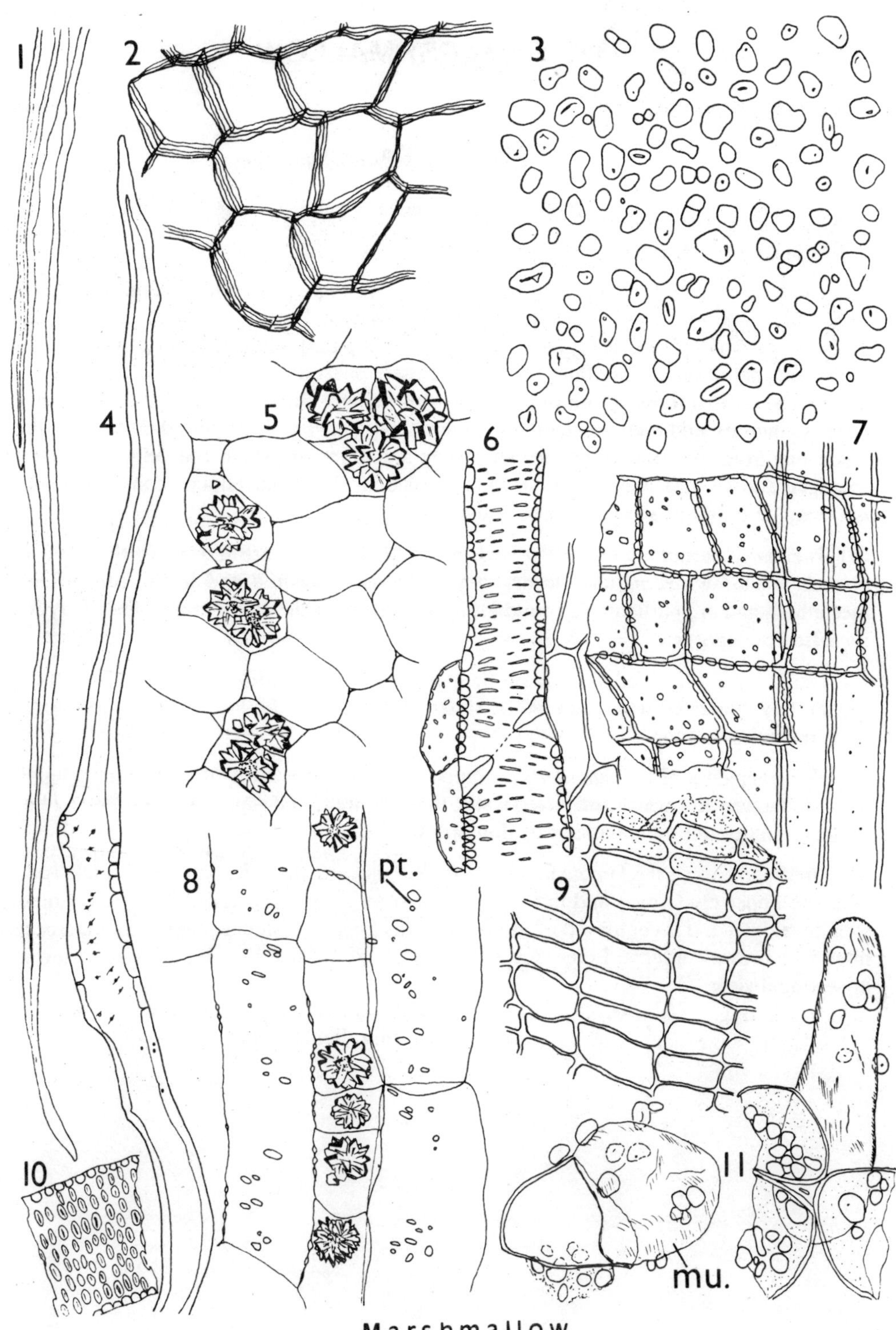

Marshmallow

×330

1 Part of a group of fibres.
2 Cork in surface view.
3 Starch granules.
4 Part of a single fibre showing pits.
5 Parenchyma in transverse section showing cluster crystals of calcium oxalate in some of the cells.
6 Scalariformly thickened vessels with adjacent xylem parenchyma.
7 Fibres and xylem parenchyma in longitudinal section.
8 Parenchyma in longitudinal section showing pits (pt.) and cluster crystals of calcium oxalate occurring in a vertical file.
9 Cork in sectional view.
10 Fragment of a bordered pitted vessel.
11 Mucilage cells containing mucilage (mu.) with adherent starch granules.

MATE

Ilex paraguariensis St. Hil. Aquifoliaceae

Paraguay Tea, Hervea

A greenish-brown powder with a faint, slightly aromatic odour and a bitter and astringent taste.

The diagnostic characters are:

(*a*) The fragments of the *lamina in surface view*. The *upper epidermis* is composed of polygonal cells with moderately and somewhat unevenly thickened walls; many of the cells contain oil globules and small prismatic crystals; the *cuticle* is irregularly striated and stomata are absent; the underlying palisade cells are fairly large and closely packed. The cells of the *lower epidermis* are much smaller than those of the upper epidermis and are thinner-walled; cuticular striations are fairly numerous and well marked; *anomocytic stomata* are very abundant. Fragments of the epidermis from over the veins are also fairly abundant, in which the cells are very regularly arranged and are nearly rectangular; very occasional short, unicellular, conical *covering trichomes* may be found attached to these fragments.

(*b*) The fairly numerous *crystals of calcium oxalate*, which are mostly in the form of *cluster crystals* but a few *prisms* also occur; they are found scattered and in the cells of the spongy mesophyll, and are particularly abundant in the cells near the endodermis. They vary in size and are often quite large.

(*c*) The groups of lignified *fibres* from the pericycle of the midrib and larger veins; the walls are moderately thickened with rounded or slit-shaped pits and the longer fibres occasionally show thin, transverse septa.

(*d*) The fragments of the *endodermis* composed of a single layer of rectangular, lignified cells with moderately thickened and pitted walls; the cells are found singly and also associated with the pericyclic fibres and other tissues of the midrib.

(*e*) The fragments of the *lamina in sectional view* showing the thick, striated cuticle (particularly over the upper epidermis) and the two to four rows of palisade cells. The spongy mesophyll is well developed and is composed of moderately thick-walled, stellate cells which are occasionally filled with brown contents. Fragments of this tissue are frequently seen in surface view as well as in sectional view.

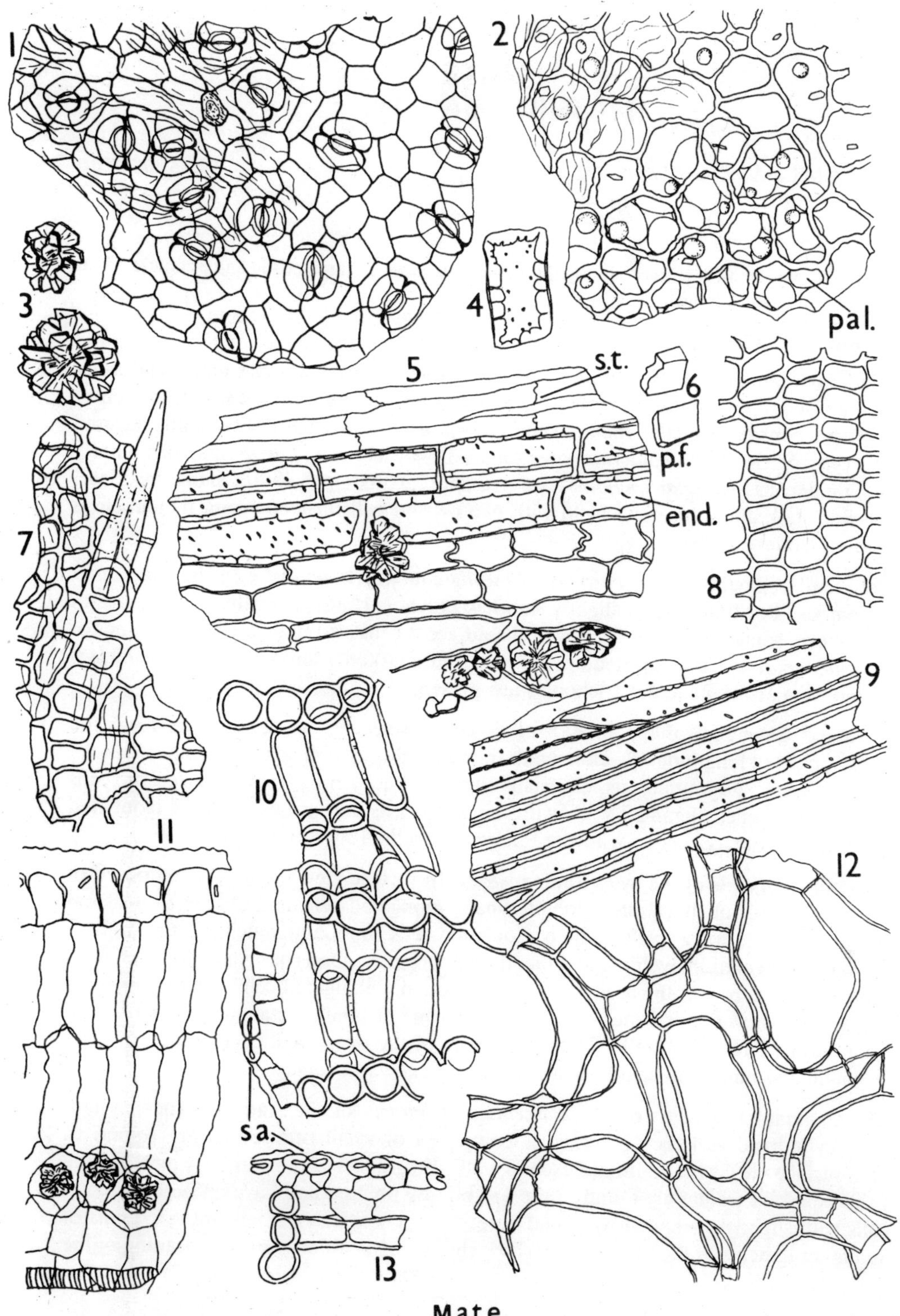

Mate

×330

1 Lower epidermis in surface view showing anomocytic stomata and cuticular striations.
2 Upper epidermis in surface view showing cuticular striations and underlying palisade cells (pal.).
3 Calcium oxalate cluster crystals.
4 Isolated cell of the endodermis.
5 Part of a vein in longitudinal sectional view showing sieve tubes (s.t.), endodermis (end.) with underlying pericyclic fibres (p.f.) and cortical cells containing prisms and cluster crystals of calcium oxalate.
6 Calcium oxalate prisms.
7 Epidermis from over a vein in surface view, with a covering trichome attached.
8 Epidermis from over a vein in surface view.
9 Part of a group of pericyclic fibres.
10 Part of the lamina in sectional view showing the lower epidermis with a stoma (sa.) and part of the spongy mesophyll.
11 Part of the lamina in sectional view showing the upper epidermis with a thick cuticle, two-layered palisade and spongy mesophyll cells containing cluster crystals of calcium oxalate.
12 Two layers of the spongy mesophyll in surface view.
13 Fragment of the lower epidermis in sectional view showing stomata (sa.) and part of the underlying spongy mesophyll.

MATRICARIA

Matricaria recutita L. (*M. chamomilla* auct.) Compositae

German Chamomile

A light brown to buff powder with a greenish tinge; it has a very strong, characteristic and aromatic odour and a slightly bitter and aromatic taste.

The diagnostic characters are:

(*a*) The abundant fragments of the *corollas of the tubular florets in surface view*. The *inner epidermis* is composed of longitudinally elongated cells with slightly thickened walls; at the centre of each lobe of the corolla, near the apex, a small group of *papillae* occurs with faintly striated margins. The cells of the *outer epidermis* are longitudinally elongated with thin, irregularly sinuous walls; numerous *glandular trichomes* are present, each composed of a short, biseriate, usually two-celled stalk and a biseriate head with two or four cells around which the cuticle is raised to form a bladder-like covering.

(*b*) The infrequent fragments of the *corollas of the ligulate florets in surface view*. The *inner epidermis* is composed of thin-walled, slightly sinuous, polygonal cells; the cells on the margins are extended to form small *papillae* and a few of the adjacent cells also show the faint outlines of papillae. The *outer epidermis* is composed of cells with thin, markedly sinuous walls; the *cuticle* is strongly striated; numerous glandular trichomes are present.

(*c*) The occasional fragments of the *involucral bracts in surface view*. Fragments from the margins are composed of longitudinally elongated, thin-walled cells with a faintly striated cuticle; *anomocytic stomata* are fairly numerous, especially near the base. In the central region the cells have considerably thickened, lignified walls with numerous pits and groups of these elongated *sclereids* occur, frequently associated with the thin-walled cells from the margins.

(*d*) The abundant fragments of the *walls of the ovaries*. In surface view the wall is composed of alternating vertical bands of thin-walled, longitudinally elongated cells and oblong to fusiform groups of about twenty to forty small, radially elongated cells containing mucilage; the walls of these groups of cells are extremely thin and difficult to distinguish; numerous glandular trichomes occur in a single vertical row in the areas of the longitudinally elongated cells. Fragments from the base of the ovary show the presence of two or three rows of small, rectangular *sclereids* with moderately thickened and pitted walls. The inner tissue of the ovary wall is composed of thin-walled cells containing numerous small *cluster crystals of calcium oxalate*.

(*e*) The very abundant fragments of the *filaments* and *anthers* of the stamens. The filament fragments are cylindrical and the epidermis is composed of small cells which are square to rectangular in surface view with slightly thickened walls. Fragments of the anthers which include the tips of the lobes are frequently found; these are bluntly pointed and have an outer layer of irregular cells with slightly thickened walls and inner tissues containing small *cluster crystals of calcium oxalate*. Fragments of the *fibrous layer* show characteristic thickening and beading of the walls.

(*f*) The fragments of the *styles* and *stigmas*; the epidermal cells at the apices of the stigmas are extended to form rounded *papillae*.

(*g*) The very abundant *pollen grains* which are fairly small, spherical with three pores and a spiny and warty exine. Groups of immature pollen grains also occur in which the markings on the exine are rather indistinct.

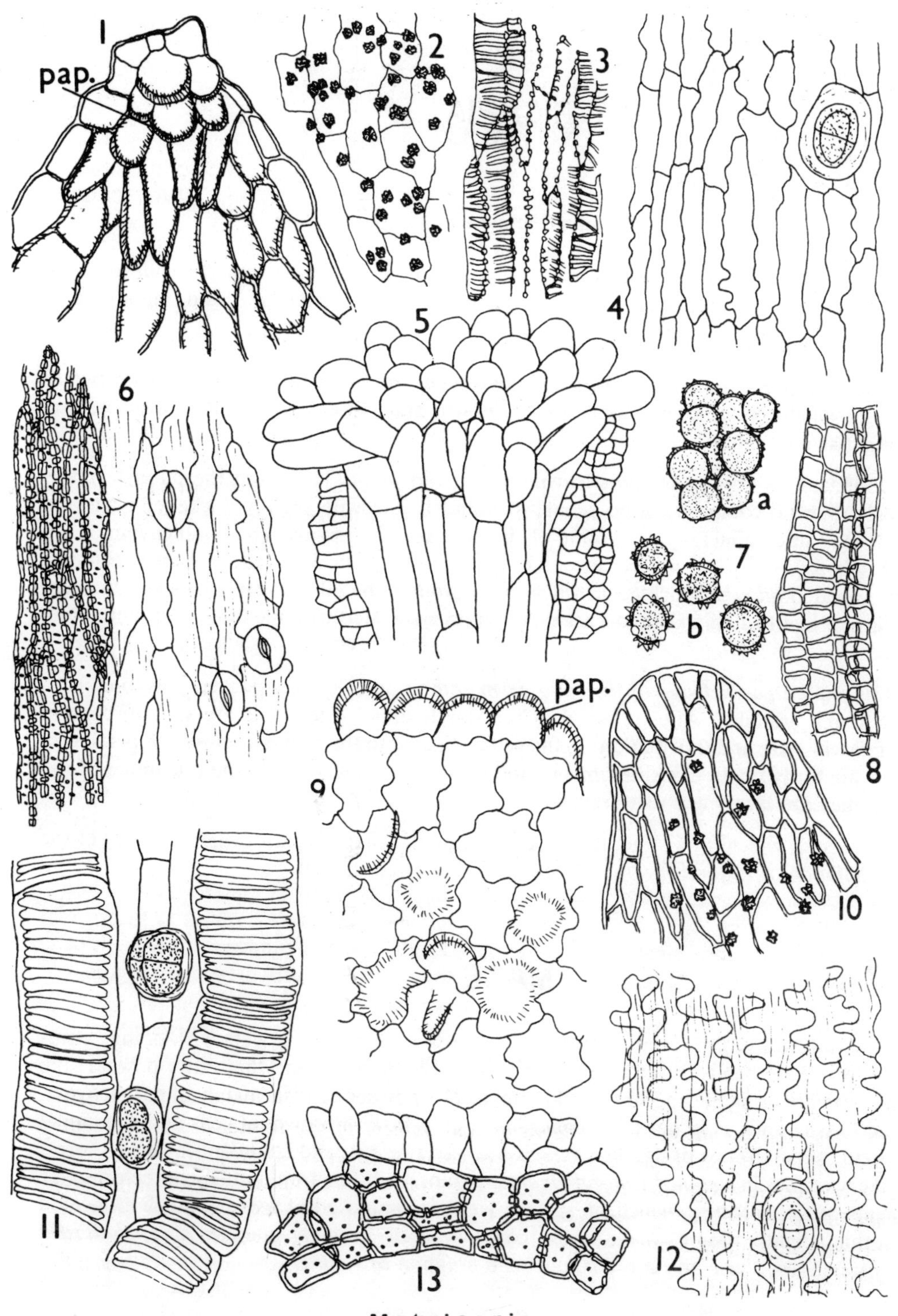

Matricaria

×330

1 Inner epidermis of a lobe of the corolla of a tubular floret in surface view showing a group of papillae (pap.) near the apex.
2 Cells from the inner tissue of the ovary wall containing cluster crystals of calcium oxalate.
3 Fibrous layer of the anther in surface view.
4 Outer epidermis of the corolla of a tubular floret in surface view showing a glandular trichome.
5 Papillose stigma and part of a style in surface view.
6 Part of a bract in surface view showing the thin-walled cells and stomata from the marginal region and elongated sclereids from the central region.
7 (a) A group of immature pollen grains; (b) mature pollen grains.
8 Part of the filament of an anther in surface view.
9 Inner epidermis of the corolla of a ligulate floret in surface view showing cells of the margin with papillae (pap.).
10 The tip of an anther lobe in surface view showing cluster crystals of calcium oxalate in the underlying tissue.
11 Part of the ovary wall in surface view.
12 Outer epidermis of the corolla of a ligulate floret showing striations and a glandular trichome.
13 Sclereids from the base of the ovary wall.

NUTMEG

Myristica fragrans Houtt. Myristicaceae

Nutmegs, Nux Moschata

A cinnamon-brown powder with a characteristic, aromatic odour and an aromatic, slightly bitter taste.

The diagnostic characters are:

(*a*) The abundant *starch granules*, some simple and spherical but mostly compound with two to eight or, occasionally, more components; they are fairly small and most granules have a central stellate or slit-shaped hilum.

(*b*) The abundant reddish-brown *parenchyma of the perisperm*. That from the outer layers is paler in colour and is composed of polygonal to rounded cells with slightly thickened walls and occasional small intercellular spaces; some of the cells contain prisms. The parenchyma of the *inner and ruminating perisperm* is composed of smaller cells with dark reddish-brown contents and large, rounded *oil cells* which occur singly or in groups; the oil cells are frequently broken. Small groups of lignified *vessels* are occasionally found associated with the inner and ruminating perisperm.

(*c*) The thin-walled *parenchyma of the endosperm* composed of closely packed polygonal cells filled with starch granules. After removal of the starch some of the cells are seen to contain crystals of varying size and distribution; in the cells adjacent to the ruminations of the perisperm the crystals are fairly small, elongated prisms and occur in groups whilst in the remainder of the endosperm they are larger and scattered.

(*d*) The *fat crystals* which form large, feathery or irregularly shaped masses when a mount of the powder in *Solution of Chloral Hydrate* is heated and allowed to cool.

MACE

The *arillus* removed from the seed of nutmeg. It occurs in commerce in yellowish-orange strips or coarsely reticulate bands, or as a yellowish- to orange-brown, somewhat gritty powder; the odour and taste are aromatic and similar to nutmeg. The powder consists mainly of parenchymatous ground tissue and, as in nutmeg, numerous large yellowish-brown oil cells and occasional crystals occur; small groups of lignified vessels are also present, and abundant fat which forms large feathery masses in a cooled *Chloral Hydrate* mount. It differs from nutmeg in the presence of fragments of the *epidermis* which, in surface view, is composed of narrow, much elongated cells with thin, slightly sinuous walls; it also contains small, irregular granules of *amylodextrin* instead of starch and these give a red colour with *Solution of Iodine*.

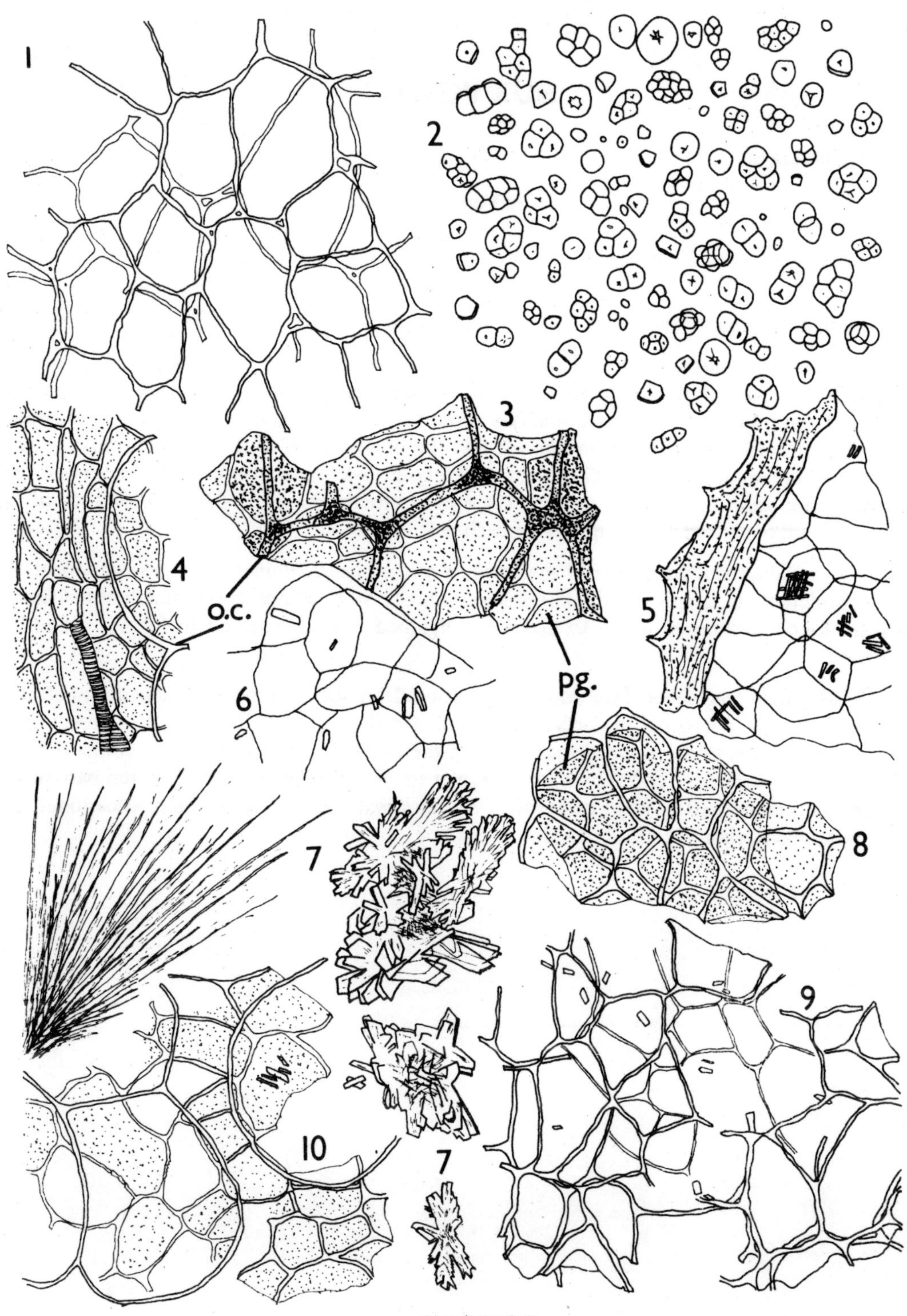

Nutmeg

×330

1 Outer layers of the perisperm in surface view.
2 Starch granules.
3 Inner or ruminating perisperm containing pigment (pg.), with part of a group of oil cells (o.c.).
4 Inner or ruminating perisperm with parts of oil cells (o.c.) and a fragment of vascular tissue.
5 Cells of the outer part of the endosperm containing crystals, with part of the adjacent ruminating perisperm.
6 Cells of the inner part of the endosperm, some containing prisms.
7 Crystalline masses of fat from a cooled Chloral Hydrate mount.
8 Layers of the perisperm containing pigment (pg.).
9 Outer layers of the perisperm with scattered prisms.
10 Inner or ruminating perisperm with oil cells.

NUX VOMICA

Strychnos nux-vomica L. Loganiaceae

Nux Vomica Seeds

A yellowish-grey to brownish-grey powder with a slightly fatty and rancid odour and an intensely bitter and persistent taste.

The diagnostic characters are:

(*a*) The *sclerenchymatous epidermis of the testa* composed of a single layer of yellowish-brown cells each of which is extended to form a trichome; the walls of the epidermal cells are strongly thickened and pitted and each trichome has about ten narrow, lignified rods running longitudinally; the trichomes are usually broken off and the broken ends of the lignified rods are seen attached to the epidermal cells. This layer is nearly always found in side view; very occasional fragments are seen in surface view with the almost circular bases of the lignified rods of the trichomes visible around the periphery of each cell.

(*b*) The very abundant fragments of the *lignified rods of the trichomes*; they are cylindrical and vary considerably in length and thickness. Occasionally more complete fragments of the trichomes are found, composed of up to about ten lignified rods aggregated to form a cylindrical structure.

(*c*) The abundant fragments of the *endosperm*. Those from the outer layer are composed of small thick-walled cells, polygonal in surface view and slightly elongated radially in sectional view; these fragments are often found associated with the pigment layer of the testa, composed of a layer of rather indistinct cells containing orange to brown pigment. The greater part of the endosperm is composed of large cells with very thick walls and a small lumen; occasional cells show faint plasmodesmata in the walls.

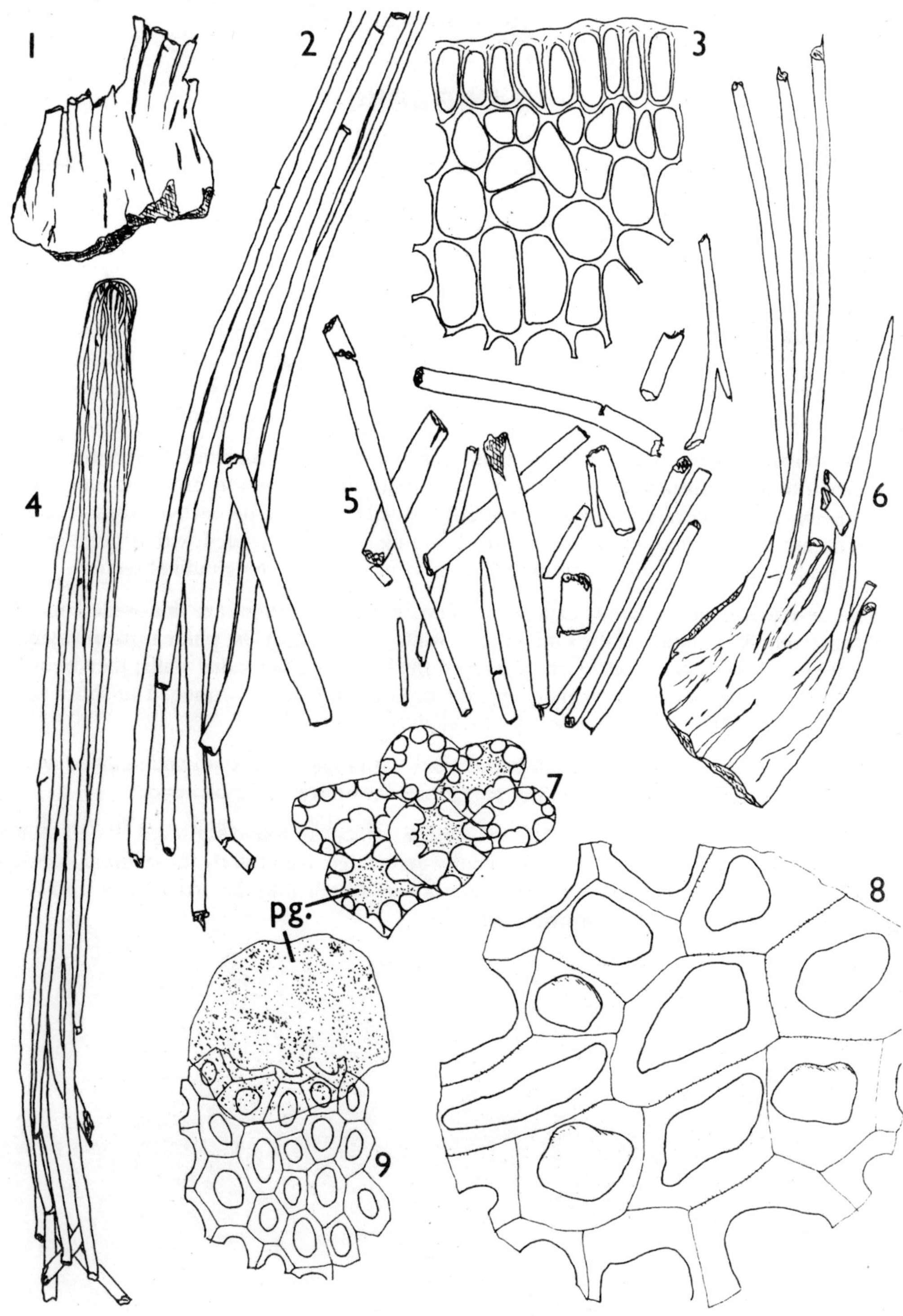

Nux Vomica

×330

1 Part of the sclerenchymatous epidermis of the testa in side view, with broken-off remains of the trichome rods attached.
2 Part of a large trichome.
3 Outer part of the endosperm in sectional view.
4 An almost complete trichome showing the rounded apex.
5 Fragments of trichome rods.
6 Part of the sclerenchymatous epidermis of the testa in side view, with parts of the trichomes attached.
7 Sclerenchymatous layer of the testa in surface view showing the bases of the lignified rods and pigment (pg.) in some of the cells.
8 Endosperm cells from the central region.
9 Outer layer of the endosperm in surface view, with associated pigment layer of the testa (pg.).

OAK BARK

Quercus robur L. and other spp. of *Quercus* — *Fagaceae*

A reddish-brown powder with a faint odour and a slightly bitter and astringent taste.

The diagnostic characters are:

(*a*) The abundant *sclereids* of two types. Those of one type are large with thick, striated walls and a small lumen and numerous branching pits; they occur in groups with adjacent parenchymatous cells some of which contain prisms and cluster crystals of calcium oxalate. The sclereids of the other type vary in size but are usually smaller; they have thinner walls with numerous simple pits and the lumen is often filled with brown contents; they also occur in groups.

(*b*) The abundant *fibres*, which occur in groups surrounded by a calcium oxalate prism sheath; individual fibres are thick-walled with a narrow, indistinct lumen and few pits; the walls are lignified (frequently more strongly in the middle lamella) and the parenchymatous cells of the crystal sheath are also frequently thick-walled and lignified. Associated with a number of the groups of fibres are short, uniseriate medullary rays in tangential longitudinal section.

(*c*) The *sieve tissue* and *medullary rays* of the phloem; the sieve tubes are thin-walled and show numerous faint sieve areas on the oblique end walls. The cells of the phloem parenchyma are mainly thin-walled but occasionally show uneven thickening on the radial walls; they frequently contain cluster crystals or, occasionally, prisms of calcium oxalate, arranged in short vertical rows. The walls of the medullary ray cells are slightly thickened.

(*d*) The abundant fragments of reddish-brown *cork* with slightly thickend and lignified walls; in surface view the cells are fairly large and polygonal; they have dense contents.

(*e*) The *prisms* and *cluster crystals of calcium oxalate*, which are found scattered as well as in the parenchymatous tissues; the prisms are frequently quite large, particularly those found associated with the larger sclereids. The cluster crystals are not so abundant as the prisms; they also vary in size and frequently have a dark brown centre.

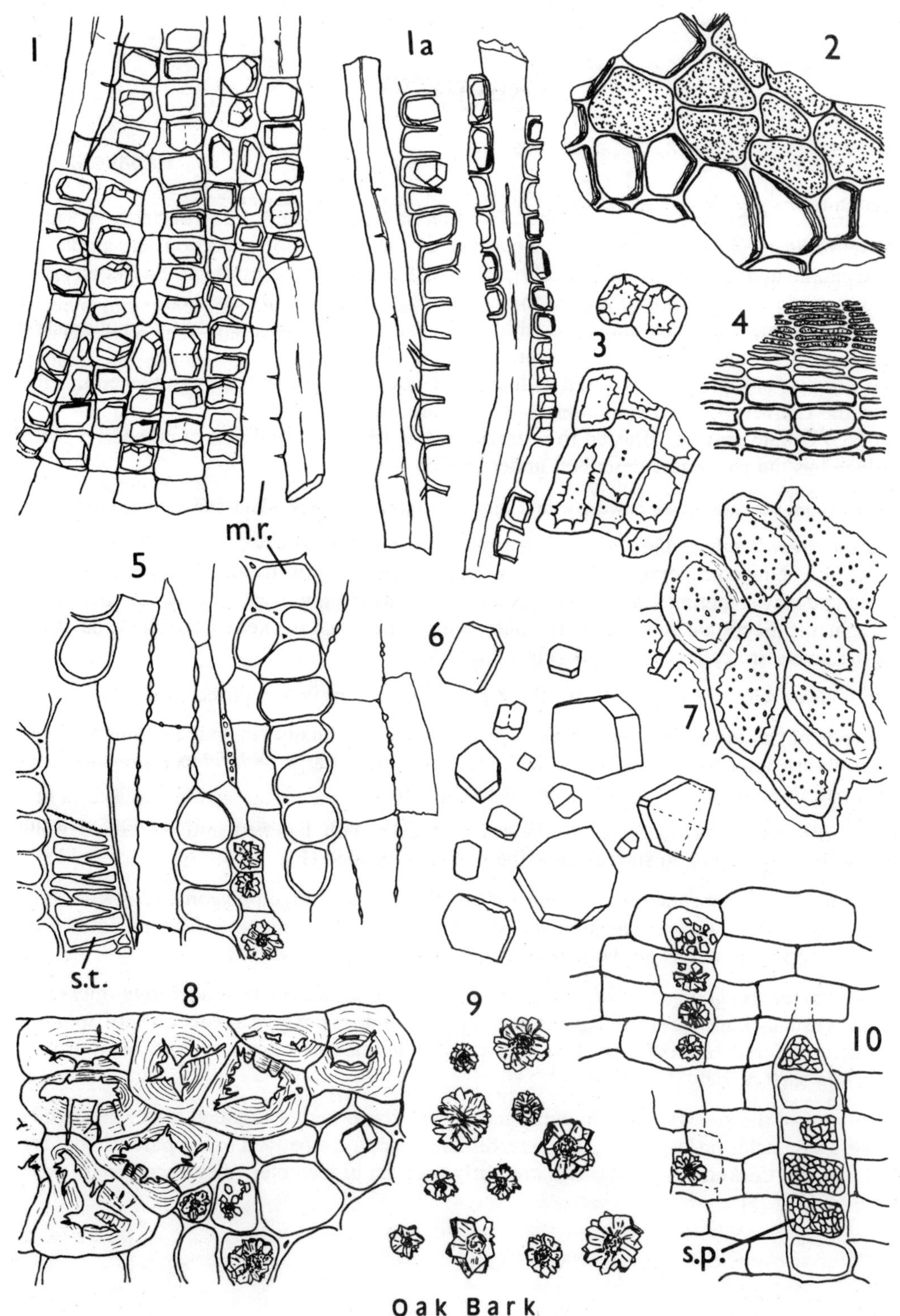

Oak Bark

×330

1 Part of a group of fibres with calcium oxalate prism sheath, associated with a medullary ray (m.r.) in tangential longitudinal section.

1a Part of a group of fibres showing the thickened walls of the parenchymatous cells.

2 Cork in surface view.

3 Groups of thin-walled sclereids.

4 Cork in sectional view.

5 Part of the phloem in tangential longitudinal section showing a sieve tube (s.t.), medullary ray (m.r.) and phloem parenchyma containing cluster crystals of calcium oxalate.

6 Prisms of calcium oxalate.

7 A group of larger, thin-walled sclereids.

8 A group of thick-walled sclereids with associated parenchyma containing calcium oxalate crystals.

9 Cluster crystals of calcium oxalate.

10 Part of the phloem in radial longitudinal section showing a medullary ray, sieve tube with sieve plates (s.p.), and parenchyma containing crystals of calcium oxalate.

OPIUM

Papaver somniferum L. **Papaveraceae**

Opium consists of the dried latex obtained from incised poppy capsules. The latex is water-soluble and has no cellular structure, but because of the method of collection all samples of Opium contain varying amounts of cell debris, the most commonly occurring being fragments of the outer capsule wall and pollen grains; these are described under (*a*) and (*b*).

If the sample has been contaminated with other parts of the capsule additional characters described under (*c*) and (*d*) may be present.

Some varieties of Opium are covered with coarsely powdered poppy leaves and when this has occurred the characters described under (*e*) will be present.

Powdered Opium may be adjusted to a standard strength by the addition of powdered cocoa husk which has the characters described under (*f*) and (*g*).

Powdered Opium is a mid-brown powder with a very characteristic, heavy odour and a bitter taste.

(*a*) The *outer epidermis of the capsule* is composed of tabular cells which in surface view are polygonal and show considerable variation in size; the anticlinal walls are somewhat unevenly thickened and may sometimes be beaded; occasional rounded *anomocytic stomata* are present on some fragments. Sectional views show the outer wall to be much thickened and the cells of the underlying layers are collenchymatous (Figs. 3 and 4).

(*b*) The *pollen grains* are spherical with three pores and a very faintly pitted exine (Fig. 6).

(*c*) The cells of the *inner epidermis of the capsule* are longitudinally elongated in surface view and the walls are lignified, conspicuously thickened and pitted. Large *undeveloped stomata* occur scattered and these do not give a reaction for lignin (Fig. 8).

(*d*) The *epidermis of the placenta* is composed of cells with lignified and thickened walls containing slit-shaped pits; in surface view the walls are beaded (Fig. 7).

(*e*) The *upper and lower epidermises of the leaf* are composed of large polygonal cells with thin, slightly sinuous walls; *anomocytic stomata* occur in the lower epidermis. The palisade cells beneath the upper epidermis are large and loosely packed (Figs. 1 and 2).

(*f*) The characteristic *layer of small, polygonal cells of cocoa husk* with moderately thickened walls; this is usually known as the sclerenchyma layer but it does not give a reaction with *Solution of Phloroglucinol* and *Hydrochloric Acid*. The cells sometimes split apart to form small groups when seen in surface view (Fig. 9).

(*g*) Fragments of the *spongy parenchyma of cocoa husk* composed of rounded cells with slightly thickened walls enclosing large, irregular intercellular spaces. Embedded in the parenchyma are lignified, spirally thickened *vessels* which are fairly uniform in diameter; they occur singly or in small groups (Fig. 5).

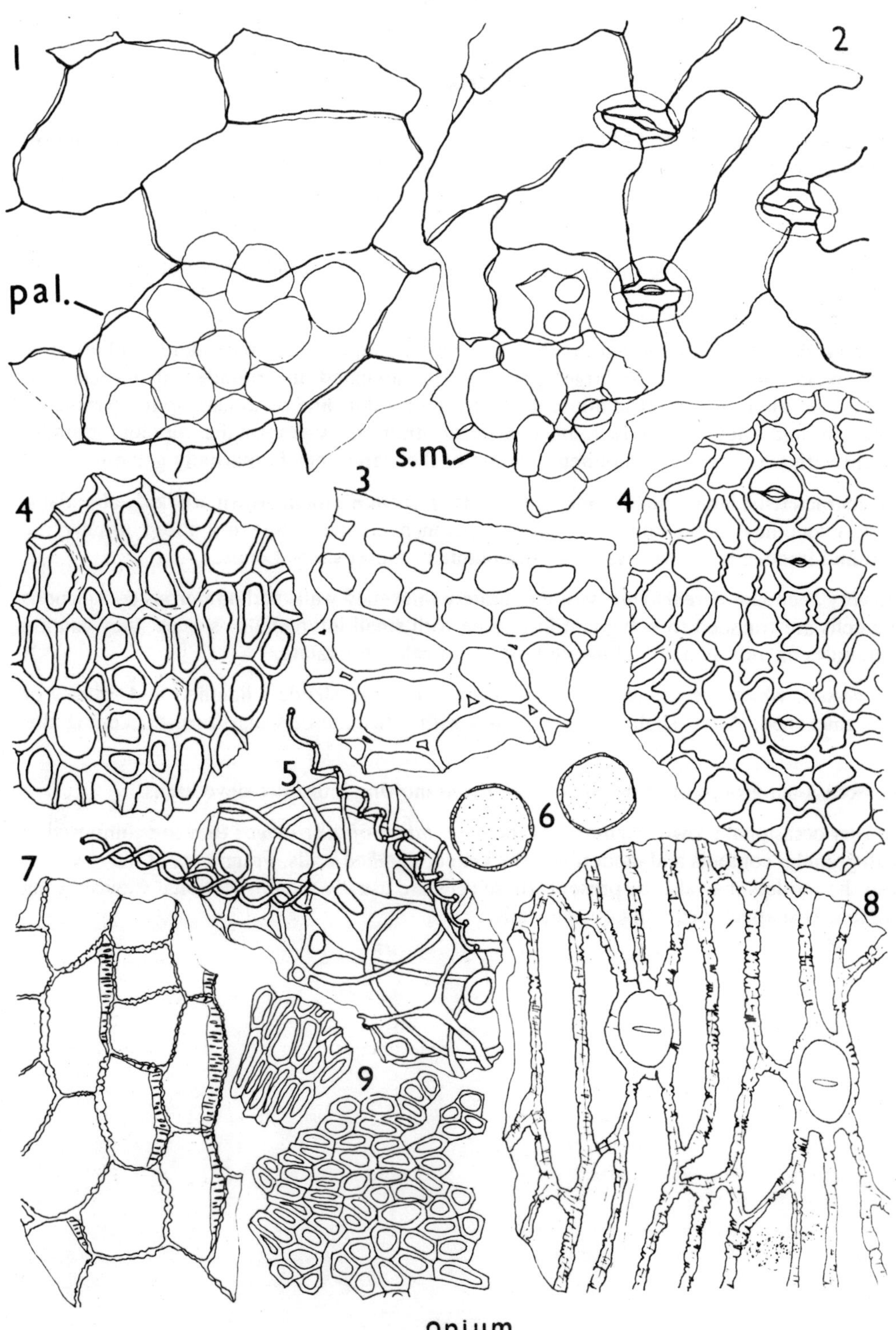

Opium

×330

1 Upper epidermis of the leaf in surface view with part of the underlying palisade (pal.).
2 Lower epidermis of the leaf in surface view showing anomocytic stomata and part of the underlying spongy mesophyll (s.m.).
3 Outer layers of the capsule in sectional view.
4 Outer epidermis of the capsule in surface view.
5 Spongy parenchyma and spiral thickenings from the middle layers of cocoa husk.
6 Pollen grains.
7 Epidermis of the placenta in oblique surface view.
8 Inner epidermis of the capsule in surface view.
9 Parts of the layer of thick-walled cells of cocoa husk in surface view.

ORRIS

Iris germanica L. var. *florentina* Dykes Iridaceae
Iris pallida Lam. and other spp. of *Iris*

Orris Rhizome

A creamish-white powder with the characteristic odour of violets and a slightly bitter and aromatic taste.

The diagnostic characters are:

(*a*) The very abundant *starch granules*; they are mostly simple, vary from almost spherical to elongated ovoid and many of the larger granules are elongated and rounded at one end and flattened at the other; an eccentric hilum in the form of a dot, line or radiate split is visible on some granules and a few also show faint, concentric striations. Occasional compound granules are present with two or three components. Some of the starch may be partially gelatinised.

(*b*) The characteristic large, much elongated *prisms of calcium oxalate* which are fairly abundant; these are sometimes found embedded in the parenchymatous tissue but more usually are scattered and fragmented. The crystals have oblique or chisel-shaped ends.

(*c*) The very abundant *parenchyma* with moderately thickened walls and numerous conspicuous pits; the cells are rounded to polygonal in outline with small intercellular spaces; they contain starch granules or, occasionally, elongated prisms of calcium oxalate.

(*d*) The *vessels*, which are usually found in groups; they are slender, lignified and spirally or annularly thickened. A few slightly larger vessels with reticulate or scalariform thickening also occur.

(*e*) The occasional groups of thin-walled *sieve tissue* showing indistinct sieve areas.

(*f*) The very occasional brown fragments of the *outer layers of the rootlets*; they are composed of cells with granular contents and moderately thickened, lignified walls. Fragments of the *endodermis* from the rootlets may also be present; these cells are usually seen in sectional view showing the lignified, U-shaped thickening on the walls.

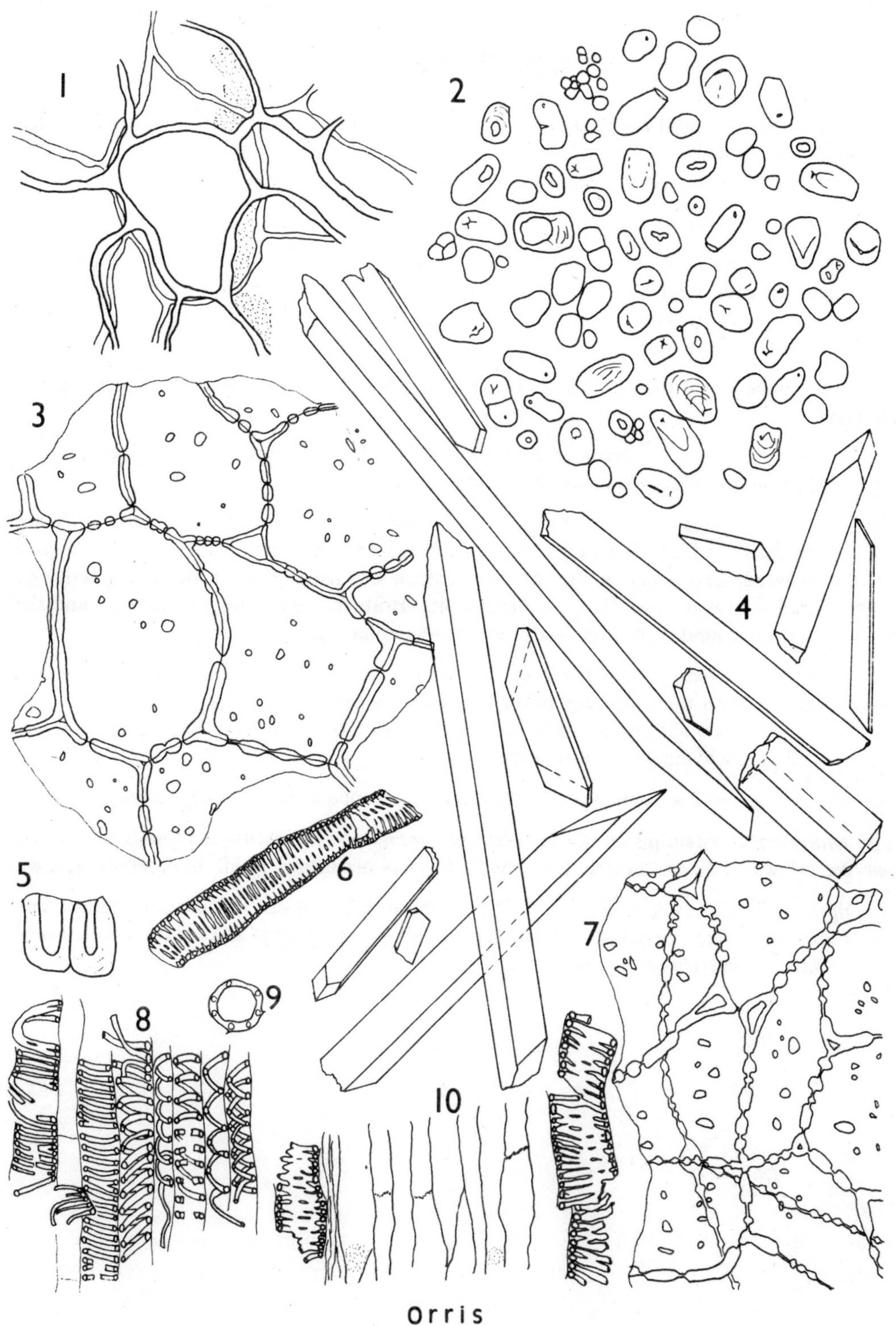

Orris

×330

1 Outer layers from the rootlets in surface view.
2 Starch granules.
3 Parenchymatous cells showing pits.
4 Elongated prisms of calcium oxalate.
5 Endodermal cells of the rootlets in sectional view.
6 Part of a vessel with scalariform thickening.
7 Parenchymatous cells showing numerous pits.
8 Part of a group of vessels with spiral and annular thickening.
9 Fragment of a reticulately thickened vessel in sectional view.
10 Sieve tissue with sieve areas and part of a reticulately thickened vessel.

PARSLEY FRUIT

Petroselinum crispum (Mill.) A.W. Hill **Umbelliferae**

A dull fawnish-brown powder with a characteristic odour and taste.

The diagnostic characters are:

(*a*) The *epicarp* composed of a layer of colourless, thin-walled cells with a faintly striated *cuticle*; in surface view the cells are arranged with six to eight rows of longitudinally elongated cells with slightly sinuous walls alternating with wider bands of straight-walled, polygonal cells; scattered *stomata* occur in the areas of polygonal cells.

(*b*) The fairly numerous brown fragments of *vittae* composed of thin-walled cells, polygonal in surface view.

(*c*) The *parenchyma of the mesocarp* composed of thin-walled, polygonal cells, some of which contain small *prism* and *cluster crystals of calcium oxalate*.

(*d*) The *reticulate parenchyma* of the mesocarp, which is not very abundant; the cells are elongated with thickened and lignified walls showing numerous conspicuous, rounded or oval pits. A few *sclereids* also occur in the mesocarp; these are usually small and elongated with moderately thickened walls and fairly numerous pits. Both the reticulate parenchyma and the sclereids are usually found associated with the fibro-vascular tissue.

(*e*) The *endocarp* consisting of a layer of thin-walled cells, elongated in surface view and arranged in groups with the long axes of adjacent groups usually more or less parallel to one another; the anticlinal walls of the cells are slightly sinuous. This layer is frequently found adherent to the parenchyma of the mesocarp.

(*f*) The *testa* composed of a single layer of irregularly thickened cells containing brown pigment.

(*g*) The *endosperm* containing numerous *aleurone grains* and *microrosette crystals of calcium oxalate*; the cell walls are moderately thickened and show occasional small, intercellular spaces.

(*h*) The lignified *fibres, vessels and tracheids* from the vascular strands; the fibres are thin-walled and occur in groups; the vessels and tracheids have small slit-shaped pits and are frequently found associated with the sclereids of the mesocarp.

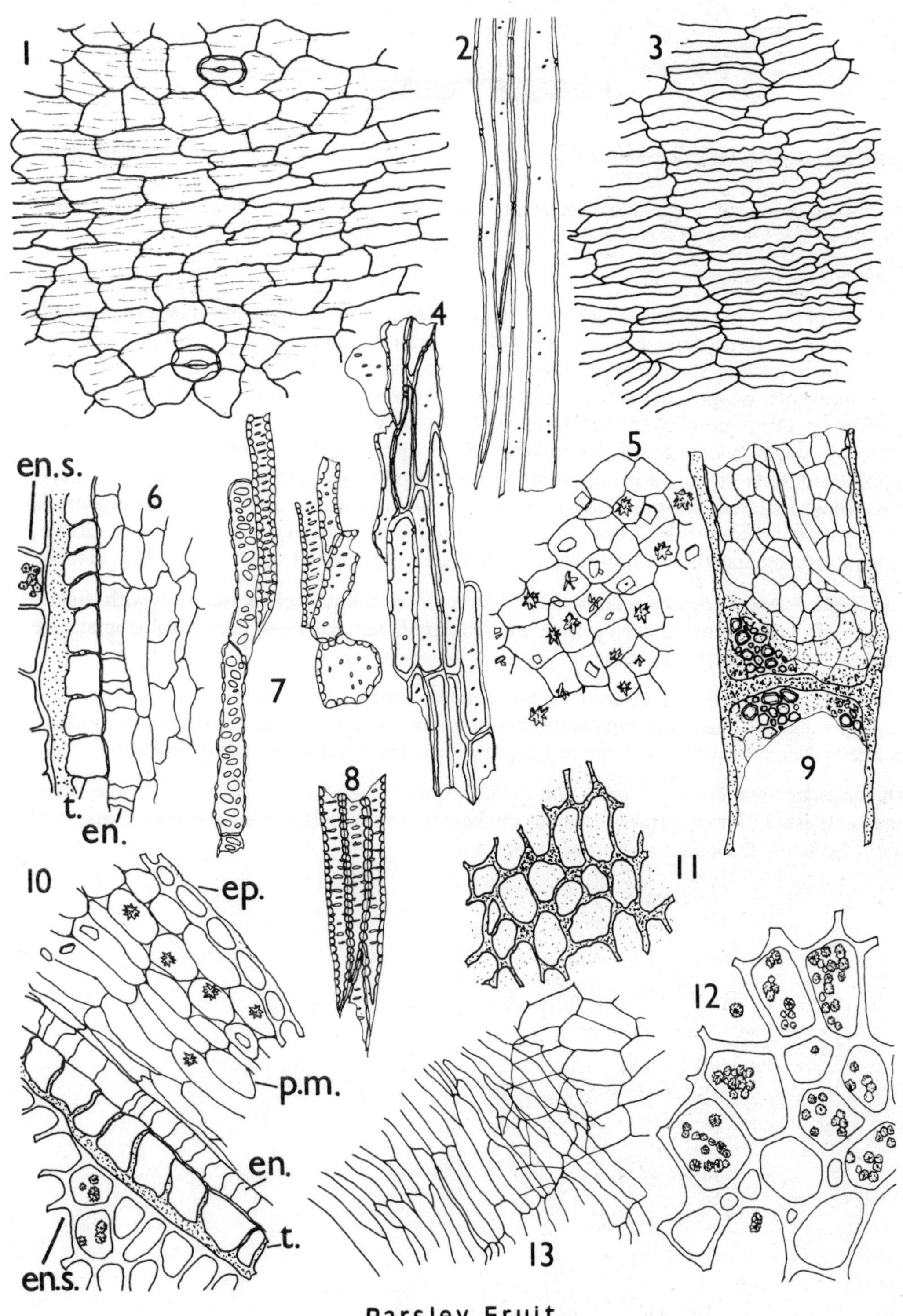

Parsley Fruit

×330

1 Epicarp in surface view showing stomata and striated cuticle.
2 A group of fibres from the fibro-vascular tissue.
3 Endocarp in surface view.
4 Part of a group of sclereids.
5 Parenchyma of the mesocarp containing prisms and cluster crystals of calcium oxalate.
6 Endosperm (en.s.), testa (t.), endocarp (en.) and part of the mesocarp in sectional view.
7 Reticulate parenchyma and sclereids associated with tracheids.
8 A group of tracheids.
9 Part of a vitta showing a transverse septum.
10 Pericarp and part of the seed in sectional view showing the epicarp (ep.), parenchyma of the mesocarp (p.m.) containing calcium oxalate crystals, endocarp (en.), testa (t.) and endosperm (en.s.) containing microrosette crystals of calcium oxalate.
11 Testa in surface view.
12 Endosperm containing microrosette crystals of calcium oxalate.
13 Endocarp and underlying parenchyma of the mesocarp in surface view.

PARSLEY LEAF

Petroselinum crispum (Mill.) A.W. Hill **Umbelliferae**

Usually occurs in commerce in the whole and fresh condition. If carefully dried it retains its bright green colour and readily breaks up to form flakes. Odour and taste are characteristic.

The diagnostic characters are:

(*a*) The cells of the *upper epidermis*, which in surface view are fairly large with thin, sinuous walls which occasionally show slight beading; stomata are absent; the underlying palisade cells are large and loosely packed. The *lower epidermis* is composed of thin-walled cells which in surface view are markedly sinuous in outline; numerous *anomocytic stomata* are present. On both epidermises, in the regions over the larger veins, each cell is extended to form a rounded, forward-projecting *papilla* and similar papillose cells occur along the marginal vein anastomosis; the papillae are fairly large, particularly on the upper epidermis, and they have a thick *cuticle* which is strongly striated. *Marginal teeth* occur on the lamina and, in surface view, the epidermal cells in these regions are smaller and straighter-walled and, if viewed from the lower surface, show abundant stomata; these marginal cells, when seen in sectional view, have a thick cuticle.

(*b*) The *epidermis of the petiole* is composed of large, longitudinally elongated cells with slightly thickened walls which show uneven pitting and beading in surface view; occasional stomata are present and the *cuticle* is finely striated.

(*c*) Abundant *parenchyma* is present in the petiole; some is composed of large cells with moderately thickened, lignified walls and fairly numerous small, rounded pits; the remainder is unlignified and may occasionally contain minute prisms and sphaerocrystalline masses.

(*d*) The *vascular tissue* from the veins and petiole contains lignified *vessels* which, in the veins, are small and usually show spiral or annular thickening; the vessels in the petiole are larger and may be reticulately thickened or bordered pitted.

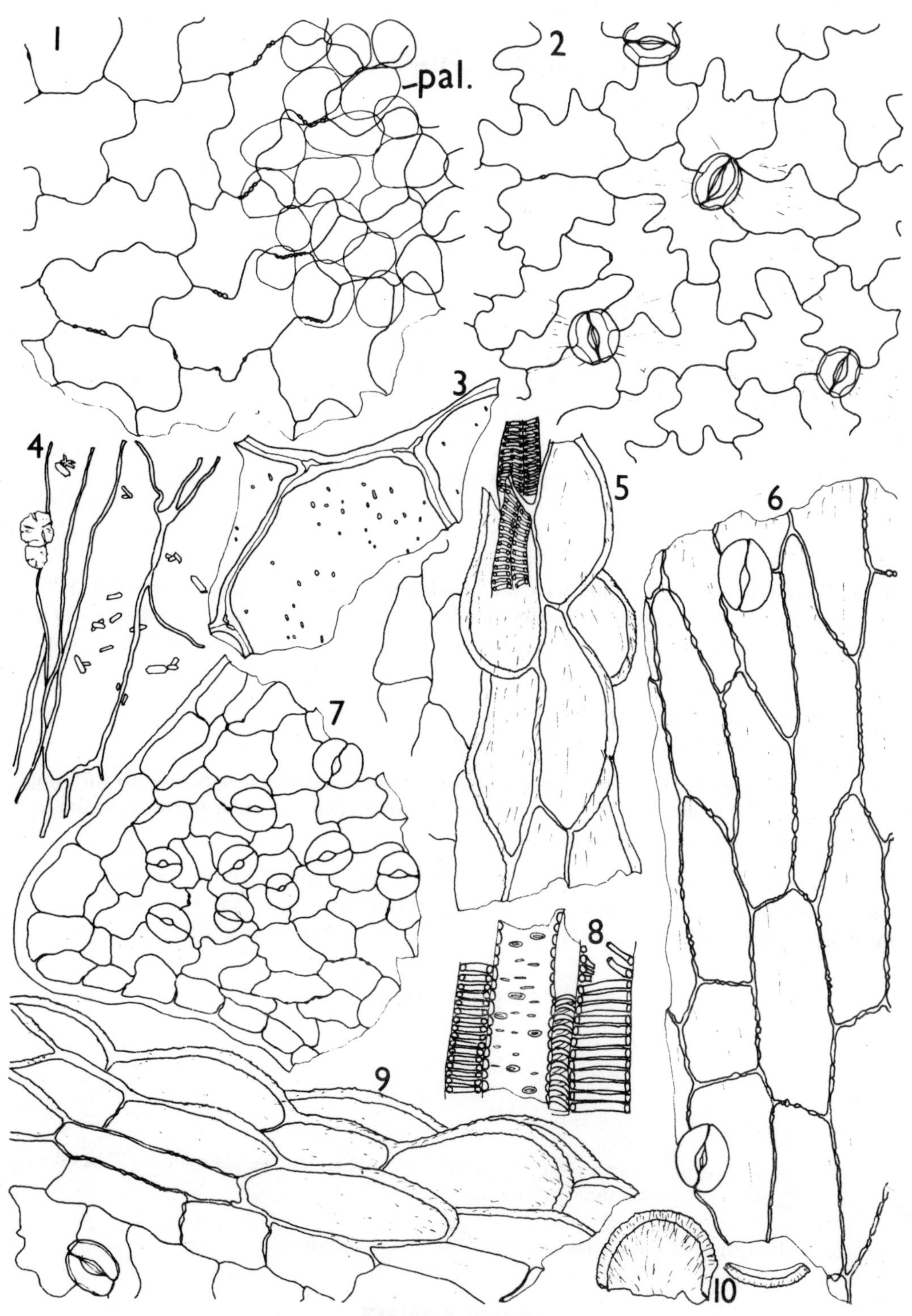

Parsley Leaf

×330

1 Upper epidermis in surface view with part of the underlying palisade (pal.).
2 Lower epidermis in surface view showing anomocytic stomata.
3 A fragment of pitted parenchyma from the petiole.
4 Thin-walled parenchyma from the inner part of the petiole, containing prism crystals and sphaerocrystalline masses.
5 Upper epidermis over a vein in surface view showing papillae.
6 Epidermis of the petiole in surface view.
7 Lower epidermis of a marginal tooth in surface view.
8 Fragment of vascular tissue from the petiole.
9 Papillose cells from the margin of the leaf in oblique surface view.
10 Fragments of papillae.

PEPPERMINT

Mentha × piperita L. Labiatae

The fresh or dried leaves and stems are a dark purplish-green (Black Peppermint) or paler green with purple patches (White Peppermint). The odour and taste are strongly aromatic and characteristic.

The diagnostic characters are:

(*a*) The *upper epidermis of the leaf* composed of large cells with thin, markedly sinuous walls in surface view which may be slightly thickened at the angles; stomata are infrequent; the cells of the underlying palisade are fairly large and loosely packed. The cells of the *lower epidermis* are smaller, slightly more sinuous in outline and uniformly thin-walled; numerous *diacytic stomata* are present. *Glandular trichomes* occur on both epidermises and are of two types; those which are more abundant, especially on the lower epidermis, are large and occur in depressions in the epidermis, each consisting of a very short unicellular stalk and a glandular head composed of eight radiating cells with a common cuticle which is raised to form a spherical, bladder-like covering; those of the second type are much smaller and composed of a short, unicellular stalk and a spherical, unicellular head. *Covering trichomes* also occur on both epidermises but they are not abundant; they are uniseriate with from three to eight cells, conical and bluntly pointed; the walls are moderately thickened and have scattered longitudinal striations. In the regions of the *leaf margins* the epidermal cells are smaller and straighter-walled and show distinct beading and pitting in the anticlinal walls; faint *cuticular striations* are present and occasional short, unicellular, thick-walled *conical trichomes*.

(*b*) The leaf is dorsiventral and *in sectional view* shows a single layer of fairly large palisade cells under the upper epidermis.

(*c*) The cells of the *epidermis of the stem* are longitudinally elongated in surface view with slightly thickened walls and a faintly striated *cuticle*. Glandular trichomes similar to those on the leaves occur, also occasional covering trichomes.

(*d*) The *vascular tissue* of the veins and the stem contains lignified *vessels* which usually have spiral or annular thickening but some of the larger elements from the stem show reticulate thickening; a small amount of *lignified parenchyma* is frequently associated with the vessels.

SPEARMINT

Garden Mint

Mentha spicata L.

The fresh or dried leaves and stems are bright green and do not have any purple colouring. The odour and taste are strong and very characteristic.

Microscopically it has all the characters described for Peppermint.

APPLEMINT

Round-leaved Mint

Mentha rotundifolia (L.) Huds.

The fresh or dried leaves and stems are greyish-green and strongly pubescent, especially on the lower surface of the leaves. The odour and taste are strong, mint-like and slightly reminiscent of apples.

Microscopically it differs from Peppermint and Spearmint in the absence of stomata from the upper epidermis of the leaves and the presence of very abundant, covering trichomes on the leaves and stems. These trichomes are uniseriate, occasionally irregularly branched and have thin, smooth or slightly warted walls; unicellular conical trichomes also occur on the upper epidermis of the leaves.

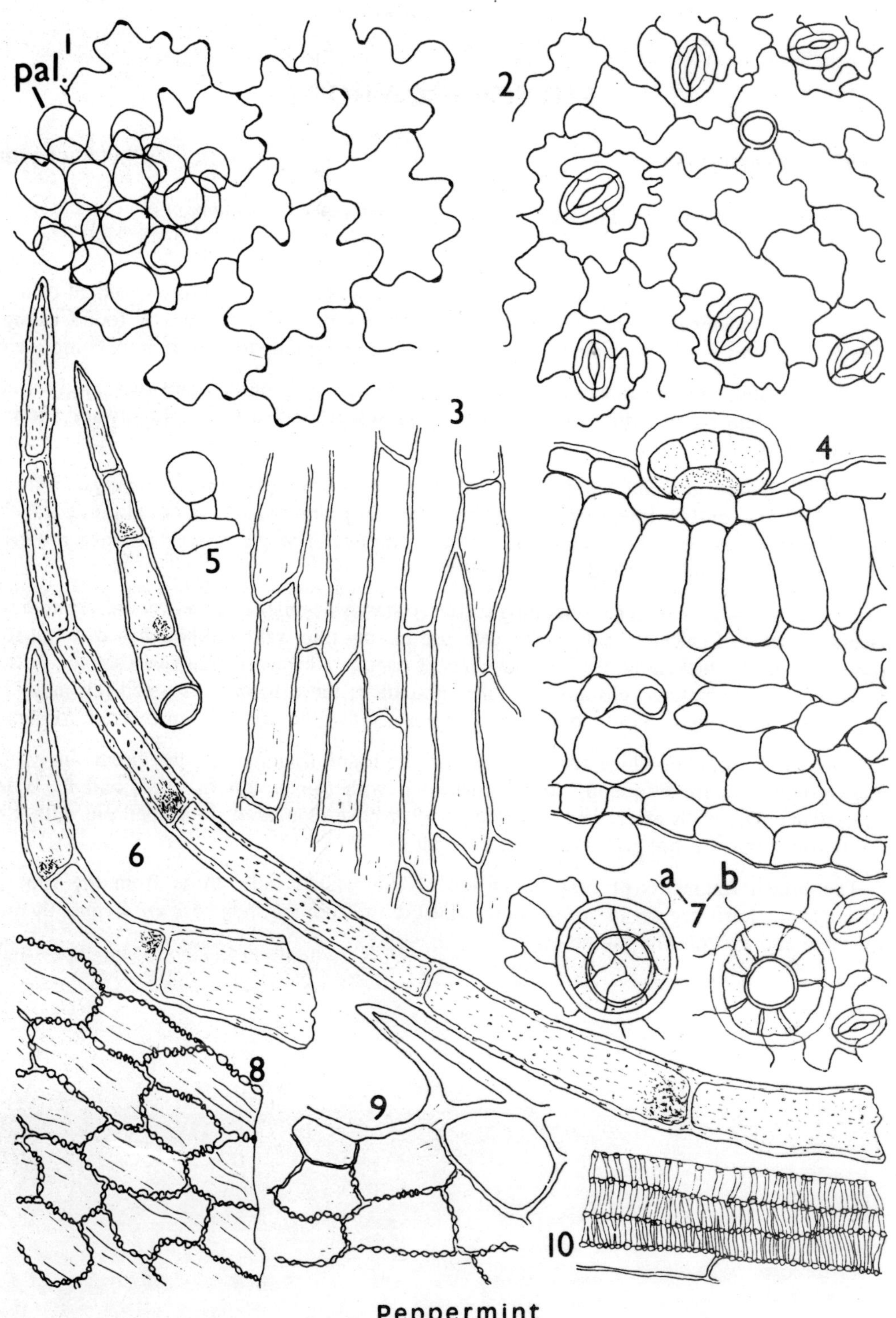

Peppermint

×330

1 Upper epidermis in surface view with part of the underlying palisade (pal.).
2 Lower epidermis in surface view showing diacytic stomata and a cicatrix.
3 Epidermis of the stem in surface view.
4 Part of the lamina in sectional view showing, in the upper epidermis, a glandular trichome with an eight-celled head and, in the lower epidermis, a glandular trichome with a unicellular head.
5 Glandular trichome with a unicellular head attached to an epidermal cell
6 Covering trichomes.
7 Multicellular-headed glandular trichomes, in surface view, attached to (a) a fragment of the upper epidermis and (b) a fragment of the lower epidermis.
8 Epidermis from near the leaf margin in surface view.
9 Epidermis from the leaf margin in surface view showing a unicellular, conical trichome.
10 Vessels and xylem parenchyma from the stem.

PHYTOLACCA ROOT

Phytolacca americana L. Phytolaccaceae

A pale brownish-buff powder with a faint odour and a slightly bitter and acrid taste.

The diagnostic characters are:

(*a*) The *starch granules*, which are fairly abundant; they are mostly simple, spherical to ovoid with a rather indistinct, point or radiate hilum. The granules are frequently found clumped together in groups and a few compound granules also occur with up to four or more components.

(*b*) The very abundant *fibres*, which occur in groups and are frequently found associated with the vessels and xylem parenchyma; they are fairly thick-walled with few, simple pits and show no reaction for lignin.

(*c*) The *idioblasts* containing bundles of *acicular crystals of calcium oxalate*; the crystals vary in size and are frequently arranged somewhat irregularly in groups which are not always parallel to the long axis of the cell; they usually fill the cell completely. Single crystals or small groups of crystals are also found scattered in the powder.

(*d*) The abundant *parenchyma* containing scattered starch granules and, occasionally, bundles of acicular crystals of calcium oxalate; the cells are mainly thin-walled although occasional fragments show slight thickening; very occasional cells contain a brownish amorphous resin. Groups of xylem parenchymatous cells are also fairly abundant; the cells are elongated rectangular in outline with moderately thickened walls and numerous pits; they give a faint reaction for lignin.

(*e*) The *vessels*, some of which are large and may be found fragmented; they occur singly or in small groups and are frequently found associated with the groups of fibres and the xylem parenchyma. The walls are reticulately thickened or have elongated slit-shaped pits with large oval borders; they do not give a reaction for lignin.

(*f*) The brown fragments of *cork* composed of thin-walled cells; those from the root are polygonal and fairly regular in surface view, whilst those from the stem base are frequently more elongated and irregular in outline.

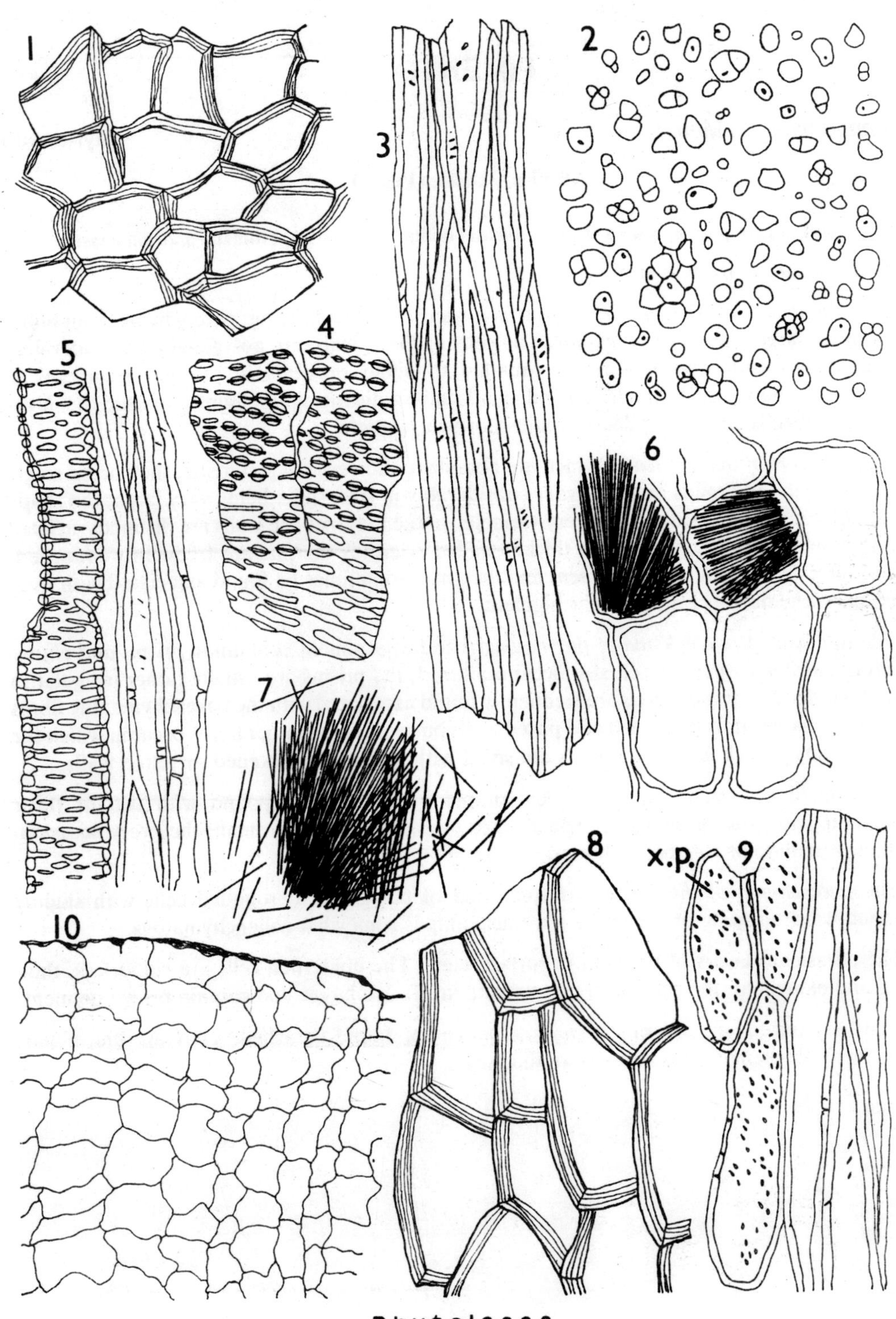

Phytolacca

×330

1 Cork from the root in surface view.
2 Starch granules.
3 Part of a group of fibres.
4 Fragment of a vessel showing bordered pits and reticulate thickening.
5 Reticulately thickened vessels and part of a group of fibres.
6 Parenchyma with two idioblasts containing acicular crystals of calcium oxalate.
7 Acicular crystals of calcium oxalate.
8 Cork from the stem base in surface view.
9 Xylem parenchymatous cells (x.p.) showing pits, and part of a group of fibres in longitudinal section.
10 Parenchyma of the phelloderm in sectional view.

PIMENTO

Pimenta dioica (L.) Merr. **Myrtaceae**

Allspice, Jamaica Pepper

A dark reddish-brown powder with a strong aromatic odour and a warm, aromatic and spicy taste.

The diagnostic characters are:

(*a*) The fragments of the *epicarp* in surface view with underlying parenchyma containing conspicuous, large, spherical *oil glands*. The cells of the epicarp are polygonal with moderately thickened walls and occasional large, rounded to ovoid *stomata* are present; fragments in sectional view show a thick *cuticle*. The oil glands have a distinct epithelium composed of a layer of thin-walled cells containing dense, reddish-brown *pigment*.

(*b*) The *sclereids of the mesocarp*, which are abundant and very characteristic; they occur singly or, more usually, in groups and they vary considerably in size, some being very large; the shape and the thickness of the walls is also very variable. In the majority the walls are distinctly striated and show numerous pits, and in the thicker-walled sclereids the pits are frequently branched. Most of the cells contain brown pigment and they may sometimes be found associated with thin-walled parenchyma containing similar pigment.

(*c*) The thin-walled *parenchyma of the mesocarp* and dissepiment containing *prisms and cluster crystals of calcium oxalate*, which also occur scattered; the prisms are usually rather irregular in shape. Lignified *fibres* and *vessels* are frequently found associated with the parenchyma; the fibres usually have moderately thickened and pitted walls but occasional larger fibres occur in which the walls are heavily thickened; the vessels are small with annularly thickened or pitted walls.

(*d*) The abundant *starch granules*, a few simple but mostly compound with two or three components; individual granules are spherical to ovoid and are fairly small; they very occasionally show a stellate or slit-shaped hilum.

(*e*) The *parenchyma of the cotyledons* composed of polygonal to rounded cells with slightly thickened walls; in some of the layers the thickening is somewhat collenchymatous.

(*f*) The occasional layers of the *testa* in surface view. The epidermal cells are colourless, thin-walled and elongated; the cells of the underlying layers are larger and contain brown pigment.

(*g*) The very infrequent *covering trichomes*, which are found detached. They are unicellular, conical, with thickened walls and a smooth cuticle.

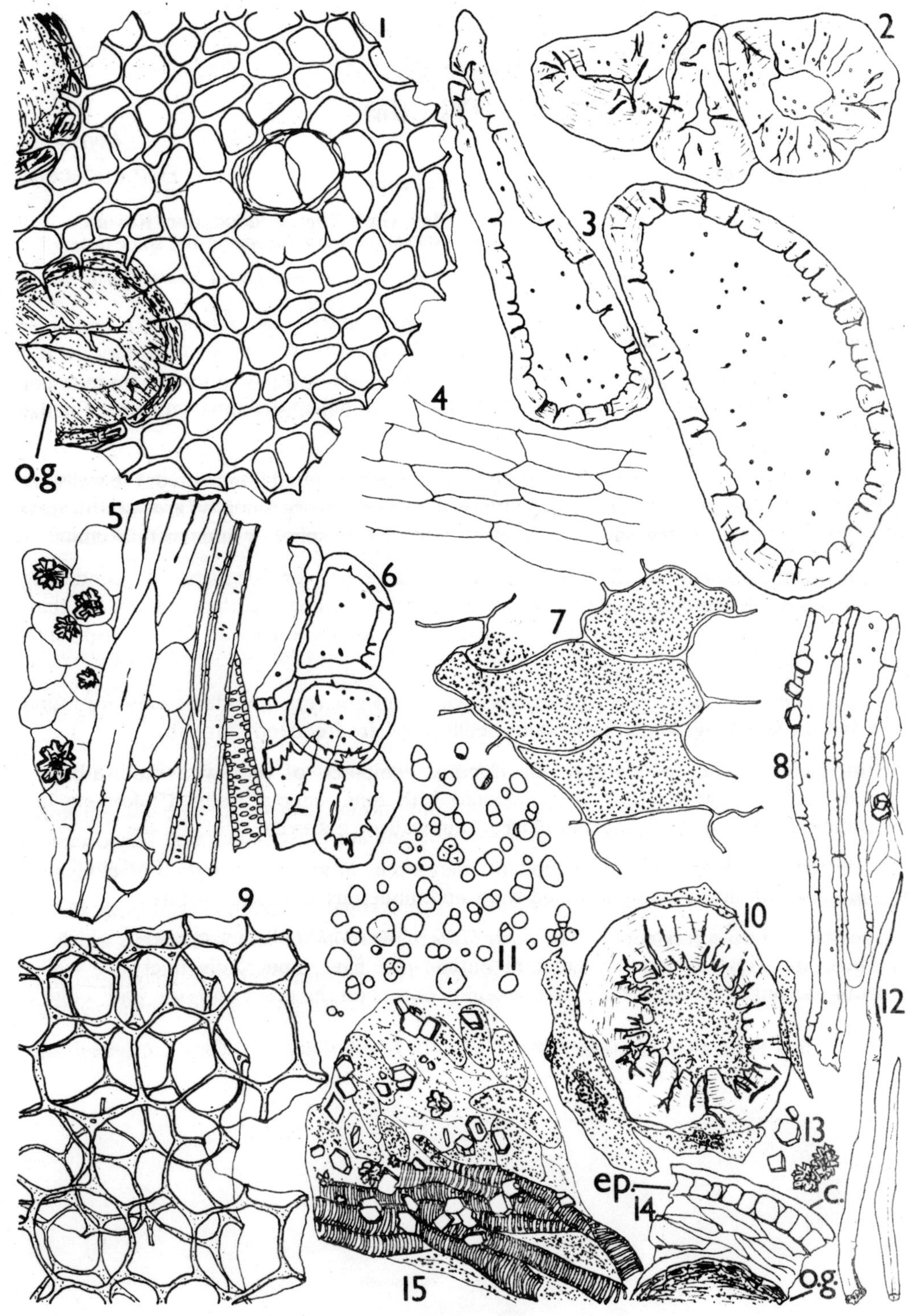

Pimento

×330

1 Epicarp in surface view showing stomata and parts of two underlying oil glands (o.g.).
2 Sclereids from the mesocarp.
3 Large, elongated sclereids from the mesocarp.
4 Epidermis of the testa in surface view.
5 Part of the mesocarp in longitudinal view showing parenchymatous cells containing cluster crystals of calcium oxalate, thick and thin-walled fibres and a pitted vessel.
6 Thinner-walled sclereids from the mesocarp.
7 Pigmented layer of the testa in surface view.
8 Fibres and parenchyma of the dissepiment with associated prism crystals of calcium oxalate.
9 Layers of a cotyledon in surface view.
10 Large sclereid in the mesocarp with associated parenchyma containing pigment.
11 Starch granules.
12 Covering trichomes.
13 Prisms and cluster crystals of calcium oxalate.
14 Outer region of the pericarp in sectional view showing the cuticle (c.), epicarp (ep.), parenchyma and part of an oil gland (o.g.).
15 Part of the dissepiment in longitudinal view showing a group of annularly thickened vessels and adjacent pigmented parenchyma containing prisms and cluster crystals of calcium oxalate.

PODOPHYLLUM

Podophyllum peltatum L. Berberidaceae

American Mandrake, American Podophyllum, May Apple Root, Podophyllum Rhizome

A pale buff to sandy coloured powder with a bitter, slightly acrid taste and a characteristic odour reminiscent of Liquorice.

The diagnostic characters are:

(*a*) The abundant *starch granules*, most of which are compound with two to four or up to ten or more components; individual granules are rather small and the majority show a distinct circular or slit-shaped hilum.

(*b*) The *vessels*, which are usually fairly large and are frequently found fragmented; the walls are lignified and have elongated slit-shaped pits with oval borders or, occasionally, are scalariformly or reticulately thickened. A few smaller vessels also occur with spiral or annular thickening.

(*c*) The abundant *parenchyma*, filled with starch granules or, very occasionally, containing cluster crystals or calcium oxalate. The cells are rounded in outline and the majority are thin-walled but occasional groups of thicker-walled cells are found and these show conspicuous pitting.

(*d*) The large *cluster crystals of calcium oxalate*; which are not very abundant; they are found scattered and, occasionally, in parenchymatous cells; they are frequently broken.

(*e*) The fragments of the *epidermis of the rhizome* composed of cells with reddish-brown contents; in surface view the cells are elongated with thin, sinuous walls. Underlying the epidermis there are two or three layers of large, thin-walled cork cells.

(*f*) The *sclereids*, which are not very abundant; they occur in groups composed of elongated rectangular cells with moderately thickened walls and numerous, conspicuous pits.

(*g*) The occasional brown fragments of the *outer layer of the rootlets* composed of cells which, in surface view, are elongated and irregular in outline and have moderately thickened walls; fragments in sectional view show that the thickening occurs on the outer and side walls only.

Compare Indian Podophyllum, page 128.

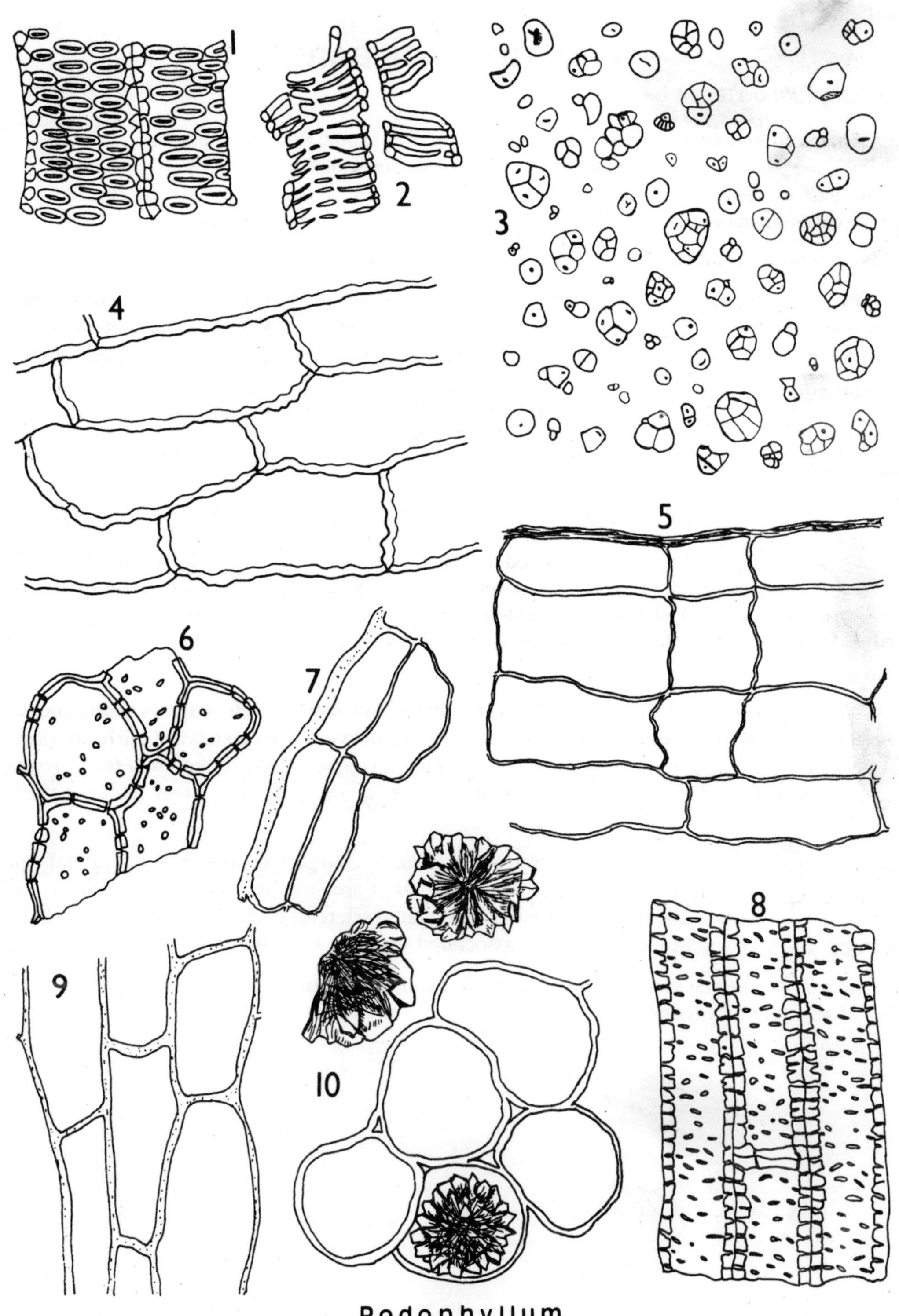

Podophyllum

×330

1 Fragments of bordered pitted vessels.
2 Fragments of reticulately thickened vessels.
3 Starch granules.
4 Epidermis of the rhizome in surface view.
5 Epidermis and underlying cork cells in sectional view.
6 Pitted parenchyma.
7 Outer layers of the rootlets in sectional view.
8 Part of a group of sclereids.
9 Outer layers of the rootlets in surface view.
10 Cluster crystals of calcium oxalate and a group of parenchymatous cells.

POMEGRANATE BARK

Punica granatum L. | Punicaceae

Pomegranate, Pomegranate Root Bark

A medium brown, somewhat gritty powder with little odour and a slightly astringent taste.

The diagnostic characters are:

(*a*) The abundant fragments of *cork*, of which there are two types. Those which are more numerous are composed of lignified cells, polygonal in surface view and moderately thickened, with pits on the inner tangential walls; in sectional view the thickening is seen to be on the inner and radial walls only. In the second type the cells are also lignified and the inner and radial walls are very heavily thickened, giving a small lumen which occurs near the unthickened, outer wall of the cell; these cells are frequently fragmented and they occur singly or in small groups; the lumen is usually filled with dense brown contents.

(*b*) The very abundant *parenchyma* of the phloem which, when seen in radial longitudinal section, consists of vertical rows of small cells each containing a single cluster crystal of calcium oxalate, alternating with more elongated parenchyma; the cells are usually thin-walled but occasional areas of thicker-walled cells occur and these give a positive reaction for lignin with *Phloroglucinol* and *Hydrochloric Acid*. Medullary rays, usually seen in tangential longitudinal section, occur with the phloem parenchyma; the cells are fairly thick-walled and show pits on the tangential walls.

(*c*) The *calcium oxalate crystals*, mainly in the form of *clusters*, which are very numerous and found scattered as well as in the cells of the phloem parenchyma; the crystals are fairly uniform in size and each one has a well marked brownish coloured centre. Also present are a few *prisms* of calcium oxalate, which are usually found scattered; these are somewhat larger than the cluster crystals.

(*d*) The *sclereids*, which are rather infrequent. These are large rectangular to polygonal cells, occurring singly or in groups of two or three; the walls are strongly thickened and have well-marked striations and oblique pits. Occasional elongated sclereids occur with very thick walls and a narrow lumen; these are usually found associated with the sieve tissue or medullary rays.

(*e*) The very occasional spherical *starch granules*, which are found scattered or, more usually, in some of the parenchymatous cells.

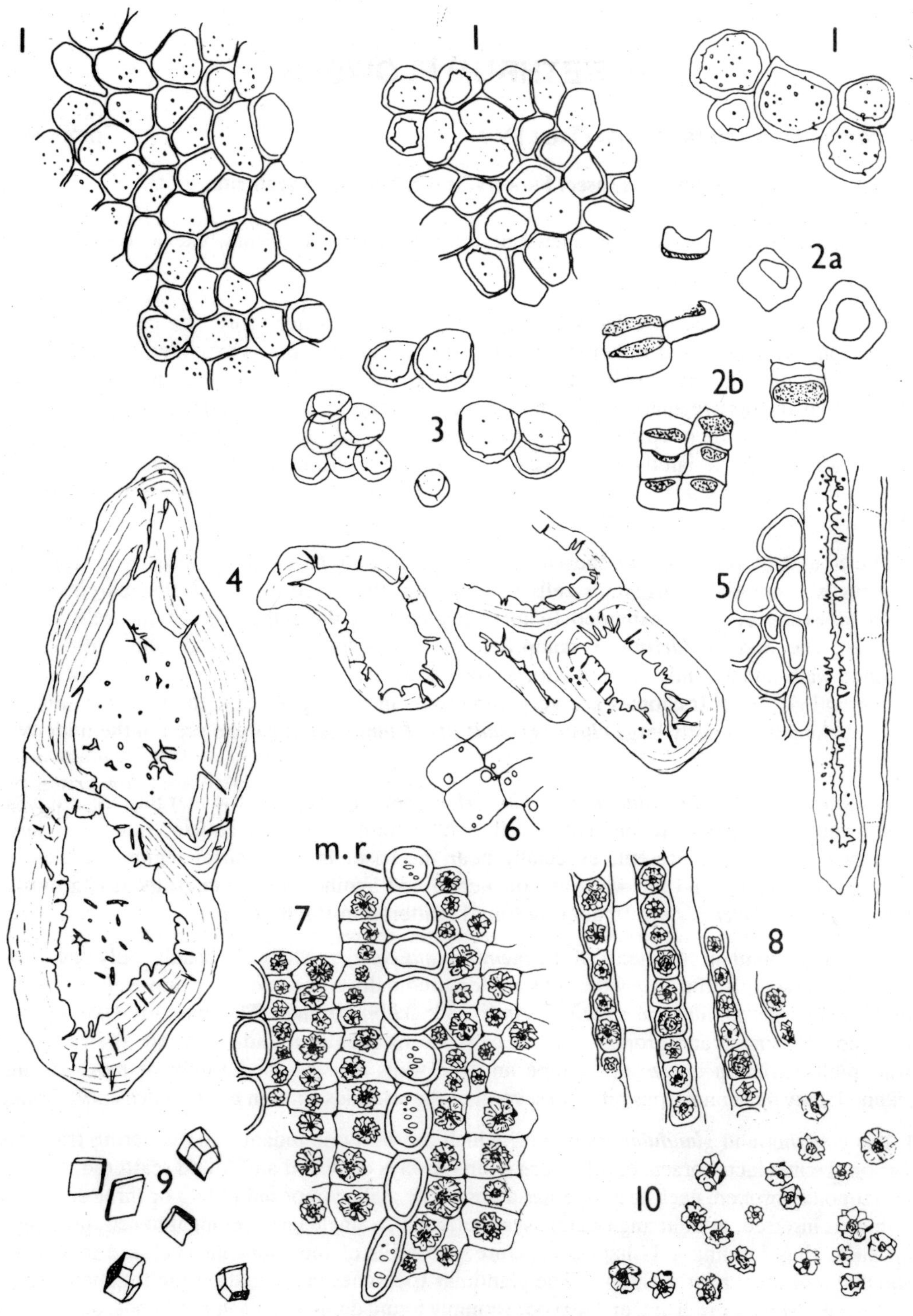

Pomegranate Bark

×330

1 Fragments of thinner-walled cork in surface view.
2a Thicker-walled cork in surface view.
2b Thicker-walled cork in sectional view.
3 Thinner-walled cork in sectional view.
4 Sclereids.
5 An elongated sclereid with associated sieve tissue and medullary ray in tangential longitudinal section.
6 Parenchyma with starch granules.
7 Phloem parenchyma with calcium oxalate cluster crystals and a medullary ray (m.r.) in tangential longitudinal section.
8 Part of the phloem in radial longitudinal section.
9 Prisms of calcium oxalate.
10 Cluster crystals of calcium oxalate.

PYRETHRUM FLOWERS

Chrysanthemum cinerariifolium (Trev.) Vis. Compositae

Dalmation Insect Flowers, Insect Flowers, Pyrethrum

A pale brown to fawn powder with a characteristic, aromatic odour and a slightly bitter and aromatic taste.

The diagnostic characters are:

(*a*) The fragments of the *corollas of the ligulate florets in surface view*. The cells of the *inner epidermis* are polygonal and rather sinuous in outline and each cell is extended to form a large *papilla*; these papillae are usually seen as a large circle on each cell but sometimes they are collapsed and appear irregularly oval to elongated in surface view; the margins of the papillae are faintly striated. The *outer epidermis* is mainly composed of thin-walled cells with a markedly sinuous outline and a striated *cuticle*; occasional glandular trichomes are present. On fragments of the outer epidermis from near the base of the corolla the walls are slightly thickened and beaded and the cuticle is less markedly striated.

(b) The abundant fragments of the *corollas of the tubular florets in surface view*. The *inner epidermis* is composed of irregular cells with slightly thickened walls; on the margins of the corolla lobes the cells are extended to form *papillae* but the remainder of the cells are not papillose. The *outer epidermis* is composed of longitudinally elongated cells with slightly thickened walls and a faintly striated cuticle; over most of the corolla the cell walls show distinct beading and glandular trichomes are very numerous; in the region near the base the walls are evenly thickened and fairly large *cluster crystals of calcium oxalate* can be seen in the underlying tissues.

(*c*) The fragments of the *involucral bracts in surface view*. Those from the margins are composed of thin-walled, polygonal to elongated cells with a faintly striated cuticle; numerous large, *anomocytic stomata* are present, especially near the base. In the central region the cells are elongated-rectangular and the walls are thickened and lignified with numerous pits; groups of these rectangular *sclereids* are frequently found scattered in the powder.

(*d*) The fairly abundant fragments of the *membranous calyces*, which are usually only one or two cells in thickness. In surface view the cells are longitudinally elongated, very thin-walled and they contain numerous *tabular, prismatic crystals of calcium oxalate*. The base of each calyx is composed of *sclereids* and groups of these cells are frequently found scattered; the cells show considerable variation in size and shape and the walls may be moderately or more strongly thickened; they have numerous pits and several of the sclereids contain *prisms of calcium oxalate*.

(*e*) The *covering* and *glandular trichomes*, which are fairly abundant. The covering trichomes occur on the involucral bracts but they are nearly always detached and found scattered; they are also frequently broken; each trichome has a uniseriate stalk composed of two or three small cells on which is inserted, at right angles and asymmetrically, a single large, elongated cell, tapering at both ends, thus forming a T-shaped structure; the walls of this elongated cell are moderately thickened and show faint striations. The glandular trichomes are found on the fragments of the corollas and the ovary wall and are also occasionally found detached; each is composed of a short, biseriate, usually two-celled stalk and a biseriate head with two or four cells; around each head the cuticle is raised to form a bladder-like covering.

(*f*) The very abundant fragments of the *filaments* and *anthers* of the stamens. The filament fragments are cylindrical and the epidermis is composed of fairly small cells which are square to rectangular in surface view with slightly thickened walls. Fragments of the anthers which include the tips of the lobes are frequently found; they are bluntly pointed and composed of thin-walled cells which in surface view appear rather similar to the cells of the membranous calyx but they do not contain calcium oxalate crystals. Fragments of the *fibrous layer* are very abundant; they are composed of elongated cells which in surface view show characteristic thickening and beading of the walls.

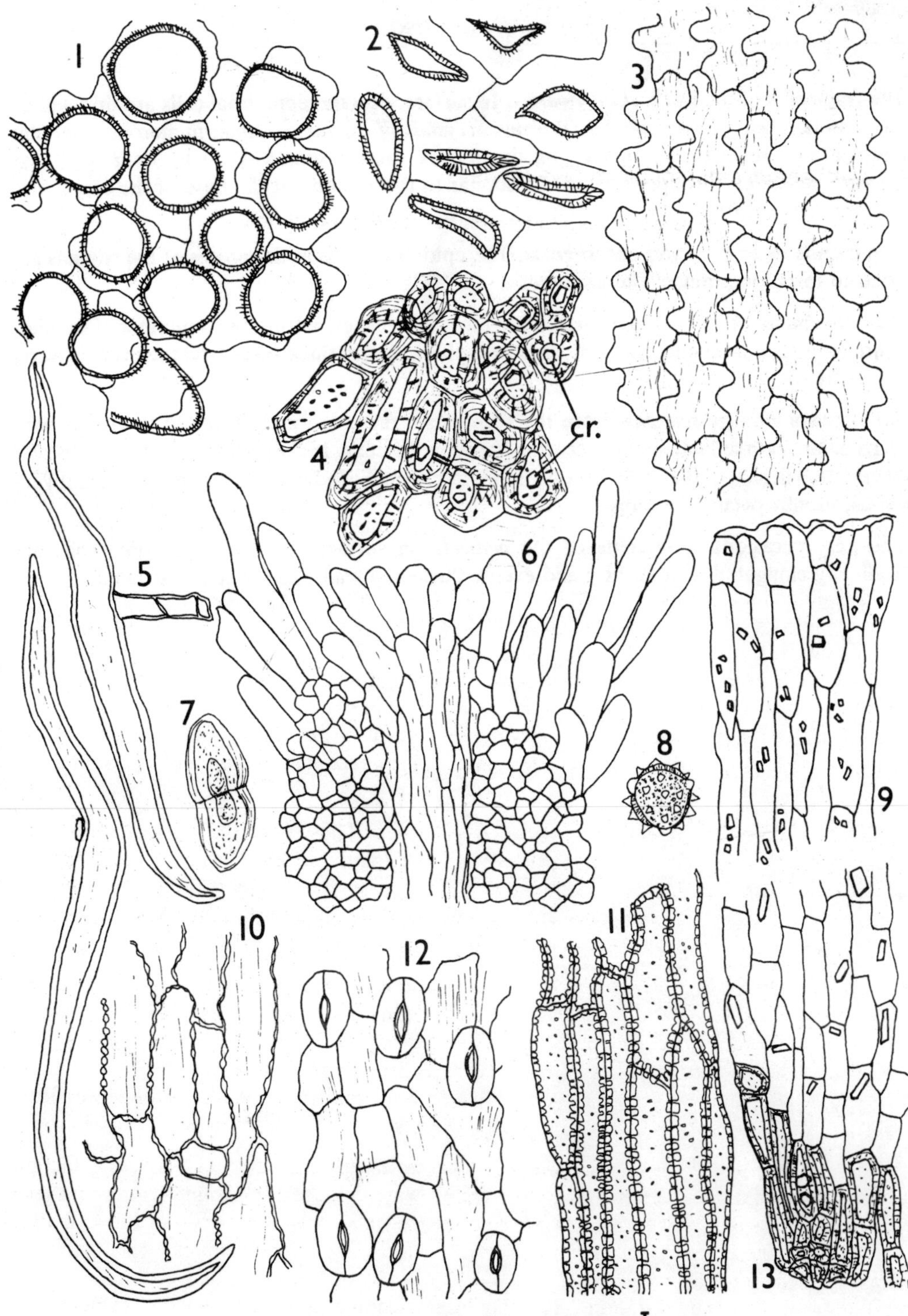

Pyrethrum Flowers I

×330

1 Inner epidermis of the corolla of a ligulate floret in surface view showing rounded papillae.
2 Inner epidermis of the corolla of a ligulate floret in surface view showing collapsed papillae.
3 Outer epidermis of the corolla of a ligulate floret showing striations.
4 A group of sclereids, some containing prisms of calcium oxalate (cr.), from the base of the calyx or the ovary.
5 Covering trichomes.
6 Papillose stigma and part of the style in surface view.
7 A glandular trichome.
8 A mature pollen grain.
9 Apical region of the calyx in surface view showing crystals of calcium oxalate in the cells.
10 Outer epidermis near the base of the corolla of a ligulate floret in surface view.
11 Elongated sclereids from the central region of an involucral bract.
12 Part of the marginal region of an involucral bract in surface view, showing stomata.
13 Part of the basal region of the calyx showing sclereids.

(*g*) The fragments of the *walls of the ovaries*. In surface view the epidermal cells are thin-walled and they contain fairly large, *tabular, prismatic crystals of calcium oxalate*; numerous glandular trichomes are present. In the underlying tissue dark brown, secretory ducts occur but these appear very indistinct. Groups of sclereids, similar to those found at the base of the calyx, also occur in the ovary wall.

(*h*) The fragments of the *styles* and *stigmas*. The epidermal cells at the apices of the stigmas are extended to form long, finger-like *papillae*.

(*i*) The very abundant *pollen grains*, which are fairly large when mature but a number of smaller, immature grains are frequently present; they are spherical with three pores and the exine is warty and distinctly spiny.

(*j*) The occasional large *sclereids* from the receptacle; these are usually found in groups with large, irregular, intercellular spaces occuring between the cells. Individual sclereids show considerable variation in shape; the walls are only moderately thickened and the pits,which are not very numerous, usually occur in groups.

(*k*) The very occasional fragments of the *pedicels*; in surface view the epidermal cells are longitudinally elongated with slightly and evenly thickened walls; the *cuticle* is striated.

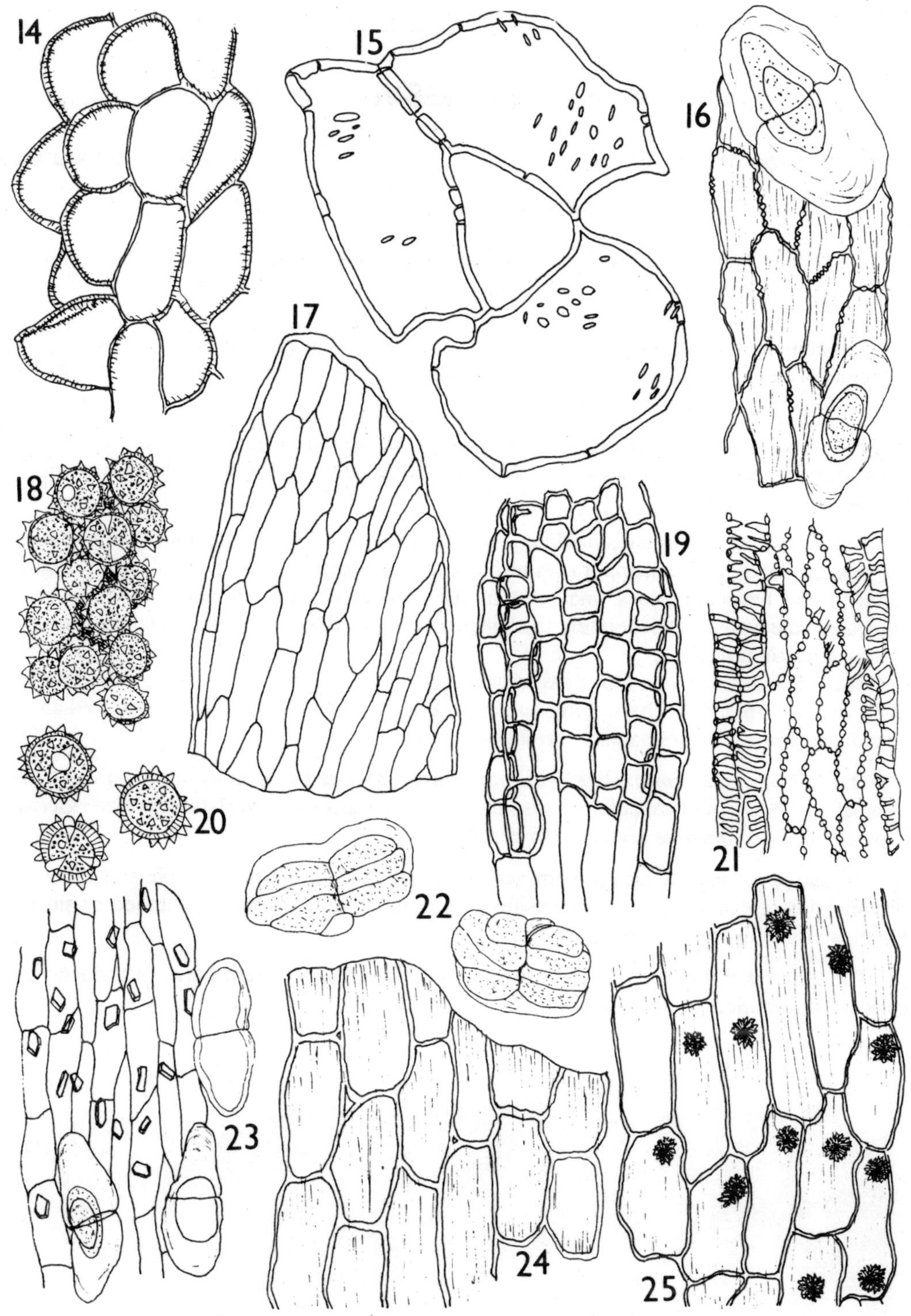

Pyrethrum Flowers II

×330

14 Inner epidermis of the corolla of a tubular floret in surface view showing marginal papillae.
15 Sclereids from the receptacle.
16 Outer epidermis of the corolla of a tubular floret in surface view showing beaded walls, striations and glandular trichomes.
17 Part of the tip of an anther lobe in surface view.
18 A group of immature pollen grains.
19 Part of the filament of an anther in surface view.
21 Fibrous layer of the anther in surface view.
22 Glandular trichomes.
23 Part of the ovary wall in surface view showing glandular trichomes and cells containing prisms of calcium oxalate.
24 Epidermis of the pedicel in surface view.
25 Outer epidermis near the base of the corolla of a tubular floret showing striations and cluster crystals of calcium oxalate in the underlying tissues.

QUASSIA

Picrasma excelsa (Sw.) Planch. Simarubaceae

Quassia Wood, Jamaica Quassia Wood

A pale, yellowish buff powder with no odour and an intensely bitter taste.

The diagnostic characters are:

(*a*) The abundant *fibres*, which occur in groups and are usually found associated with the other elements of the xylem; they are lignified, with moderately thickened walls and few pits. A few slightly larger fibres may be present, from the adherent bark.

(*b*) The *vessels*, which occur singly or in small groups and are frequently found fragmented or associated with other xylem elements. They are fairly large, lignified and have very numerous minute, bordered pits.

(*c*) The *medullary rays* in tangential and radial longitudinal views; the majority are multiseriate but a small number of uniseriate rays also occur. In tangential view the cells are polygonal to rounded and have numerous small pits in the tangential walls; in radial view the cells are elongated; the walls are moderately thickened and lignified; occasional cells contain fairly large prisms of calcium oxalate.

(*d*) The *xylem parenchyma*, found associated with the vessels and fibres; the cells are moderately thick-walled, lignified and have fairly numerous pits; they are longitudinally elongated and often contain prisms of calcium oxalate, arranged in vertical files.

(*e*) The *prisms of calcium oxalate*, which are found scattered as well as in the parenchymatous cells of the xylem and medullary rays; they show considerable variation in size. Occasional *twinned* and *conglomerate crystals* also occur.

(*f*) The *starch granules*, which are not very abundant; they are mostly simple and spherical but occasional compound granules occur with two or three components; a rounded or slit-shaped hilum is visible in some of the granules.

(*g*) The occasional fragments of dark brown *cork*, from the adherent bark. In surface view the cells are thin-walled and polygonal.

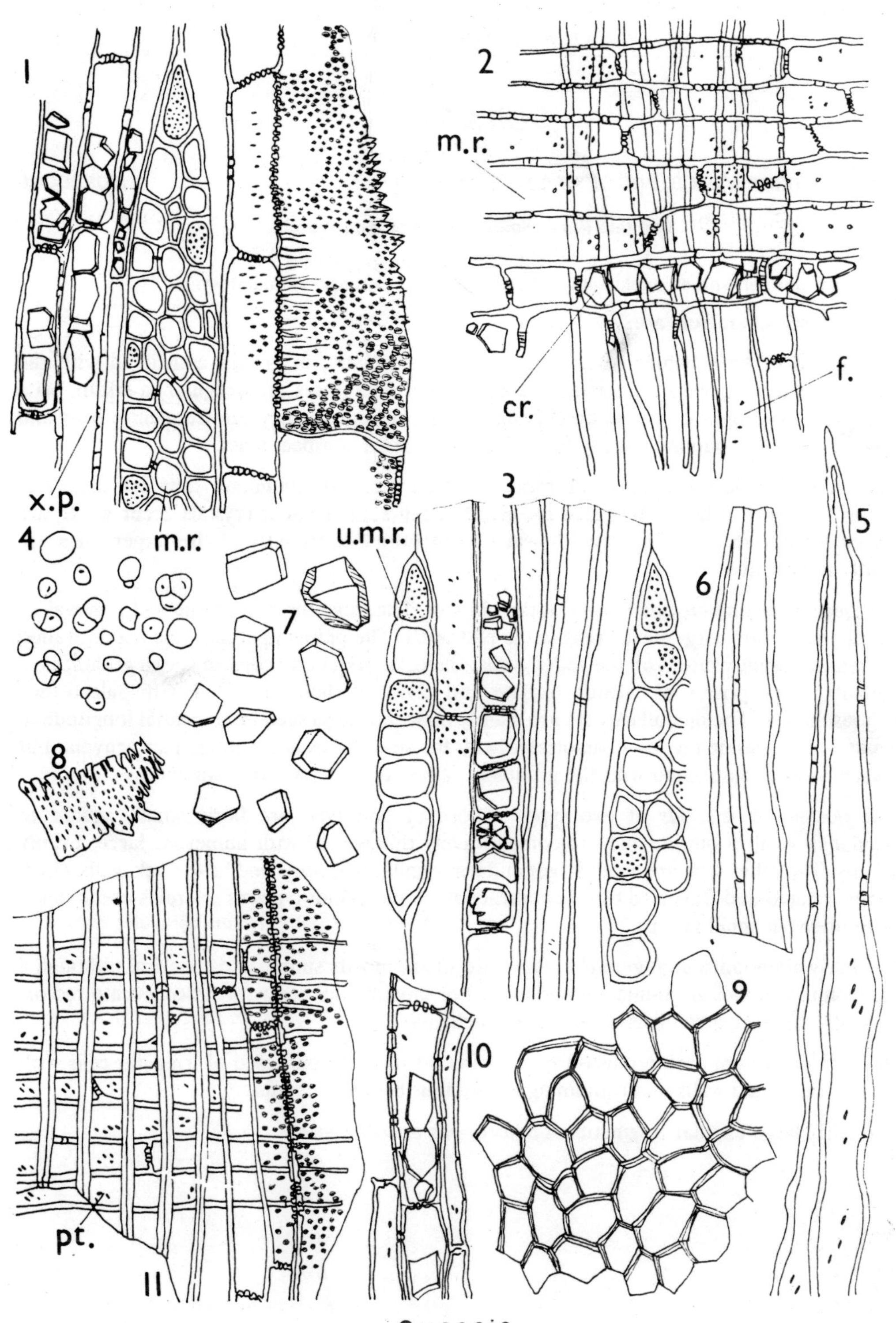

Quassia

×330

1 Part of the xylem in tangential longitudinal section showing xylem parenchymatous cells (x.p.), some containing prisms of calcium oxalate, part of medullary ray (m.r.) and a bordered pitted vessel.
2 Part of the xylem in radial longitudinal section showing medullary ray cells (m.r.), some containing prisms of calcium oxalate (cr.), with underlying fibres (f.) and xylem parenchyma.
3 Part of the xylem in tangential longitudinal section showing a uniseriate medullary ray (u.m.r.), xylem parenchyma with prisms of calcium oxalate, fibres and part of a multiseriate medullary ray.
4 Starch granules.
5 Fibres from the phloem.
6 Xylem fibres.
7 Calcium oxalate prisms.
8 Fragment of a bordered pitted vessel.
9 Cork in surface view.
10 Xylem parenchyma.
11 Part of a group of fibres with xylem parenchyma and a bordered pitted vessel, and underlying medullary ray cells showing pits (pt.), in radial longitudinal section.

QUILLAIA

Quillaja saponaria Molina, and other spp. of *Quillaja* *Rosaceae*

Quillaia Bark, Soap Bark, Panama Wood

A pinkish-buff powder with an unpleasant and acrid taste; it is strongly sternutatory.

The diagnostic characters are:

(*a*) The abundant *fibres* which occur singly or, more usually, in groups associated with the medullary rays in tangential longitudinal section. Individual fibres are irregular in outline with lignified walls varying in thickness and giving an uneven lumen; they are frequently bent and adjacent fibres in a group are usually intertwined to form a compact mass.

(*b*) The characteristic *calcium oxalate crystals*, which are very abundant; they are most frequently in the form of large elongated *prisms* although some smaller crystals occur which are *cubical* or *lozenge-shaped*. The crystals usually are found scattered and the larger ones are frequently fragmented.

(*c*) The *sieve tissue* and *medullary rays* of the phloem. The sieve tubes are large and thin-walled and occasionally show large sieve areas in the end walls. The phloem parenchyma is thin-walled and sometimes slightly pitted on the radial walls; the cells frequently contain starch granules or, occasionally, large prisms of calcium oxalate and many of them are filled with pale brown amorphous matter. The medullary rays are mainly multiseriate as seen in tangential longitudinal section and are occasionally found associated with the sieve tubes and phloem parenchyma, but more usually occur associated with the groups of fibres; the cells are thin-walled.

(*d*) The occasional *sclereids* of two types. Those of one type are fairly small, square to rectangular or oval in outline and are comparatively thin-walled with numerous large, evenly spaced pits. The other type are much larger and less regular in outline and have thick walls which are faintly striated and traversed by a few, rather small pits. Both types of sclereids occur singly or, more often, in small groups.

(*e*) The fairly abundant *starch granules*; these are small, mostly simple and spherical although a few compound granules are found with up to four or more components; they occur scattered or, more usually, as compacted masses in the parenchyma.

(*f*) The very occasional dark reddish-brown fragments of *cork* composed of irregular cells with moderately thickened walls and containing amorphous brown contents.

(*g*) The fairly large angular fragments of *amorphous brown matter*.

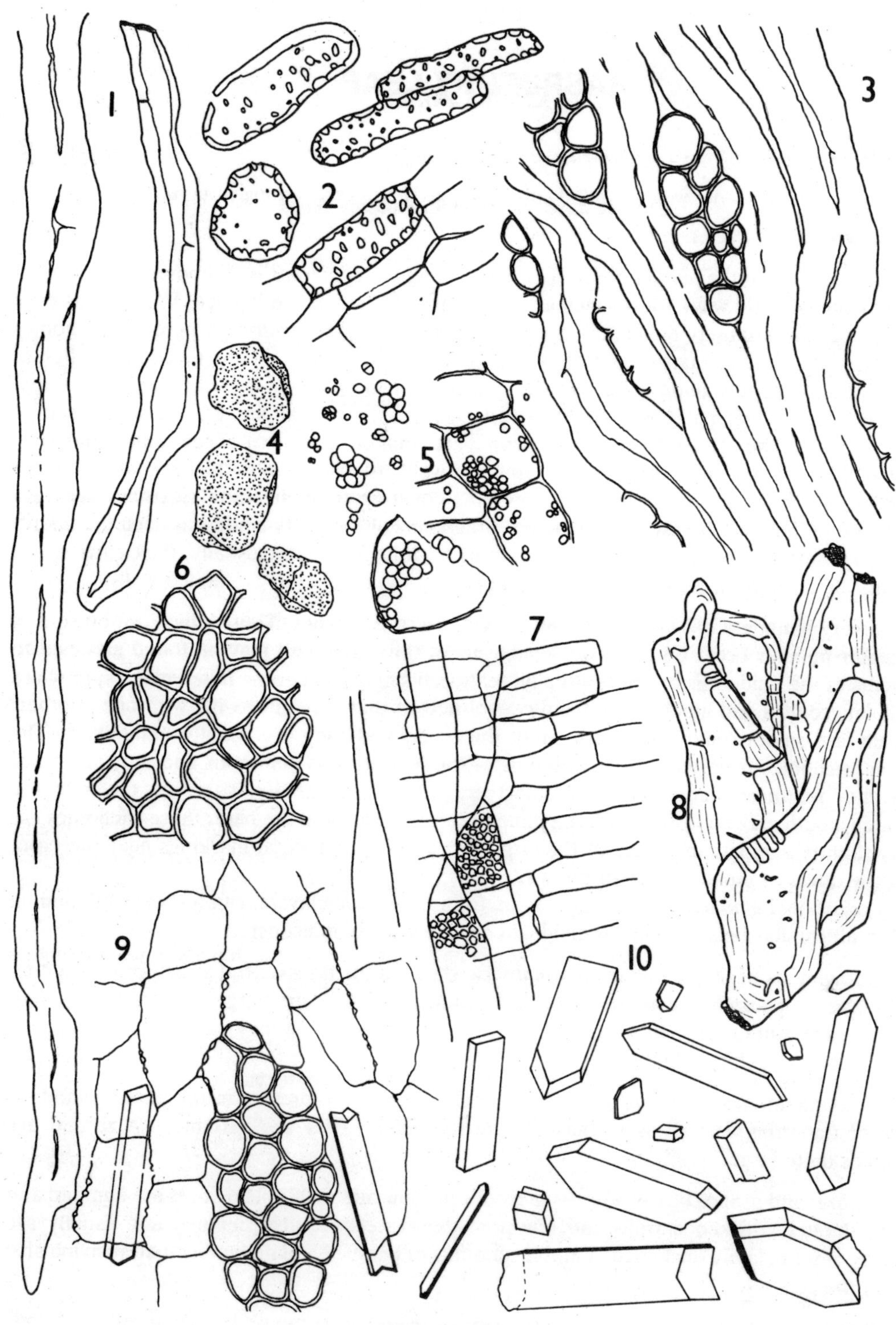

Quillaia

×330

1 Parts of single fibres.
2 Smaller sclereids with thin walls and large pits.
3 Part of a group of fibres and medullary rays in tangential longitudinal section.
4 Fragments of amorphous brown matter.
5 Starch granules, some contained in parenchyma.
6 Cork in surface view.
7 Sieve tubes with sieve areas and part of a medullary ray in radial longitudinal section.
8 Larger sclereids with thick walls and few pits.
9 Phloem parenchyma and part of a medullary ray in tangential longitudinal section.
10 Calcium oxalate crystals.

RASPBERRY LEAF

Rubus idaeus L. Rosaceae

A pale greyish-green powder with a faint odour and a slightly bitter and astringent taste.

The diagnostic characters are:

(*a*) The fragments of the *lamina in surface view*. The *upper epidermis* is composed of polygonal cells with very slightly wavy walls which are irregularly thickened and beaded; in the areas over the veins the cells are more elongated; covering trichomes, or the *cicatrices* where the trichomes have been attached, are fairly numerous and some of these give a faint reaction for lignin; stomata are absent; the underlying palisade cells are small and closely packed and occasional idioblasts occur in the palisade composed of larger cells each containing a cluster crystal of calcium oxalate. The cells of the *lower epidermis* are smaller than those of the upper epidermis and they have rather indistinct, slightly sinuous walls which are not thickened or beaded; numerous small *anomocytic stomata* are present; covering trichomes and cicatrices are very numerous and these are occasionally lignified. Fragments of the lower epidermis from the midrib and larger veins also show very numerous covering trichomes or, more usually, the cicatrices left by them; the cells from these regions are elongated and have slightly thickened walls.

(*b*) The very abundant *covering trichomes*, which are of two types. Those which are present in the greater number occur on the lower epidermis of the leaves and may be found attached to fragments of the epidermis or, more usually, scattered singly or in dense felted masses; they are unicellular, conical and much twisted and convoluted so that they intertwine with one another; the walls are smooth and only moderately thickened and they are usually unlignified. The covering trichomes from the upper epidermis of the leaf are less numerous and they are much larger; they are unicellular, conical and almost straight, tapering gradually towards the apex; the walls are smooth and very thick so that a lumen is absent except at the base; these trichomes are usually slightly lignified and some of the larger ones show faint spiral markings near the base, giving the effect of crossed lines on the wall.

Very occasional *glandular trichomes* may be found; they are clavate with a short stalk and an ovoid, multicellular head, but the individual cells are usually indistinct.

(*c*) The fragments of the *lamina in sectional view* showing the dorsiventral structure with a one- or two-layered palisade; scattered irregularly in the palisade are large, spherical or ovoid idioblasts each containing a cluster crystal of calcium oxalate. The spongy mesophyll is composed of small, irregular, thin-walled cells.

(*d*) The abundant *cluster crystals of calcium oxalate*, which are present in the parenchymatous tissues of the veins as well as in the palisade idioblasts. They are variable in size and are sometimes quite large.

(*e*) The *fibres* and groups of *vascular tissue* from the veins and rachis. The fibres are lignified and have moderately thickened walls and few pits; the vessels are also lignified and usually are annularly or reticulately thickened. Varying amounts of lignified and unlignified parenchyma also occur in the powder.

(*f*) The occasional fragments of the *fibrous layer of the anthers* composed of small cells with rods of lignified thickening on the side walls which appear as beads in surface view.

(*g*) The *pollen grains* which are small, subspherical with three pores and an almost smooth exine.

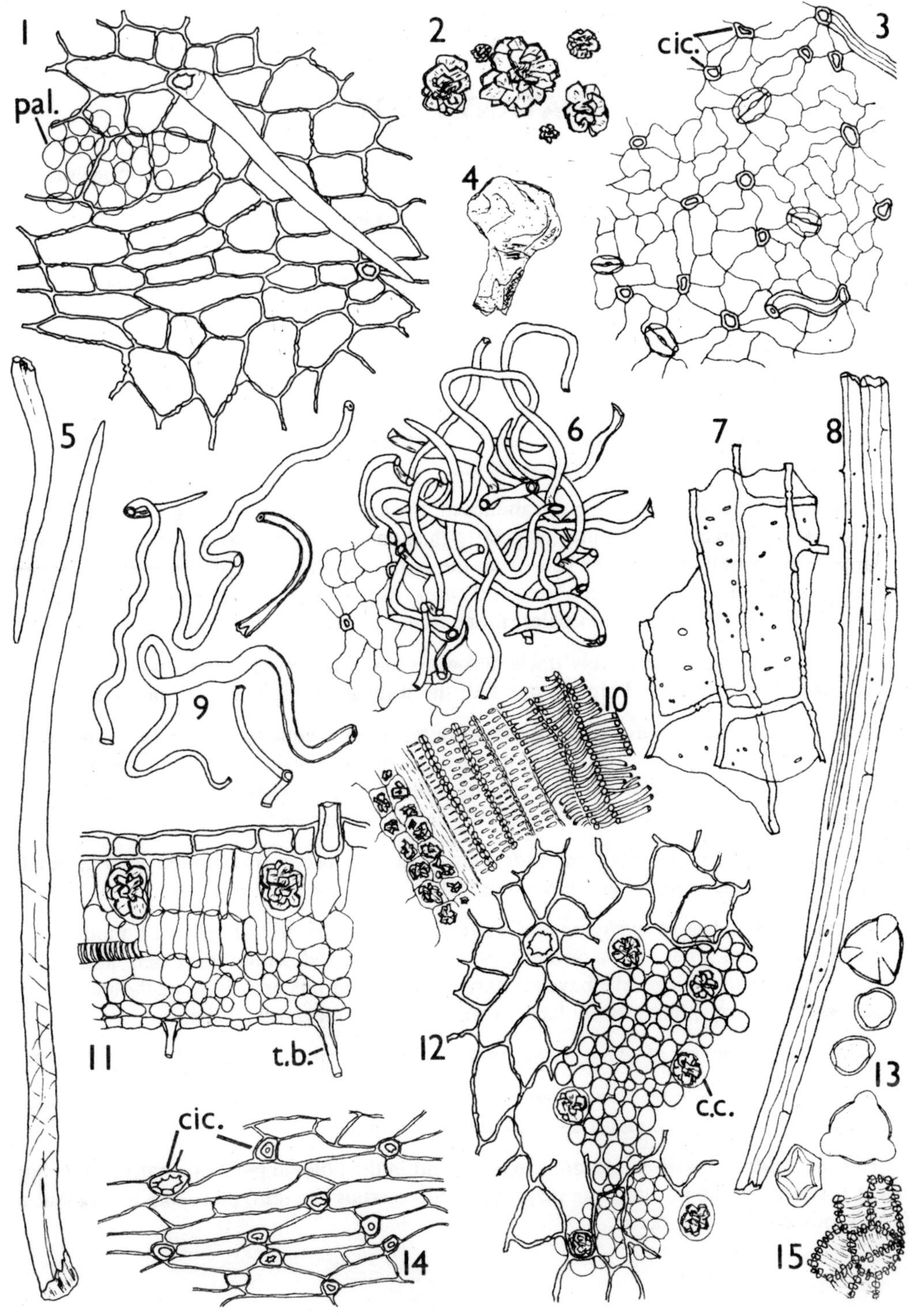

Raspberry Leaf

×330

1 Upper epidermis in surface view showing an attached covering trichome, a cicatrix, the elongated cells over a small vein and part of the underlying palisade (pal.).
2 Cluster crystals of calcium oxalate.
3 Lower epidermis in surface view showing stomata, cicatrices (cic.) and parts of attached covering trichomes.
4 A glandular trichome.
5 Thick-walled covering trichomes.
6 Felted mass of thin-walled covering trichomes attached to part of the lower epidermis.
7 Lignified pitted parenchyma.
8 Fibres.
9 Thin-walled covering trichomes.
10 Part of the vascular tissue of a vein with associated parenchymatous cells containing cluster crystals of calcium oxalate.
11 Part of the lamina in sectional view showing trichome bases (t.b.) and two-layered palisade with idioblasts containing cluster crystals of calcium oxalate.
12 Part of the upper epidermis in surface view, with underlying palisade showing idioblasts (c.c.) containing cluster crystals of calcium oxalate.
13 Pollen grains.
14 Epidermis from the midrib in surface view showing numerous cicatrices (cic.).
15 Fibrous layer of the anther in surface view.

RHATANY ROOT

Krameria triandra Ruiz and Pavon — Leguminosae

Krameria, Peruvian Rhatany

A dark reddish-brown, fibrous powder with no odour and an intensely astringent taste, imparting a red colour to the saliva.

The diagnostic characters are:

(*a*) The fairly abundant *starch granules*, which are simple and compound with two or three and, less commonly, four or five components. Individual granules vary considerably in shape from subspherical to irregularly polyhedral and a slit or stellate hilum is sometimes visible; very occasional granules show faint concentric striations.

(*b*) The fragments of *cork*, which are quite abundant; the cells are relatively large and, in surface view, polygonal to elongated with thin, irregularly thickened walls; fragments in sectional view show a large number of layers. All the cells from the outer region contain dense, reddish-brown pigment which sometimes becomes separated and occurs as large masses scattered in the powder; the cells from the inner layers contain paler, more transparent, pinkish-brown pigment.

(*c*) The phloem *fibres* with moderately thickened walls and a lumen of varying width; they are somewhat tortuous in outline and bluntly pointed; the walls are unlignified and pits are absent.

(*d*) The *parenchyma and medullary rays* of the phloem, which frequently occur associated with the fibres; the parenchymatous cells adjacent to the fibres are thin-walled and often contain small prisms or sandy crystals of calcium oxalate; the medullary rays are mostly uniseriate as seen in tangential longitudinal view and the cell walls are slightly thickened.

(*e*) The abundant *vessels and fibre-tracheids*, which usually occur fragmented and in small groups; the elements are lignified and have small, slit-shaped bordered pits.

(*f*) The fragments of *xylem parenchyma and medullary rays* composed of cells with moderately thickened and lignified walls; these sometimes occur associated with the vessels and fibre-tracheids. The parenchymatous cells have scattered, slit-shaped pits and those of the medullary rays have more numerous, large, irregularly ovoid pits in the tangential walls.

(*g*) The occasional fragments of *collenchyma* from the phelloderm composed of fairly large cells.

(*h*) The masses of dark *reddish-brown pigment* which occur scattered as well as associated with the cork; some of the masses contain embedded starch granules.

(*i*) The *calcium oxalate crystals* which are usually found in the phloem parenchymatous cells but may occur scattered in the powder; the majority of the crystals are thin, plate-like prisms but a few small sandy crystals also occur.

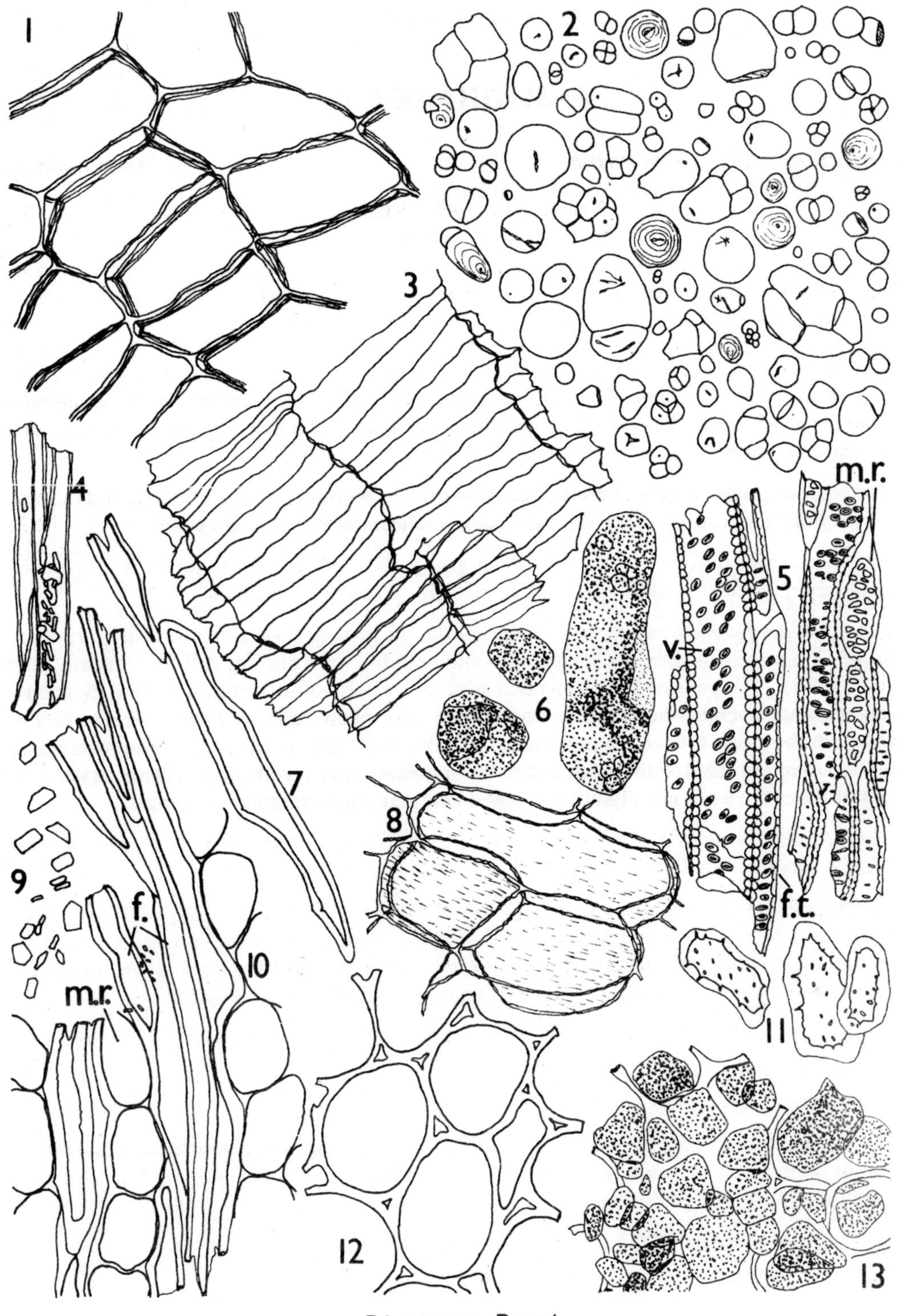

Rhatany Root

×330

1 Cork layers in surface view.
2 Starch granules.
3 Part of the cork in sectional view.
4 Fragment of phloem parenchyma containing small prisms of calcium oxalate.
5 Fragments of the xylem showing vessels (v.) and fibre-tracheids (f.t.) with bordered pits and part of a uniseriate medullary ray (m.r.) with associated fibre-tracheids, in tangential longitudinal view.
6 Isolated masses of pigment from the cork.
7 Phloem fibres.
8 Inner cork layers, in surface view, containing pigment.
9 Prisms of calcium oxalate.
10 Part of the phloem in tangential longitudinal view showing fibres (f.), medullary rays (m.r.) and scattered sandy crystals of calcium oxalate.
11 Isolated xylem parenchymatous cells.
12 A group of cells from the phelloderm.
13 Fragments of the outer cork cells with dense masses of pigment.

RHUBARB

Rheum palmatum L. or *Rheum officinale* Baillon, or possibly hybrids or mixtures of these two spp. — Polygonaceae

Chinese Rhubarb, Rhubarb Rhizome

A yellowish-brown to reddish-brown, somewhat gritty powder with a characteristic, empyreumatic odour; the taste is bitter and astringent.

The diagnostic characters are:

(*a*) The abundant *starch granules*, which are simple and spherical or, more usually, compound with from two to five components; most granules have a distinct, central hilum in the form of a cleft or radiating split.

(*b*) The fairly abundant *cluster crystals of calcium oxalate* which are found scattered and in some of the parenchymatous cells. They are very large and are frequently fragmented.

(*c*) The *vessels*, which occur singly or in small groups and are frequently found in fragments. They are large, reticulately thickened and do not give a reaction for lignin.

(*d*) The abundant *parenchyma of the medullary rays* and *ground tissue*. The medullary rays are composed of cells with slightly thickened walls and both the walls and the cell contents are deep brownish-yellow. The parenchyma associated with the vessels consists of thin-walled, elongated cells tapering at the ends when seen in longitudinal view; these cells are filled with starch. The remainder of the ground tissue is composed of cells varying from rounded to oval to rectangular in outline; they are filled with starch granules or, occasionally, with large cluster crystals of calcium oxalate; the walls are slightly thickened and may show irregular swellings.

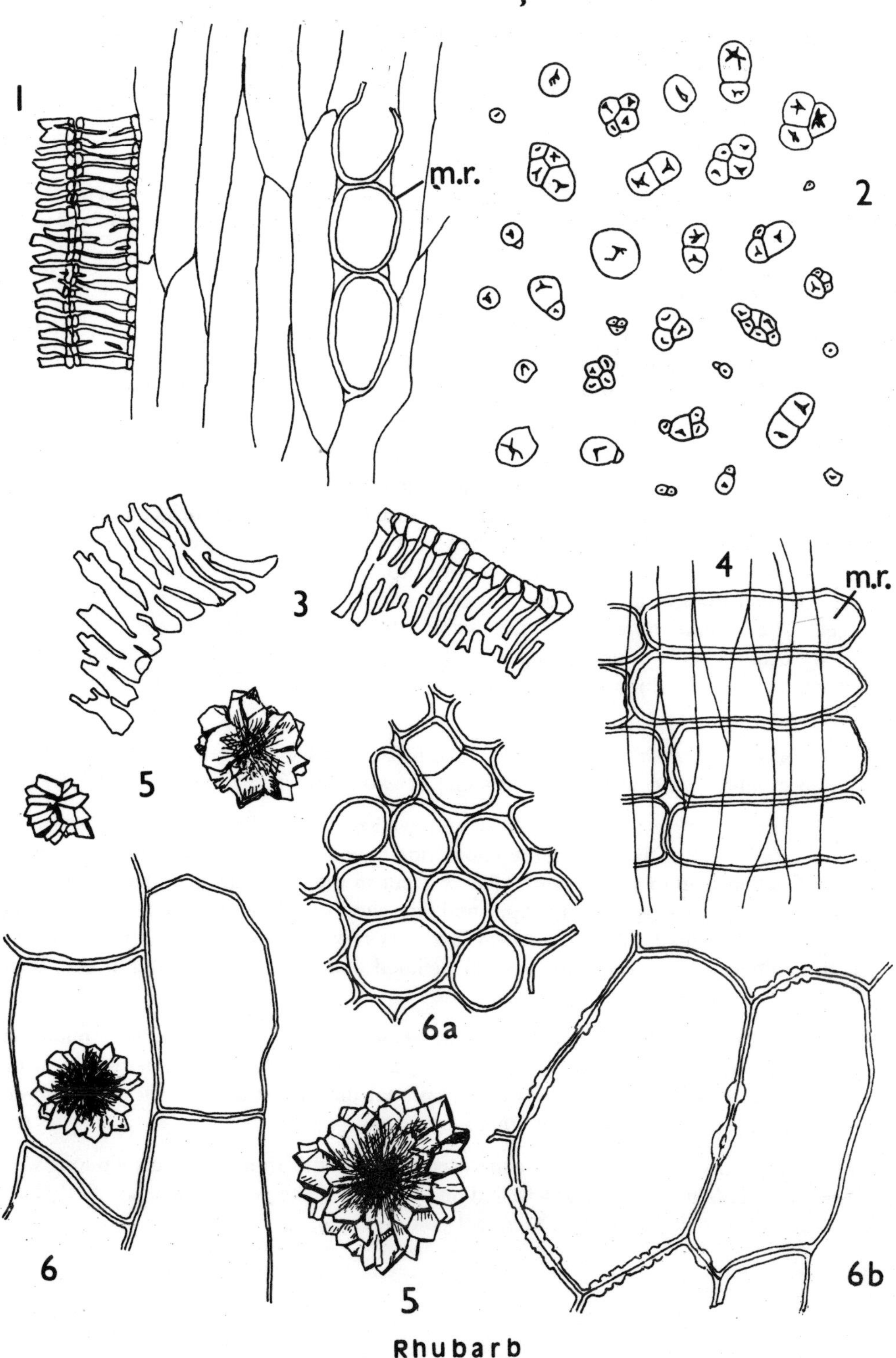

Rhubarb

1 Reticulately thickened vessels associated with parenchyma and a medullary ray (m.r.) in tangential longitudinal section.
2 Starch granules.
3 Fragments of reticulately thickened vessels.
4 Medullary ray (m.r.) in radial longitudinal section underlying parenchymatous cells.
5 Cluster crystals of calcium oxalate.
6 Parenchyma of the ground tissue containing a calcium oxalate crystal.
6a Small-celled, rounded parenchyma of the ground tissue.
6b Parenchymatous cells of the ground tissue showing irregular thickening.

ROSEMARY

Rosmarinus officinalis L. Labiatae

Usually occurs in commerce as the dried whole or broken greyish-green leaves with fragments of stem and occasional small blue flowers. It has a characteristic aromatic odour and an aromatic, pungent and slightly bitter taste.

The diagnostic characters are:

(*a*) The *upper epidermis of the leaf* composed of a layer of tabular cells, which, in surface view, are polygonal to irregular with slightly thickened walls and occasional pits; stomata are absent. The underlying *hypodermis* is composed of from one to several layers of large, irregularly rounded to ovoid cells with thickened anticlinal walls; in surface view the walls appear distinctly beaded.

(*b*) The *lower epidermis of the leaf* has very abundant covering trichomes interspersed with glandular trichomes so that the epidermal cells are usually obscured in surface view; they are polygonal with straight to slightly sinuous walls and *diacytic stomata* occur frequently. The *covering trichomes*, which form dense, felted masses, are uniseriate, thin-walled, much branched structures with each branch arising from a slightly swollen joint and terminating in a single, tapering cell. The *glandular trichomes* are mainly of the typical labiate type with a short, unicellular stalk and a radiate head composed of eight cells with a common cuticle forming a bladder; a few smaller glandular trichomes with a unicellular stalk and a spherical unicellular head also occur.

(*c*) The *leaf lamina in sectional view* shows that the *palisade*, which underlies the hypodermis, is arranged to form large, crescent-shaped areas one or two layers in thickness.

(*d*) The *epidermis of the stem* is composed of thin-walled, longitudinally elongated cells with occasional diacytic stomata; the cells of the underlying *hypodermis* are thick-walled and conspicuously beaded when seen in surface view. *Fibres* occur in the pericycle; they have moderately thickened walls with numerous slit-shaped pits and they show only a faint reaction for lignin. The vascular tissue contains small, lignified *tracheids* and *vessels* with spiral or annular thickening and small-celled, lignified parenchyma; large-celled lignified and pitted parenchyma occurs in the pith.

(*e*) The *outer epidermis of the calyx*, like the lower epidermis of the leaf, has very numerous, branched, covering trichomes and abundant glandular trichomes. The *inner epidermis*, in surface view, is composed of wavy-walled cells with occasional diacytic stomata; *unicellular, conical covering trichomes* occur scattered on the inner epidermis.

(*f*) The *outer epidermis of the corolla* is composed of cells with thin, markedly sinuous walls; those of the *inner epidermis* are straight-walled and *papillose*. The *pollen grains* are fairly large, spherical, with six pores and furrows and a finely pitted exine.

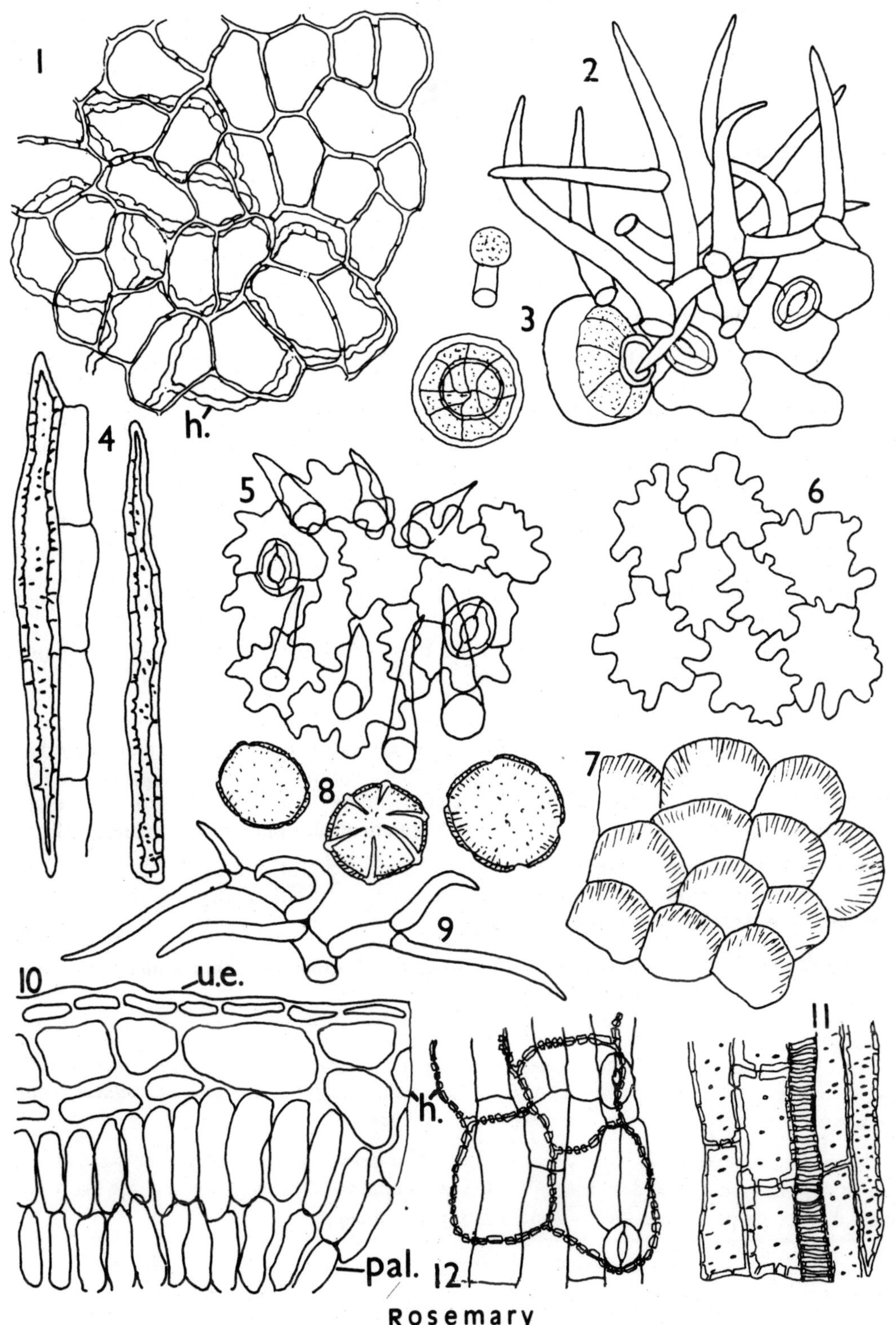

Rosemary

×330

1 Upper epidermis of the leaf in surface view with part of the underlying hypodermis (h.).
2 Lower epidermis of the leaf in surface view with stomata and trichomes.
3 Glandular trichomes.
4 Pericyclic fibres and parenchyma of the stem.
5 Inner epidermis of the calyx in surface view with unicellular trichomes.
6 Outer epidermis of the corolla in surface view.
7 Inner epidermis of the corolla showing papillae.
8 Pollen grains.
9 A branched covering trichome.
10 Part of the lamina in sectional view showing the upper epidermis (u.ep.), hypodermis (h.) and palisade (pal.).
11 Vascular tissue of the stem with associated larger-celled parenchyma of the pith.
12 Epidermis of the stem in surface view with underlying hypodermis (h.).

SAGE

Salvia officinalis L   Labiatae

Sage Leaves

Usually occurs in commerceas small fragments of the dried leaves which are greyish-green and densely pubescent, especially on the lower surface; it has a strong, aromatic and very characteristic odour and taste.

The diagnostic characters are:

(*a*) The *upper epidermis*, which, in surface view, is composed of polygonal, slightly sinuous cells with thickened and markedly beaded walls and a faintly striated *cuticle*; the underlying palisade cells are loosely packed. The cells of the *lower epidermis* are thin-walled and more sinuous in outline but they are difficult to discern owing to the dense covering of trichomes. *Diacytic stomata* are present on both epidermises.

(*b*) The very abundant *covering trichomes*, which occur on both epidermises and also on the petiole; they are particularly numerous on the lower epidermis. Individual trichomes are uniseriate composed of two, or occasionally three cells, and usually have a short basal cell and a very long, undulating, whip-like terminal cell which tapers to a blunt apex; the walls are smooth and moderately thickened.

Very occasional short, unicellular covering trichomes also occur; they are conical with a thick wall and a finely warted cuticle.

(*c*) The abundant *glandular trichomes*, which also occur on both epidermises; those found most frequently are the typical labiate type consisting of a very short, rounded stalk and a glandular head composed of eight radiating thin-walled cells with a common cuticle which is raised to form a spherical, bladder-like covering. Other glandular trichomes are smaller and of the capitate type, composed of a one- or two-celled stalk and a spherical, unicellular or bicellular head.

(*d*) The *lamina in sectional view* shows the leaves to be dorsiventral with a palisade composed of two layers, and small groups of vascular tissue in the spongy mesophyll; the *vessels* are lignified, narrow, and show spiral or annular thickening.

(*e*) The *epidermis of the petiole* composed of longitudinally elongated, thin-walled cells with a faintly striated cuticle and numerous covering trichomes.

The vessels of the petiole are larger than those in the veins of the leaves and show reticulate thickening.

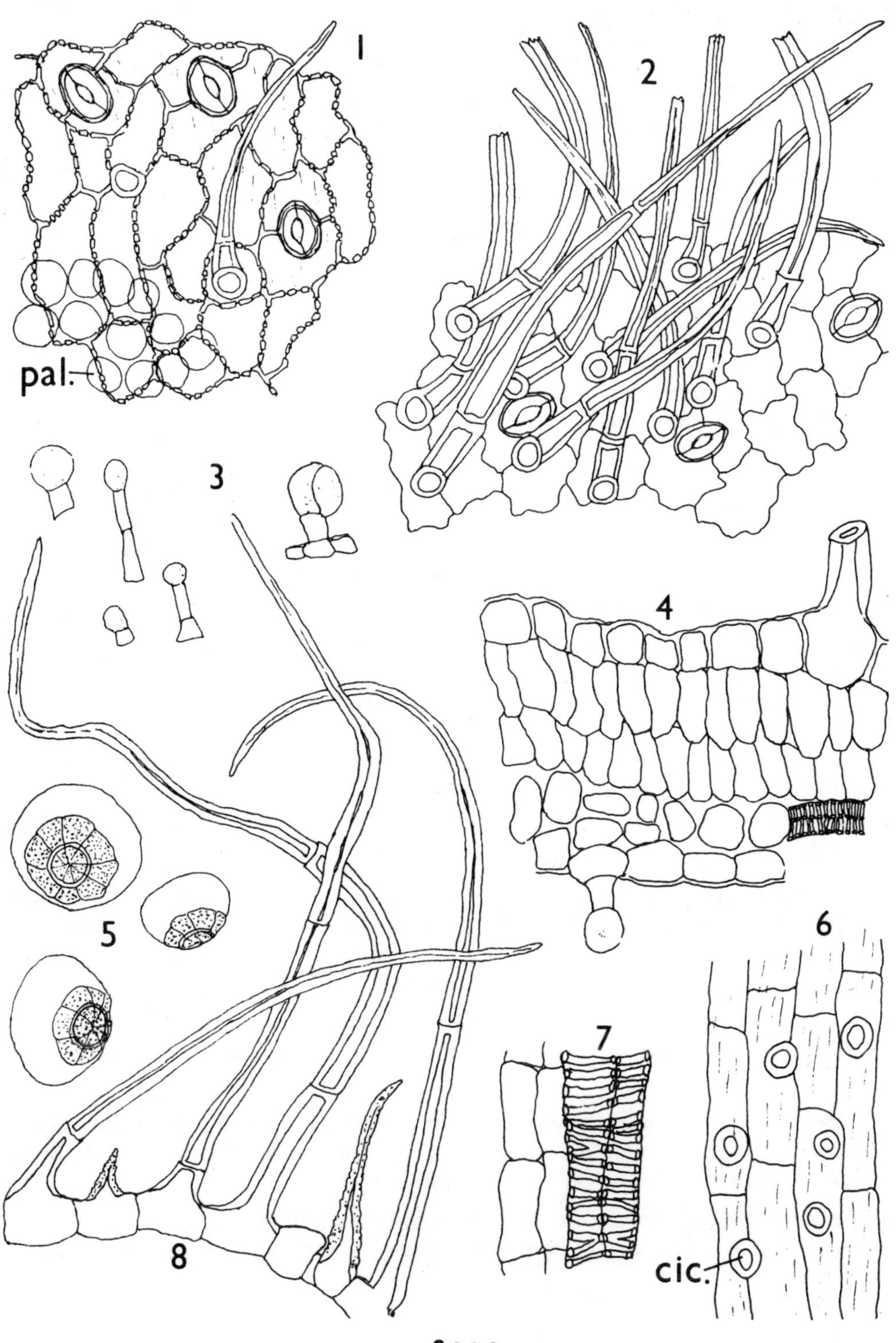

Sage

×330

1 Upper epidermis in surface view showing diacytic stomata, covering trichomes and part of the underlying palisade (pal.).
2 Lower epidermis in surface view showing diacytic stomata and numerous covering trichomes.
3 Capitate glandular trichomes.
4 Part of the lamina in sectional view showing the base of a covering trichome in the upper epidermis and a capitate glandular trichome in the lower epidermis.
5 Multicellular-headed glandular trichomes in side and surface views.
6 Epidermis of the petiole in surface view showing cicatrices (cic.).
7 Vessels and parenchyma from the petiole.
8 Part of the epidermis from near the margin, in sectional view, showing covering trichomes.

SARSAPARILLA

Smilax ornata Lam., *Smilax regelii* Killip and Morton and other spp. of *Smilax* — Liliaceae

Sarsaparilla Root

A pale pinkish-fawn powder, odourless and with a slightly bitter taste.

The diagnostic characters are:

(*a*) The abundant *starch granules*, which are mostly compound with two, three or up to six or more components; individual granules are polyhedral and fairly small; a point hilum is visible in some of the granules.

(*b*) The *piliferous layer* composed of a single layer of pale yellowish-brown cells which frequently contain masses of brown granular material; the cells are fairly large and occasionally show the remains of *root hairs*. This layer is nearly always found associated with the underlying cells of the exodermis.

(*c*) The *exodermis* composed of two or three layers of cells which, in transverse sectional view, are strongly thickened on the outer and anticlinal walls and only moderately thickened on the inner walls; the walls are yellowish in colour and only the middle lamella gives a reaction for lignin. In longitudinal view the cells are axially elongated with oblique or bluntly pointed ends; a few conspicuous pits occur, particularly in the outer and anticlinal walls. These cells may be found singly or as a layer associated with either the cells of the piliferous layer or with the parenchymatous cells of the outer part of the cortex.

(*d*) The *acicular crystals of calcium oxalate*, which are fairly large and are found scattered or in bundles in some of the parenchymatous cells of the cortex.

(*e*) The *endodermis* consisting of a single layer of cells, rather similar in appearance to those of the exodermis but with evenly thickened walls and numerous pits; these cells do not give a reaction for lignin. This layer is frequently found associated with the fibrous cells of the pericycle or with the pitted cells of the inner part of the cortex.

(*f*) The *vessels*, which are fairly large and are usually found fragmented; the walls are lignified and the majority show scalariform or reticulate thickening; a small number of bordered pitted vessels also occur.

(*g*) The *fibrous cells*, which are generally found in groups; they vary in shape but are usually narrow and elongated with bluntly pointed ends. The walls may be moderately or heavily thickened; they are lignified and have numerous pits.

(*h*) The *xylem parenchyma*, composed of fairly large cells which are elongated rectangular in longitudinal view with moderately thickened, lignified walls and numerous conspicuous pits.

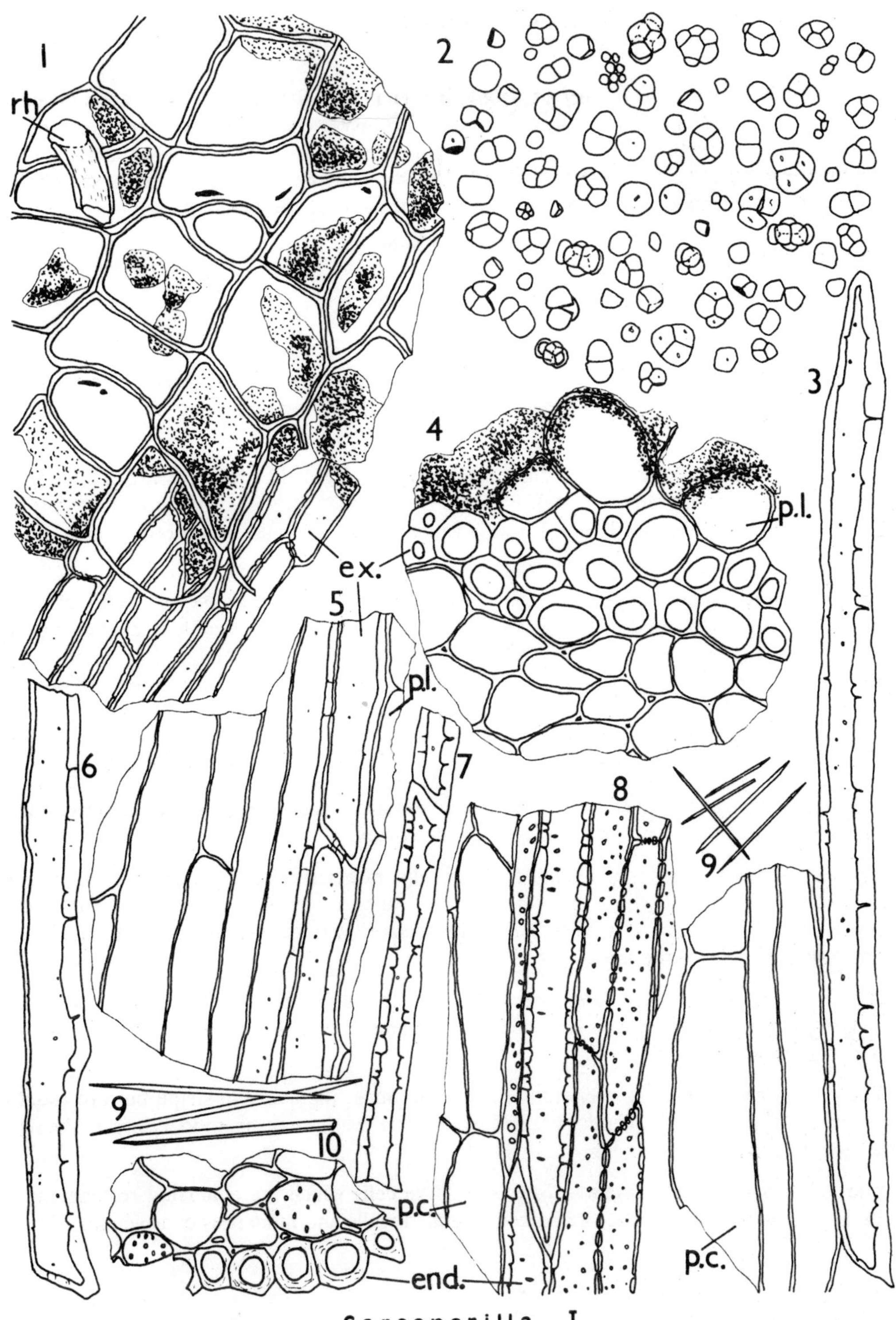

Sarsaparilla I

×330

1 Piliferous layer in surface view showing granular contents, the remains of a root hair (r.h.) and part of the underlying exodermis (ex.).
2 Starch granules.
3 A cell of the exodermis in longitudinal view with associated parenchymatous cells of the cortex (p.c.).
4 Piliferous layer (p.l.), exodermis (ex.) and parenchyma of the cortex in transverse section.
5 Part of the piliferous layer (p.l.), exodermis (ex.) and cortex in longitudinal view.
6 Part of a cell of the exodermis in longitudinal view.
7 Cells of the endodermis in longitudinal view.
8 Endodermis (end.) with associated parenchyma of the cortex (p.c.) and fibrous cells of the pericycle, in longitudinal view.
9 Acicular crystals of calcium oxalate.
10 Endodermis (end.) and pitted parenchyma of the cortex (p.c.) in transverse section.

(*i*) The abundant *parenchyma of the cortex and pith*. That from the cortex is mainly composed of fairly large, thin-walled cells which appear rounded in transverse sectional view and elongated in longitudinal view; the cells from the innermost region of the cortex are somewhat smaller, have slightly thicker walls and are occasionally pitted. The parenchyma of the pith is composed of cells with moderately thickened walls and numerous pits; these cells are lignified.

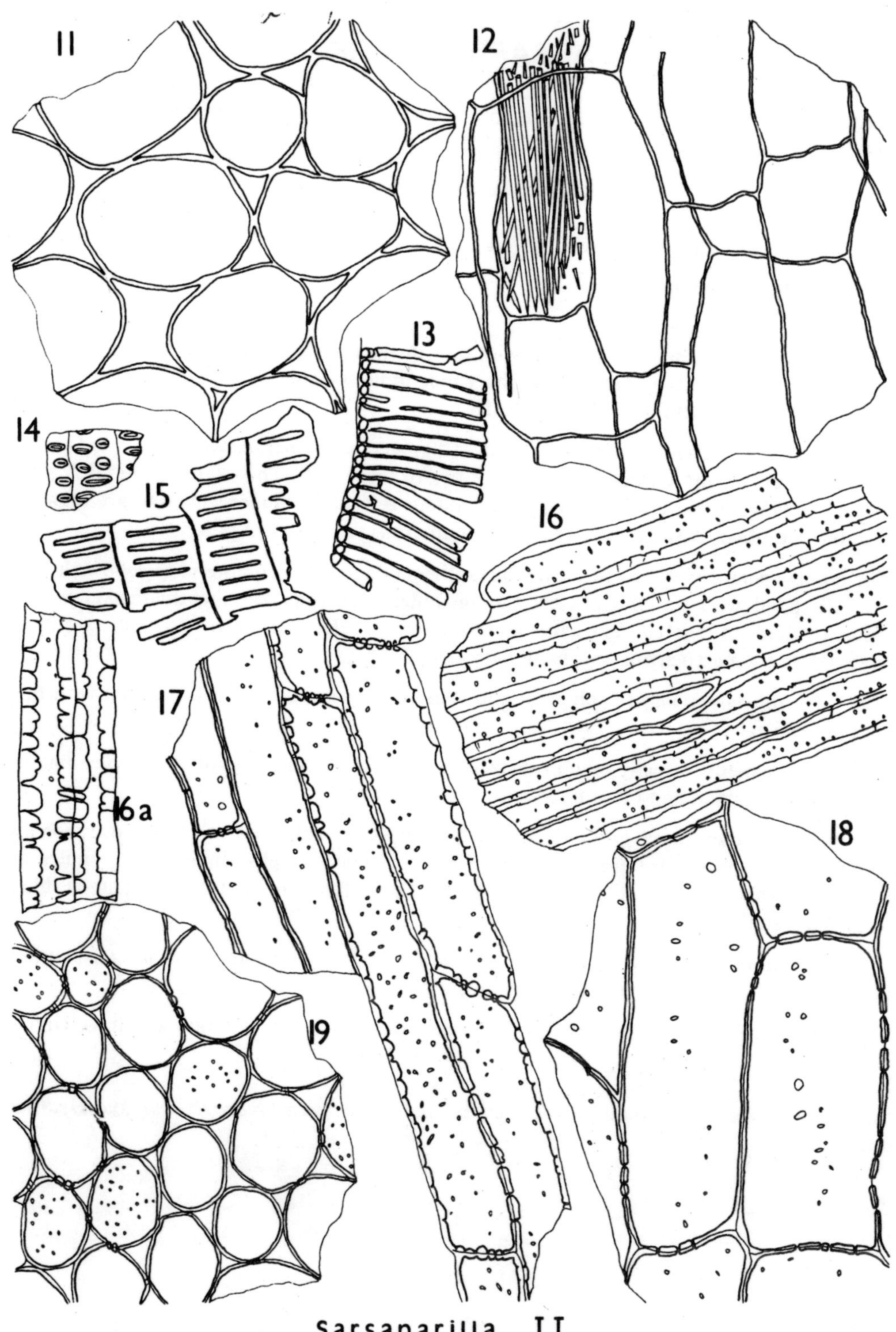

Sarsaparilla II

×33(

11 Parenchyma of the cortex in transverse section.
12 Parenchyma of the cortex in longitudinal view showing a bundle of acicular crystals of calcium oxalate in one of the cells.
13 Part of a reticulately thickened vessel.
14 Fragment of a bordered pitted vessel.
15 Part of a scalariformly thickened vessel.
16 Part of a group of fibrous cells.
16a Part of a group of thicker-walled fibrous cells
17 Xylem parenchyma in longitudinal view.
18 Parenchyma of the pith in longitudinal view.
19 Parenchyma of the pith in transverse section.

SASSAFRAS BARK

Sassafras albidum (Nutt.) Nees (*Sassafras officinale* Nees and Eberm.) and *Sassafras variifolium* (Salisb.) O. Kuntze Lauraceae

Sassafras, Sassafras Root Bark

A light brown powder with a characteristic, aromatic odour and taste.

The diagnostic characters are:

(*a*) The abundant large *fibres* which occur singly or, very occasionally, in groups of two or three; the walls are much thickened and lignified with few, distinct pits and a narrow lumen. Several of the fibres have forked ends and many also show indentations on the side walls corresponding to the outlines of the adjacent medullary ray cells.

(*b*) The occasional *sclereids* and more abundant lignified *pitted parenchymatous cells*, both of which occur singly or, more rarely, in groups of two or three cells. The sclereids are fairly thick-walled and rectangular in outline; the parenchymatous cells have thinner walls and are square to rectangular in outline; both types of cells have numerous well-marked pits.

(*c*) The *phloem parenchyma* and *medullary rays*; the parenchyma is composed of yellowish, thin-walled cells filled with starch granules; the medullary ray cells are slightly thicker walled. Occasional strands of *crushed sieve tissue (ceratenchyma)*, yellowish-brown in colour, are found associated with the parenchyma and medullary rays.

(*d*) The large *oil cells*, ovoid to spherical and thin-walled, usually found associated with thin-walled parenchyma.

(*e*) The *cork* fragments, usually seen in surface view when the cells are polygonal to elongated, thin-walled and lignified and often filled with brown contents.

(*f*) The fairly abundant *starch granules*, simple or compound with two to three or, occasionally, four components, found scattered and in the parenchymatous cells. Individual granules are spherical to polyhedral and many show a central point or cleft hilum; faint striations are visible in some of the granules.

(*g*) The *calcium oxalate crystals*, which are not very abundant; they are small, *acicular* and are found in some of the parenchymatous cells of the phloem.

(*h*) The very infrequent *vessels* from the adherent wood; they are lignified and have circular bordered pits.

The powder gives an immediate, overall cherry-red colour with *Phloroglucinol and Hydrochloric Acid*.

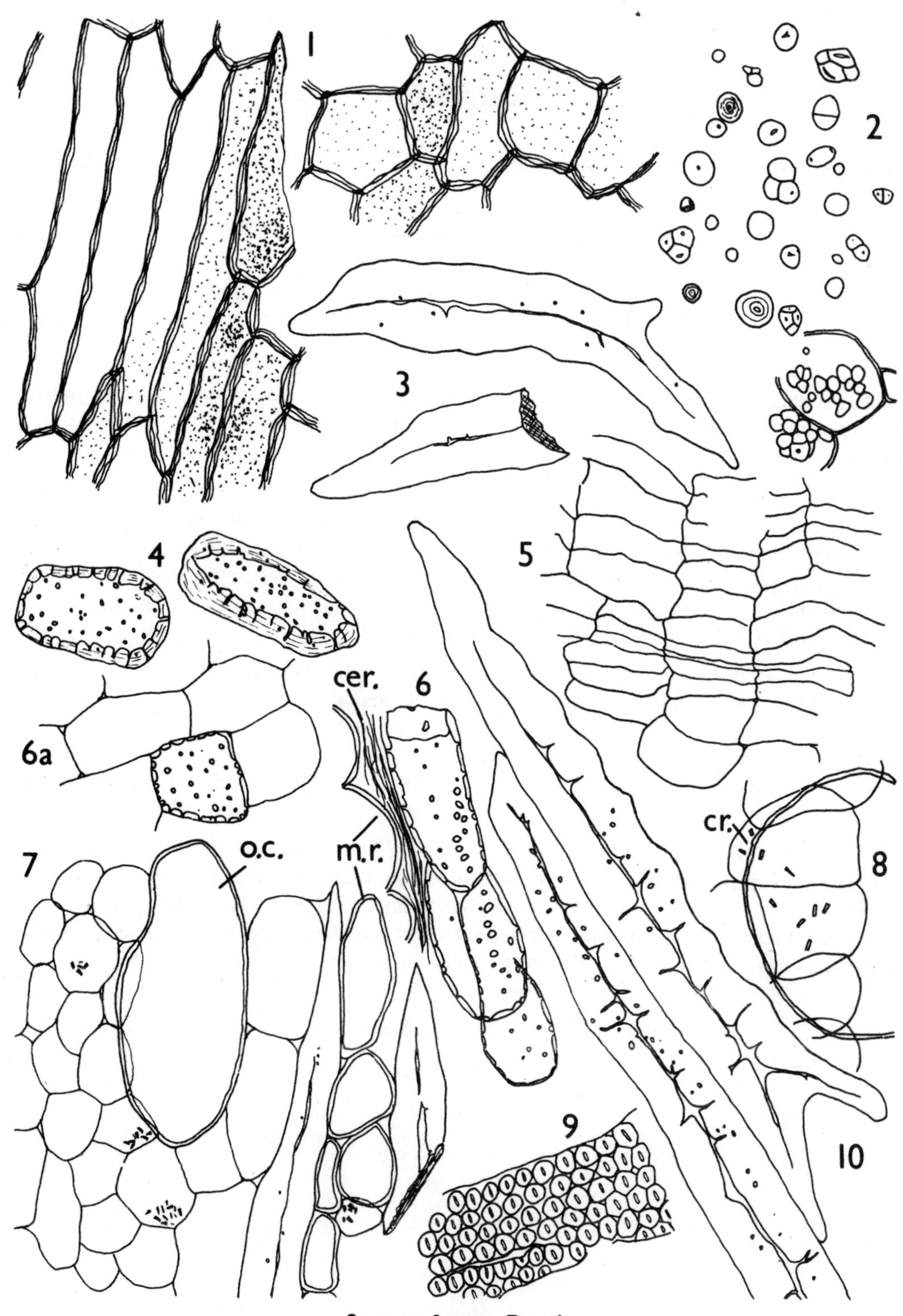

Sassafras Bark

×330

1 Cork in surface view.
2 Starch granules, some contained in parenchyma.
3 Short fibre with a forked end and part of another fibre.
4 Sclereids.
5 Cork, phellogen and phelloderm in sectional view.
6 Pitted parenchyma with ceratenchyma (cer.) and part of a medullary ray (m.r.).
6a A single pitted parenchymatous cell with unlignified parenchyma.
7 Part of the phloem in tangential longitudinal section showing parenchyma containing acicular crystals of calcium oxalate, an oil cell (o.c.), parts of fibres and medullary ray cells (m.r.).
8 Parenchyma with acicular crystals of calcium oxalate (cr.) and part of an oil cell.
9 Fragment of a bordered pitted vessel.
10 Two typical fibres.

SENEGA

Polygala senega L. or certain closely related spp. of *Polygala* — Polygalaceae

Seneca Snakeroot, Senega Root

A pale grey to brown powder with a characteristic, somewhat aromatic odour reminiscent of wintergreen and a taste which is sweet at first, then becoming bitter and acrid; it is very irritant to mucous membranes.

The diagnostic characters are:

(*a*) The very abundant *parenchyma* containing globules of fixed oil; the cells vary in size and have slightly thickened walls. In transverse sectional view the cells are rounded to oval and have triangular or rectangular intercellular spaces; in longitudinal view they are elongated and frequently taper at the ends.

(*b*) The fragments of yellowish-brown *cork* composed of thin-walled cells, many of which have brown granular contents; the majority of the cells are elongated rectangular in surface view but occasional fragments occur from the crown of the root in which the cells are polygonal and more or less isodiametric in surface view. Fragments of the cork are also frequently found in sectional view, composed of from four to eight or more layers of cells.

(*c*) The *vessels* and *tracheids*, which are usually found in groups; they are lignified, and the larger vessels show reticulate thickening; the smaller vessels and the tracheids have numerous slit-shaped pits and some of the vessels show oval perforations in the lateral walls. A small amount of lignified *xylem parenchyma* is found, usually associated with the groups of vessels and tracheids; the cells are elongated in longitudinal view and have moderately thickened walls with numerous pits.

(*d*) The occasional fragments of the *scale leaves in surface view*; these are frequently purplish in colour. The epidermis is composed of large cells with thin, sinuous walls and they may show faint cuticular striations; *anomocytic stomata* occur very rarely. Fragments from the margins of the leaves are composed of smaller, straight-walled cells and they show the presence of small, unicellular *covering trichomes* with moderately thickened and striated walls; these trichomes are also occasionally found scattered in the powder.

(*e*) The fragments of *sieve tissue* composed of very thin-walled longitudinally elongated cells, with occasional sieve plates visible on the end walls.

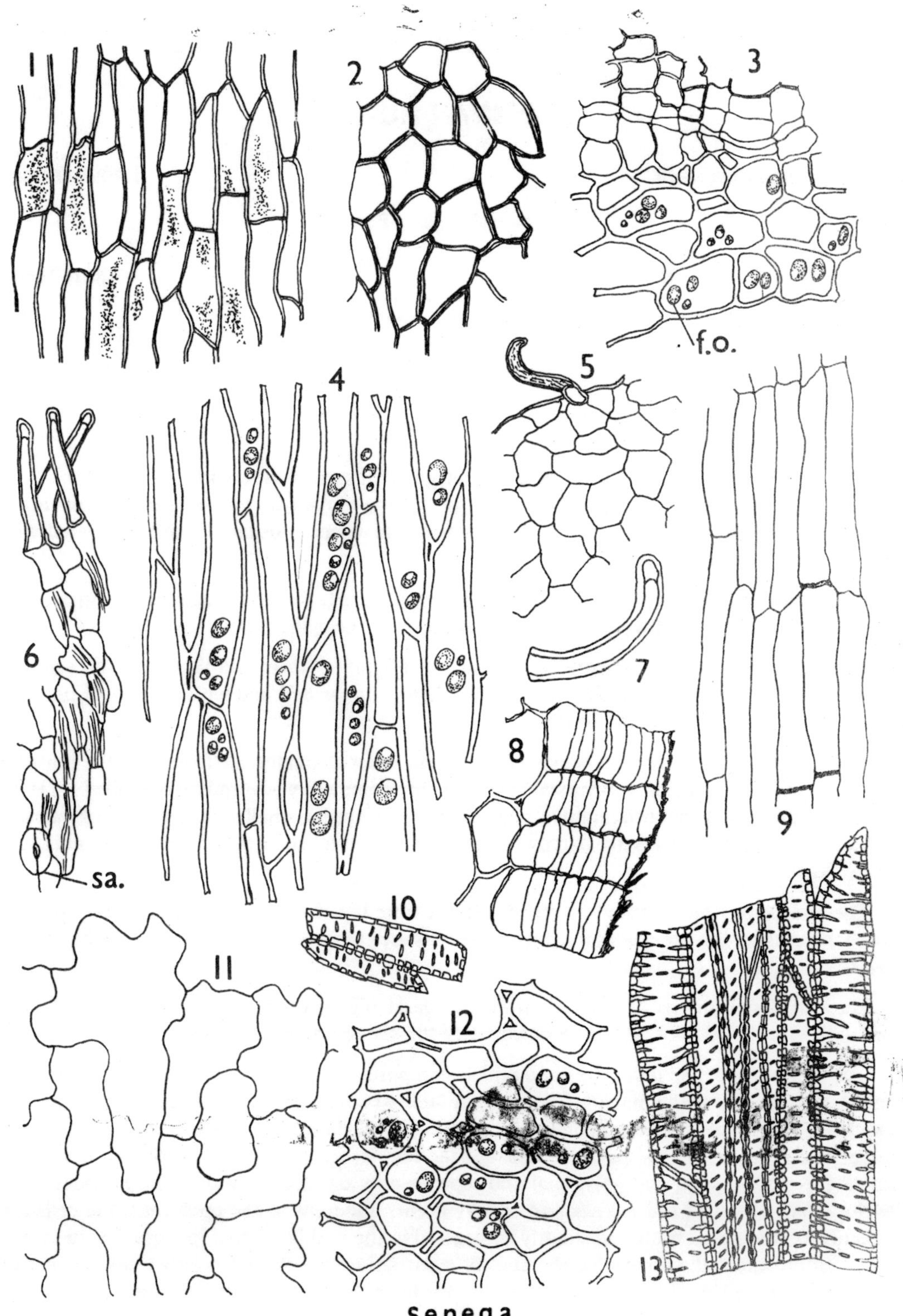

Senega

×330

1 Cork in surface view showing granular material in some of the cells.
2 Cork from the crown of the root in surface view.
3 Part of the cork and phelloderm in sectional view with globules of fixed oil (f.o.) in the cells of the phelloderm.
4 Parenchyma in longitudinal view.
5 Fragment of the epidermis of the scale leaves in surface view with an attached trichome.
6 Fragment of the epidermis from the margin of a scale leaf in surface view showing cuticular striations, a stoma (sa.) and attached trichomes.
7 A detached trichome.
8 Cork in sectional view.
9 Sieve tissue in longitudinal view.
10 Xylem parenchyma in longitudinal view.
11 Epidermis of the scale leaves in surface view.
12 Parenchyma in transverse section.
13 Part of a group of vessels and tracheids.

SENNA FRUIT

Cassia angustifolia Vahl. Leguminosae

Tinnevelly Senna Pod

Cassia senna L. Leguminosae

Alexandrian Senna Pod

A brown to greenish-brown powder with a faint odour and a mucilaginous, somewhat bitter and unpleasant taste.

The diagnostic characters are:

(*a*) The *epicarp* composed of a layer of cells, polygonal in surface view with thin walls which are sometimes slightly beaded. Very occasional *paracytic* or *anomocytic stomata* occur; fragments in sectional view show the presence of a thick *cuticle*. This layer is usually found associated with parenchyma of the hypodermis.

(*b*) The occasional *covering trichomes*, which occur scattered; they are unicellular, conical, with thick and distinctly warted walls and are sometimes bent near the base.

(*c*) The *parenchyma of the pericarp*, with associated lignified *fibres* and *vessels* of the vascular tissue which are not abundant. The fibres are narrow, thin-walled and with occasional pits; the vessels show annular thickening or irregularly arranged pits.

(*d*) The lignified *fibres of the mesocarp* which are the most characteristic feature of the powder; they are usually arranged in two crossed layers and are completely covered on one side by a layer of small, thin-walled parenchymatous cells each containing a small *prism crystal of calcium oxalate*. The individual fibres are narrow with moderately thickened walls, occasional pits and a distinct lumen.

(*e*) The *endocarp*, which is usually adherent to the fibre layers of the mesocarp on the opposite side to the calcium oxalate-containing layer; the cells are elongated in surface view and have thin, unlignified walls.

(*f*) The occasional groups of *sclereids* from the basal region of the fruit; individual cells are irregularly ovoid in outline and have moderately thickened and pitted walls.

(*g*) The fragments of the *testa*; the *epidermis* is composed of a layer of palisade cells which are conical, thick-walled with a narrow lumen at the base which tapers towards the apex; fragments in sectional view show the presence of a thick cuticle. In surface view, when viewed from above, the very small lumens of the palisade cells appear very irregular; when viewed from below the lumens are more regular and polygonal and separated by the thinner walls. The hypodermis is developed as a layer of *bearer cells* and usually occurs adherent to the epidermis; the cells are thickened on the radial walls and slightly contracted in the middle so that in surface view, when viewed from below, the lumens of the central constriction and those on either side appear as concentric rings; when viewed from above the pits in the walls are partially visible.

(*h*) The abundant fragments of the *cotyledons* composed of thin-walled parenchymatous cells differentiated into epidermis, palisade and spongy mesophyll, with a palisade layer under both epidermises.

(*i*) The occasional fibres, sclereids and parenchyma from the *pedicel*; the *fibres and sclereids* are larger than those occurring in the pericarp and part of a *calcium oxalate prism sheath* may be associated with the fibres; the parenchymatous cells have slightly thickened walls and frequently contain fairly large *cluster crystals of calcium oxalate* arranged in short vertical files. Some of these larger prisms and cluster crystals also occur scattered.

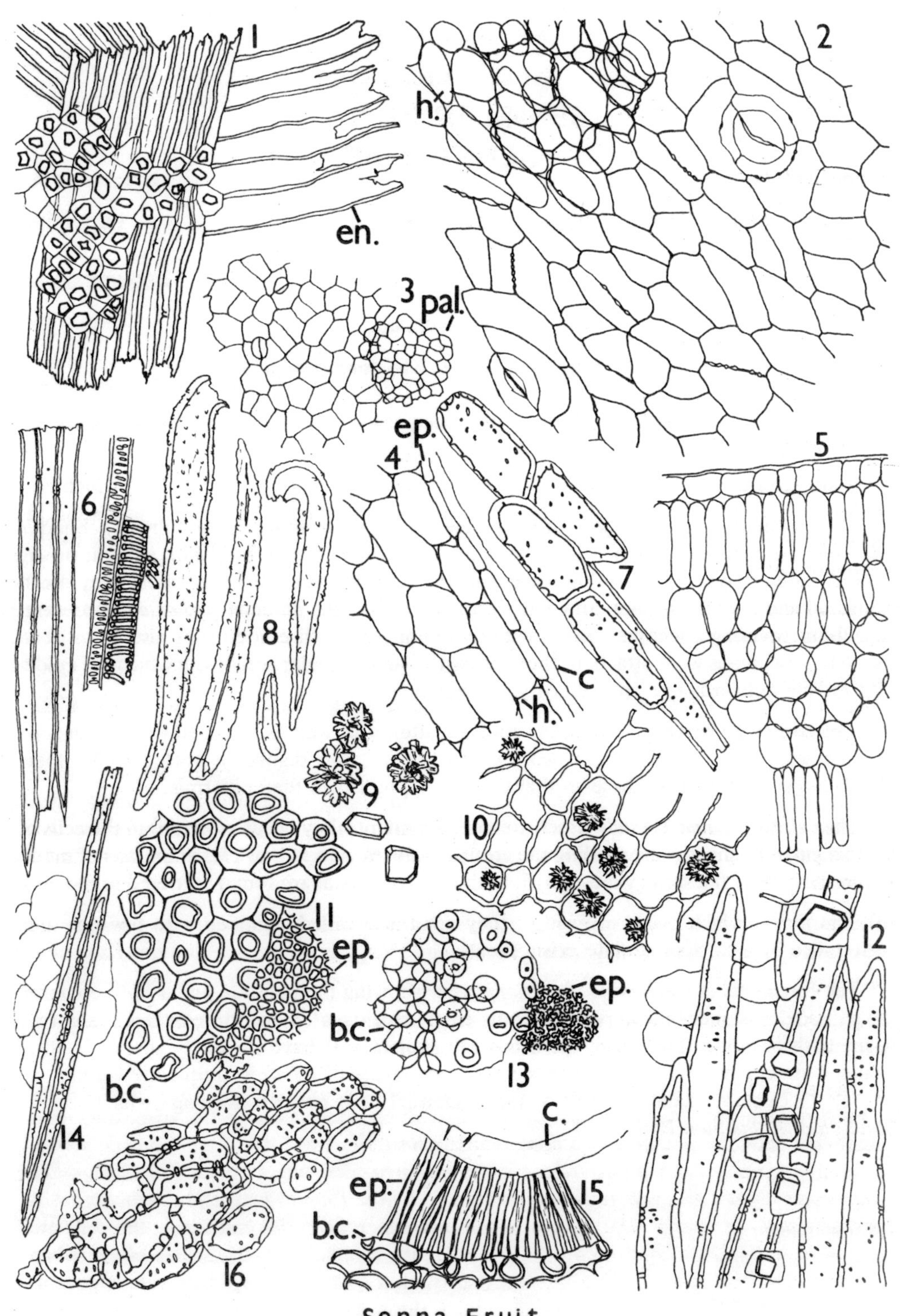

Senna Fruit

×330

1 Layers of fibres of the mesocarp in surface view with overlying parenchymatous cells containing prisms of calcium oxalate, and part of the underlying endocarp (en.).
2 Epicarp in surface view showing stomata and part of the underlying hypodermis (h.).
3 Epidermis and underlying palisade layer (pal.) of the cotyledon in surface view.
4 Outer part of the pericarp in sectional view showing cuticle (c.), epicarp (ep.) and parenchyma of the hypodermis (h.).
5 Part of a cotyledon in sectional view.
6 Fibres and vascular elements from the pericarp.
7 Sclereids and part of a fibre from the pedicel.
8 Covering trichomes.
9 Prisms and cluster crystals from the pedicel.
10 Parenchyma from the pedicel containing cluster crystals of calcium oxalate.
11 Part of the testa in surface view showing the bearer cells (b.c.) seen from below, with underlying palisade cells of the epidermis (ep.).
12 Fibres with crystal sheath from the pedicel.
13 Part of the testa in surface view showing the palisade epidermis (ep.) and bearer cells (b.c.) in two planes of focus.
14 Fibres and parenchyma of the pericarp.
15 Part of the testa in sectional view showing the cuticle (c.), the palisade epidermis (ep.) and the underlying layer of bearer cells (b.c.).
16 A group of sclereids from the base of the fruit.

SENNA LEAF

Cassia angustifolia Vahl. Leguminosae

Tinnevelly Senna Leaves

Cassia senna L. Leguminosae

Alexandrian Senna Leaves, Khartoum Senna Leaves

A greyish-green or yellowish-green powder with a faint, characteristic odour and a mucilaginous, slightly bitter taste.

The diagnostic characters are:

(*a*) The fragments of the *lamina in surface view*. The leaf is isobilateral and the *upper* and *lower epidermises* are similar in appearance; they are composed of cells with thin, straight or slightly sinuous walls, polygonal in outline except in the regions over the veins where they are more elongated and may show faint cuticular striations. Numerous *paracytic stomata* are present and unicellular covering trichomes are also fairly abundant. Both epidermises also have *cicatrices* where the trichomes were attached; these consist of small circular scars from which the epidermal cells radiate outwards in a characteristic arrangement.

(*b*) The *covering trichomes*, which are found scattered as well as attached to fragments of the epidermises; they are unicellular, conical, with thick and distinctly warted walls; they are sometimes curved near the base so that they lie appressed to the epidermis.

(*c*) The *calcium oxalate crystals* which are very abundant; they occur as *prisms* in the cells of the parenchymatous sheath surrounding the groups of fibres, and also as *cluster crystals* of moderate size in the cells of the spongy mesophyll; both types of crystal are found scattered in the powder.

(*d*) The *fibres*, which occur in groups; they are thick-walled, lignified with few pits and are surrounded by a calcium oxalate prism sheath.

(*e*) The fragments of the *lamina in sectional view* showing the palisade under both epidermises; the palisade cells under the upper epidermis are much elongated and more or less straight-walled whereas those under the lower epidermis are shorter and have distinctly sinuous walls. The rounded spongy mesophyll cells between the two layers of palisade frequently contain cluster crystals of calcium oxalate. Many of the epidermal cells contain mucilage which stains with *Solution of Ruthenium Red*.

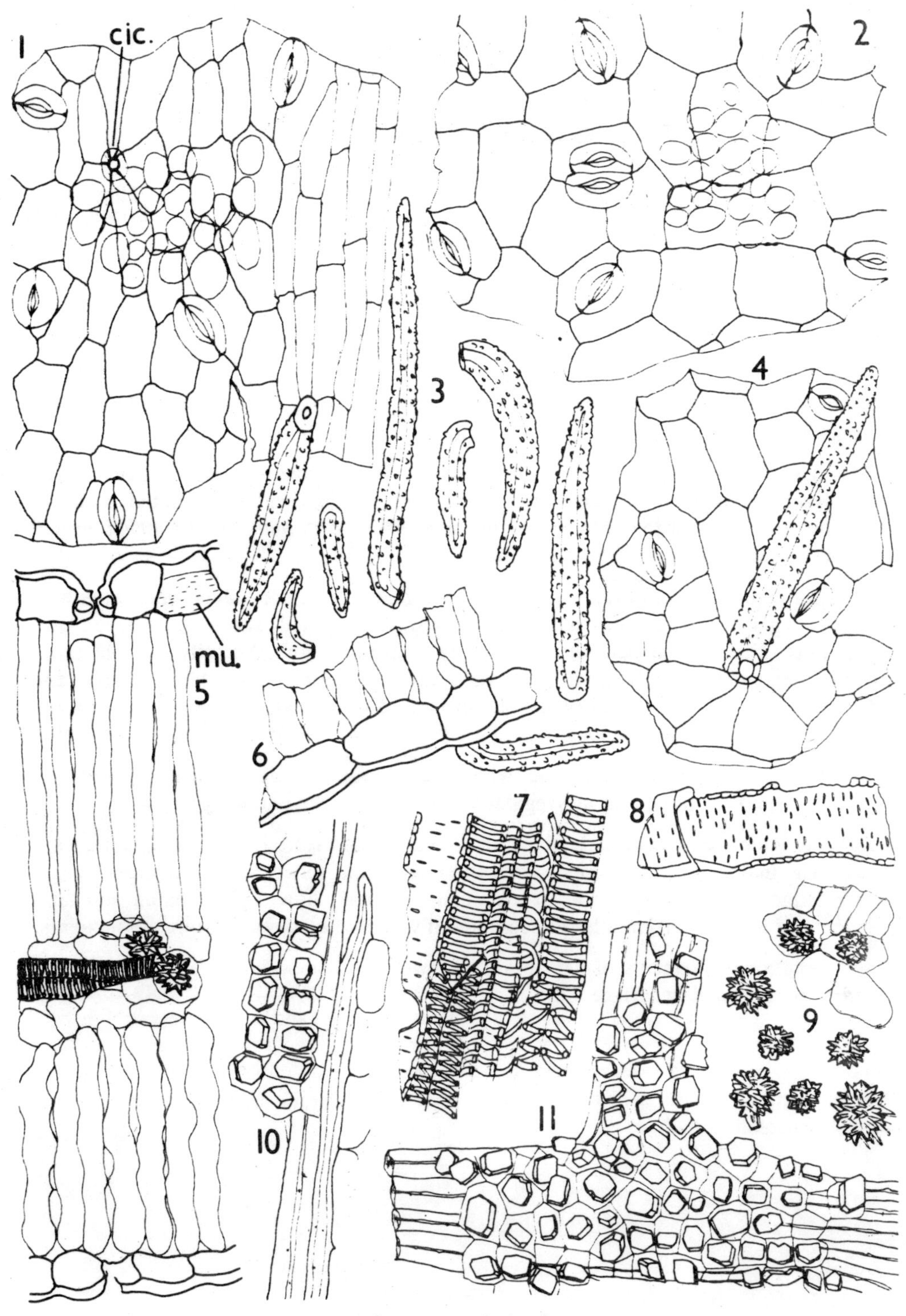

Senna Leaf

×330

1 Epidermis in surface view showing paracytic stomata, a cicatrix (cic.), underlying palisade cells and the elongated cells over a vein with striated cuticle and an attached trichome.

2 Epidermis in surface view showing paracytic stomata and underlying palisade cells.

3 Covering trichomes.

4 Epidermis in surface view with paracytic stomata and an attached trichome.

5 Part of the lamina in sectional view showing the upper epidermis containing mucilage (mu.), the upper and lower palisade, spongy mesophyll cells containing cluster crystals of calcium oxalate and the lower epidermis.

6 Part of the lamina in sectional view with a trichome attached to the lower epidermis.

7 Xylem elements from one of the larger veins.

8 Part of a pitted vessel from one of the larger veins.

9 Cluster crystals of calcium oxalate.

10 Part of a group of fibres with calcium oxalate prism sheath.

11 Groups of fibres with calcium oxalate prism sheaths at the junction of two small veins.

SLIPPERY ELM

Ulmus rubra Muhl. (*Ulmus fulva* Michaux) Ulmaceae

Slippery Elm Bark

A pale buff powder with a characteristic, spicy odour and a mucilaginous taste.

The diagnostic characters are:

(*a*) The very abundant *fibres*, which generally occur in groups and are frequently broken; individual fibres are twisted and irregular in outline with blunt ends and an uneven lumen; the walls are thick but only the middle lamella and primary wall are lignified.

(*b*) The abundant *mucilage*, which occurs as large masses, in mucilage cells or as fragments. The mucilage cells occur singly or adhering in groups and are frequently associated with the parenchyma or sieve tubes of the phloem; the mucilage stains with *Solution of Ruthenium Red* and sometimes shows distinct concentric lamellations.

(*c*) The numerous fragments of *sieve tissue* composed of fairly large, thin-walled sieve tubes with sieve areas forming a coarse network on the side walls and occasionally showing the sieve plates on the end walls. The phloem parenchyma is fairly thin-walled and the cells are sometimes unevenly thickened and have small swellings on the walls; these cells contain starch granules and prisms of calcium oxalate. The *medullary rays* are also found associated with the parenchyma and the sieve tubes, usually in tangential longitudinal section; they are composed of thin-walled cells.

(*d*) The abundant *prisms of calcium oxalate*, which vary in size and are frequently quite large. The crystals are found scattered and in irregular vertical files in the parenchyma.

(*e*) The *starch granules*, which are fairly abundant and are found scattered and in the parenchymatous cells. The majority of the granules are rather small and spherical but occasional larger granules are found which are spherical to lenticular and may show a point hilum and faint striations; some of the smaller granules are compound with two or three or more components.

(*f*) The very occasional fragments of dark orange-brown *cork* composed of fairly thick-walled cells, rounded to polygonal in surface view.

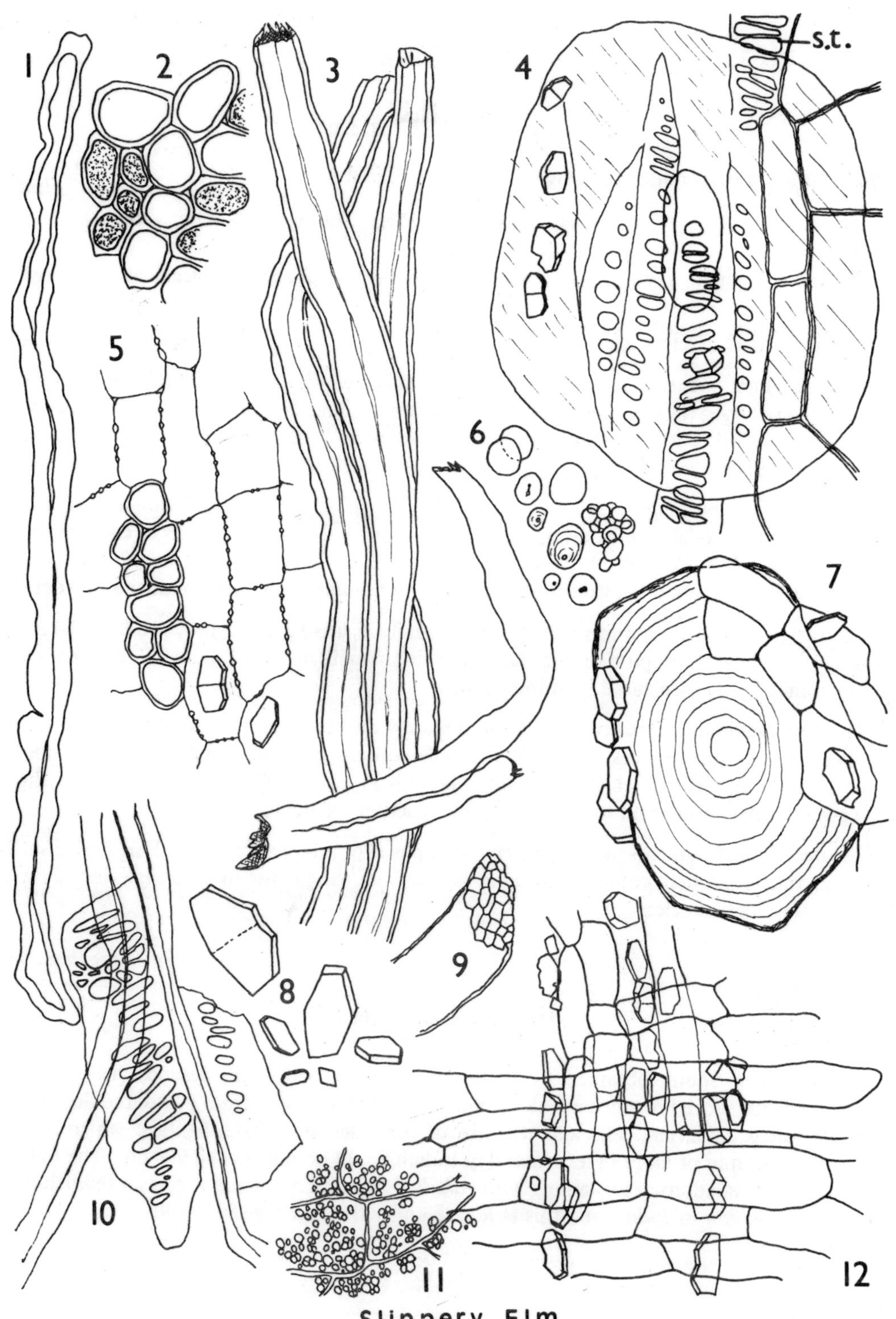

Slippery Elm

×330

1 A single fibre.
2 Cork in surface view.
3 Part of a group of fibres.
4 A mass of mucilage (as seen in a Cloral Hydrate mount), with underlying sieve tubes (s.t.), phloem parenchyma and calcium oxalate prisms.
5 A medullary ray and phloem parenchyma in tangential longitudinal section.
6 Larger starch granules.
7 A mucilage cell (as seen in a Ruthenium Red mount) showing the lamellations in the mucilage, with adhering parenchyma and calcium oxalate prisms.
8 Prisms of calcium oxalate.
9 Part of a sieve tube showing a sieve plate in surface view.
10 Sieve tubes showing sieve areas on the side walls, and adjacent fibres.
11 Parenchyma containing small starch granules.
12 Part of the phloem showing phloem parenchymatous cells containing prisms of calcium oxalate and part of a medullary ray in radial longitudinal section.

SQUILL

Drimia maritima (L.) Stearn [Urginea maritima (L.) Baker] Liliaceae

Scilla, Squill Bulb, White Squill

An off-white to pale buff, very hygroscopic powder with a slight odour and a mucilaginous, intensely bitter and acrid taste.

The diagnostic characters are:

(*a*) The very abundant *acicular crystals of calcium oxalate* which vary considerably in size and are frequently very large; they occur in bundles embedded in mucilage in the parenchymatous cells and are also found scattered throughout the powder in broken groups or as single, much fragmented crystals.

(*b*) The abundant *mucilage cells*, some of which are intact and contain bundles of acicular crystals of calcium oxalate whilst others are broken open and show fragments of calcium oxalate crystals or the impressions left by them; the mucilage stains with *Alkaline Solution of Corallin*. Irregularly shaped fragments of mucilage are also found scattered throughout the powder.

(*c*) The *vessels*, which are found singly or more usually in small groups; they are fairly large with lignified walls which have spiral or annular thickening. Small groups of thin-walled *phloem tissue* are sometimes found associated with the vessels.

(*d*) The very abundant *parenchyma* composed mainly of thin-walled rounded to elongated cells with small intercellular spaces; many of the cells contain spheroidal masses of fine radiating needle crystals of *sinistrin* which are pale yellowish in colour. Occasional groups of slightly thicker-walled cells occur and these give a faint reaction for lignin.

(*e*) The occasional fragments of the *epidermis* composed of thin-walled cells, elongated in surface view with very infrequent rounded, *anomocytic stomata*; fragments in sectional view show the presence of a thick cuticle.

INDIAN SQUILL

Powdered Indian Squill, obtained from *Drimia indica* (Roxb.) J.P. Jessop, (*Urginea indica* Kunth) is slightly more brownish in colour and can be distinguished from powdered Squill by the more elongated epidermal cells and the size of the calcium oxalate crystals, which in Squill measure up to 1 mm or more in length and in Indian Squill do not exceed 900 μm. The mucilage in Indian Squill, in addition to staining with *Alkaline Solution of Corallin*, gives a reddish-purple colour with *Solution of Iodine* and this is not given by the mucilage in Squill.

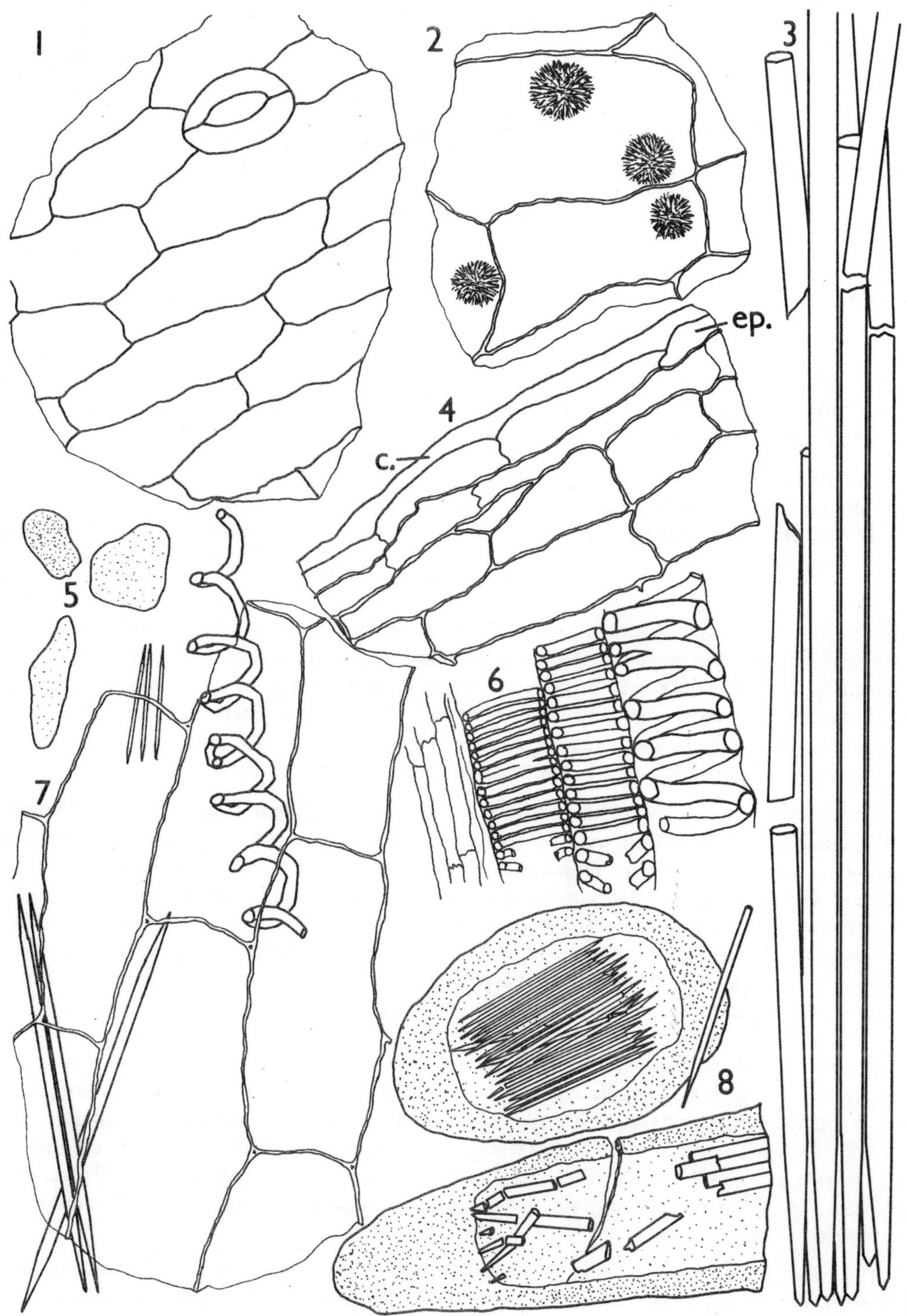

Squill

×330

1 Epidermis in surface view showing a stoma.
2 Parenchymatous cells containing spheroidal masses of sinistrin.
3 Part of a group of very large acicular crystals of calcium oxalate.
4 Cuticle (c.), epidermis (ep.) and parenchyma in sectional view.
5 Fragments of mucilage.
6 Fragments of vessels with spiral and annular thickening associated with thin-walled phloem tissue.
7 Parenchyma with associated acicular crystals of calcium oxalate and a fragment of a spirally thickened vessel.
8 Mucilage cells containing acicular crystals of calcium oxalate.

STAR ANISE

Illicium verum Hook. *f.* *Magnoliaceae*

Star Anise Fruits

A dark, reddish-brown powder with an aromatic, characteristic odour and a sweet, warming and characteristic taste.

The diagnostic characters are:

(*a*) The fragments of the *epicarp* in surface view composed of irregular, brown, polygonal cells with slightly thickened walls which may show occasional beading; large, circular, *anomocytic stomata* are fairly frequent and the cuticle shows well marked irregular striations.

(*b*) The columnar cells of the *endocarp*, which are usually seen in sectional view. They are very large and are found in small groups but the individual cells are frequently broken; the walls are slightly thickened and lignified with a few, slit-shaped pits and are mainly colourless, although brown pigment is present in the end walls; some of the cells contain a few small, scattered prisms.

(*c*) The *outer epidermis of the testa*, which is very characteristic. It consists of a single layer of radially elongated cells with thick, striated, lignified walls with numerous irregular, frequently branched pits; the inner tangential wall is usually not thickened; the lumen is small and irregular and usually filled with dark brown pigment. When seen in surface view the cells are polygonal and, if viewed from above, the walls are sinuous and the lumen appears much branched due to the abundant pitting in the outer region; on focusing down the walls become almost straight and the lumen appears smaller and less markedly irregular.

(*d*) The very abundant *sclereids* which show considerable variation in size, shape and the degree of thickening and pitting of the walls. The sclereids of the pedicel and mesocarp are very large and usually are found singly or embedded in unlignified parenchyma; they may be markedly branched with finger-like projections or may have shorter, sharply pointed projections; others are relatively smooth in outline; the walls are usually heavily thickened, striated and have few pits; many of these cells contain brown pigment. Other sclereids of the mesocarp are found in groups but are frequently broken; these also are very large and they are much elongated, forming *fibrous sclereids*; the walls are heavily thickened and striated and have numerous simple pits. The *inner sclerenchymatous layer of the testa* is composed of two or more rows of brownish cells which, in surface view, are irregularly elongated-rectangular and show irregular intercellular spaces; they are fairly large but the walls are only moderately thickened and striated; pits are present and, in surface view, these frequently are seen in an approximately circular arrangement. Other types of sclereids are also present in the testa near the hilar region; these generally are found in small groups and may be fairly small and rounded, with moderately thickened walls and fairly numerous pits, or larger with only slightly thickened walls and few pits; some of the larger cells may contain scattered prisms.

(*e*) The *parenchyma of the mesocarp* composed of brown, irregular cells with slightly thickened somewhat uneven walls and small intercellular spaces; some of the cells may contain small prisms. Embedded in the parenchyma are large spherical, thin-walled *oil cells*.

(*f*) The inner *epidermis of the testa* composed of a single layer of thin-walled parenchymatous cells which in surface view are elongated-rectangular and fairly regular; the walls may show slight beading. These cells contain numerous *rhomboidal to rectangular tabular crystals of calcium oxalate*, which vary in size but are frequently quite large; these crystals are also found scattered in the powder.

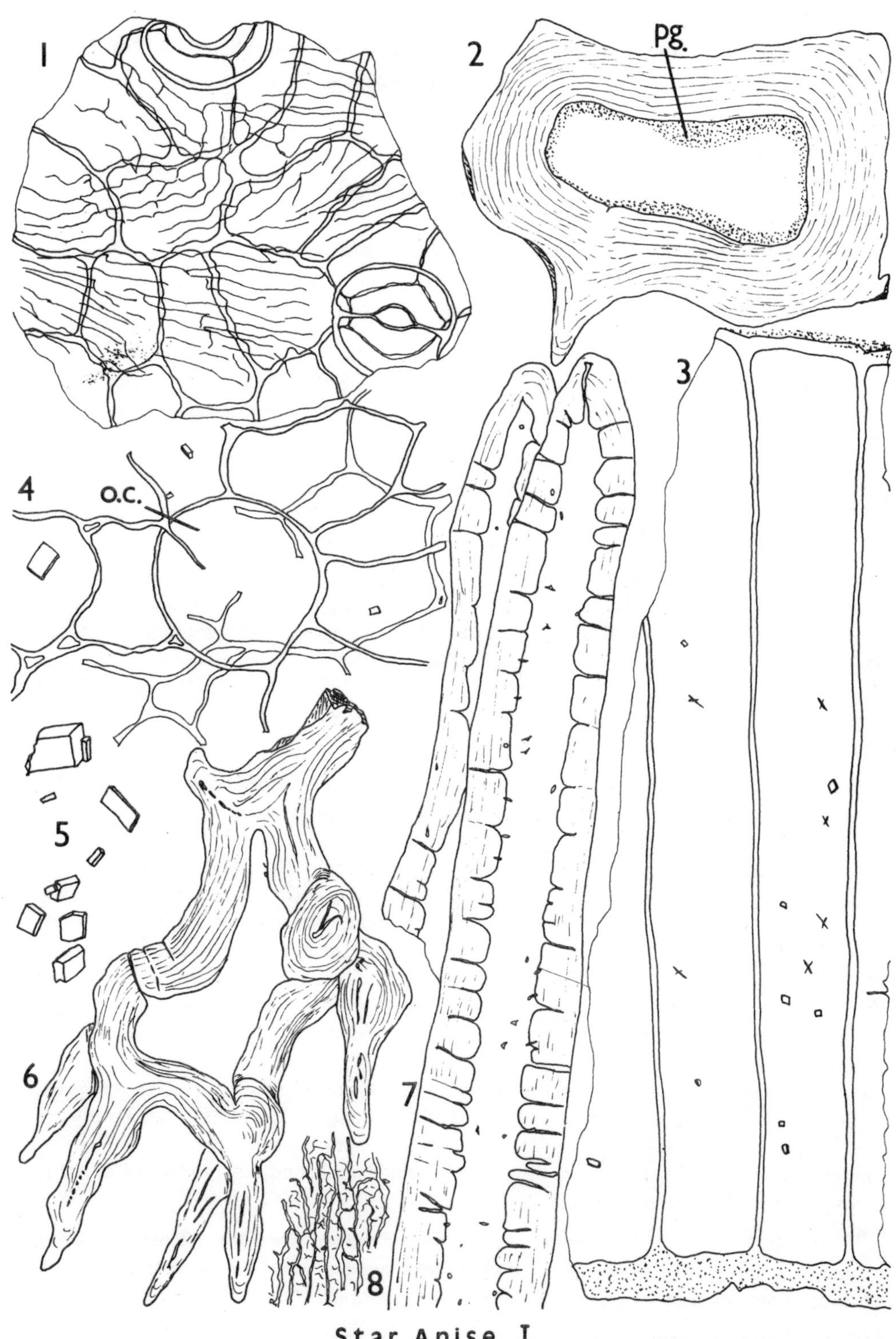

Star Anise I

×330

1 Epicarp in surface view showing stomata and straited cuticle.

2 An isolated sclereid from the pedicel or mesocarp, containing pigment (pg.).

3 Cells of the endocarp in sectional view showing pigment in the end walls.

4 Parenchyma of the mesocarp with an oil cell (o.c.).

5 Tabular crystals of calcium oxalate.

6 An isolated sclereid from the pedicel or mesocarp.

7 Fibrous sclereids from the mesocarp.

8 A fragment of cuticle from the epicarp.

(*g*) The fragments of the *endosperm* composed of colourless, polygonal cells with slightly thickened walls.

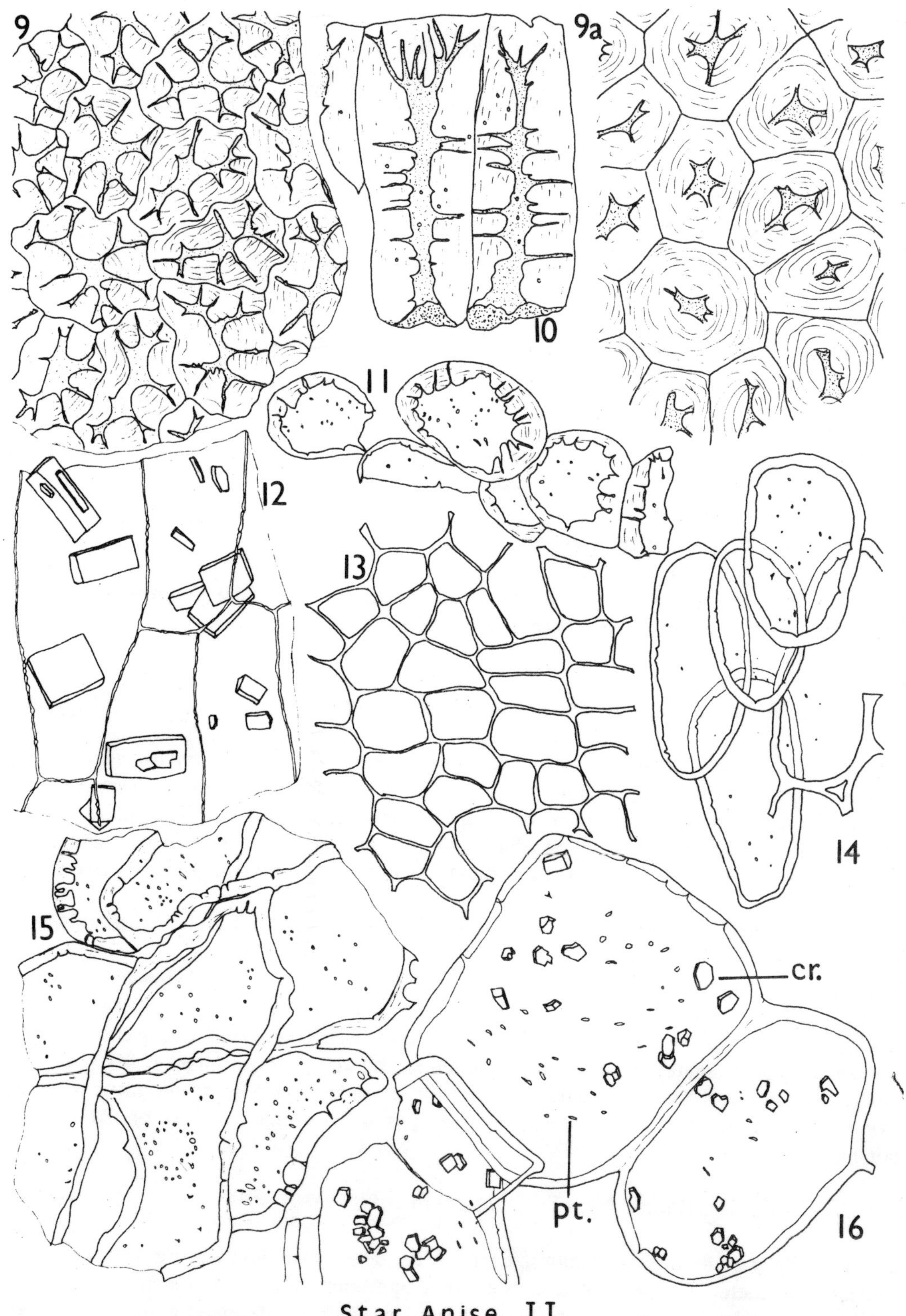

Star Anise II

×330

9 Outer epidermis of the testa in surface view, seen from above.
9a As 9, but focused down to a lower level.
10 Outer epidermis of the testa in sectional view.
11 Sclereids from the hilar region of the testa.
12 Inner epidermis of the testa in surface view showing cells containing tabular crystals of calcium oxalate.
13 Parenchyma of the endosperm.
14 Sclereids from the hilar region of the testa.
15 Inner sclerenchymatous layers of the testa.
16 Sclereids from the hilar region of the testa showing crystals (cr.) and pits (pt.).

STARCHES

White to pale creamish or greyish-white powders or irregular masses which crepitate when crushed; odourless and almost tasteless.

MAIZE STARCH obtained from *Zea mays* L. — Gramineae

Simple granules, approximately 5 to 30 μm in diameter, polyhedral to subspherical with a central hilum occurring as an irregular split or, more usually, as a cleft with three to five rays. Striations are not visible. (*Synonym*: Corn Starch.)

MARANTA STARCH obtained from *Maranta arundinacea* L. — Marantaceae

Simple granules, approximately 7 to 50 μm in length, irregularly ovoid to ellipsoidal and occasionally showing small tuberosities; the hilum is usually slit-shaped and is slightly eccentric, in ovoid granules being situated nearer the broader end. Fine concentric striations are visible in most granules. (*Synonym*: Arrowroot Starch.)

RICE STARCH obtained from *Oryza sativa* L. — Gramineae

Simple granules or aggregations from compound granules; individual granules are approximately 2 to 10 μm in diameter, polyhedral or subspherical. A small central point hilum is visible in a few of the granules; there are no striations. (*Synonym*: Rice Starch.)

POTATO STARCH obtained from *Solanum tuberosum* L. — Solanaceae

The granules are mostly simple with occasional compound granules having two or three components; they show great variation in size, the larger granules measuring up to approximately 100 μm in length. Individual granules are ovoid to subspherical and frequently show tuberosities; they have an eccentric point hilum which is situated near the narrower end in ovoid granules. Most of the granules show well-marked concentric striations. (*Synonym*: English Arrowroot.)

TAPIOCA STARCH obtained from *Manihot esculenta* Crantz — Euphorbiaceae

Single granules, many of which show one or more flattened surfaces indicating that they were originally parts of compound granules; some of the compound granules are still intact, with two or three components. A few rounded or subspherical simple granules also occur. Individual granules are approximately 5 to 30 μm in diameter. The large central hilum is linear or, more usually, an irregularly stellate cleft. Some of the granules show faint concentric striations. (*Synonyms*: Cassava Starch, Manihot or Manioc Starch, 'Brazilian' or 'Rio' or 'Para' Arrowroot.)

WHEAT STARCH obtained from *Triticum aestivum* L. — Gramineae

Mainly simple granules of two distinct size ranges; the larger granules measure approximately 25 to 45 μm in diameter and the smaller ones measure approximately 3 to 15 μm in diameter; a few granules intermediate in size are also found. A small number of compound granules with two or three components are also present. Individual granules are lenticular and they appear oval, circular or biconvex in outline, depending on their orientation. The central point hilum appears as a line when the granules are seen in edge view. Faint concentric striations are visible in some of the larger granules.

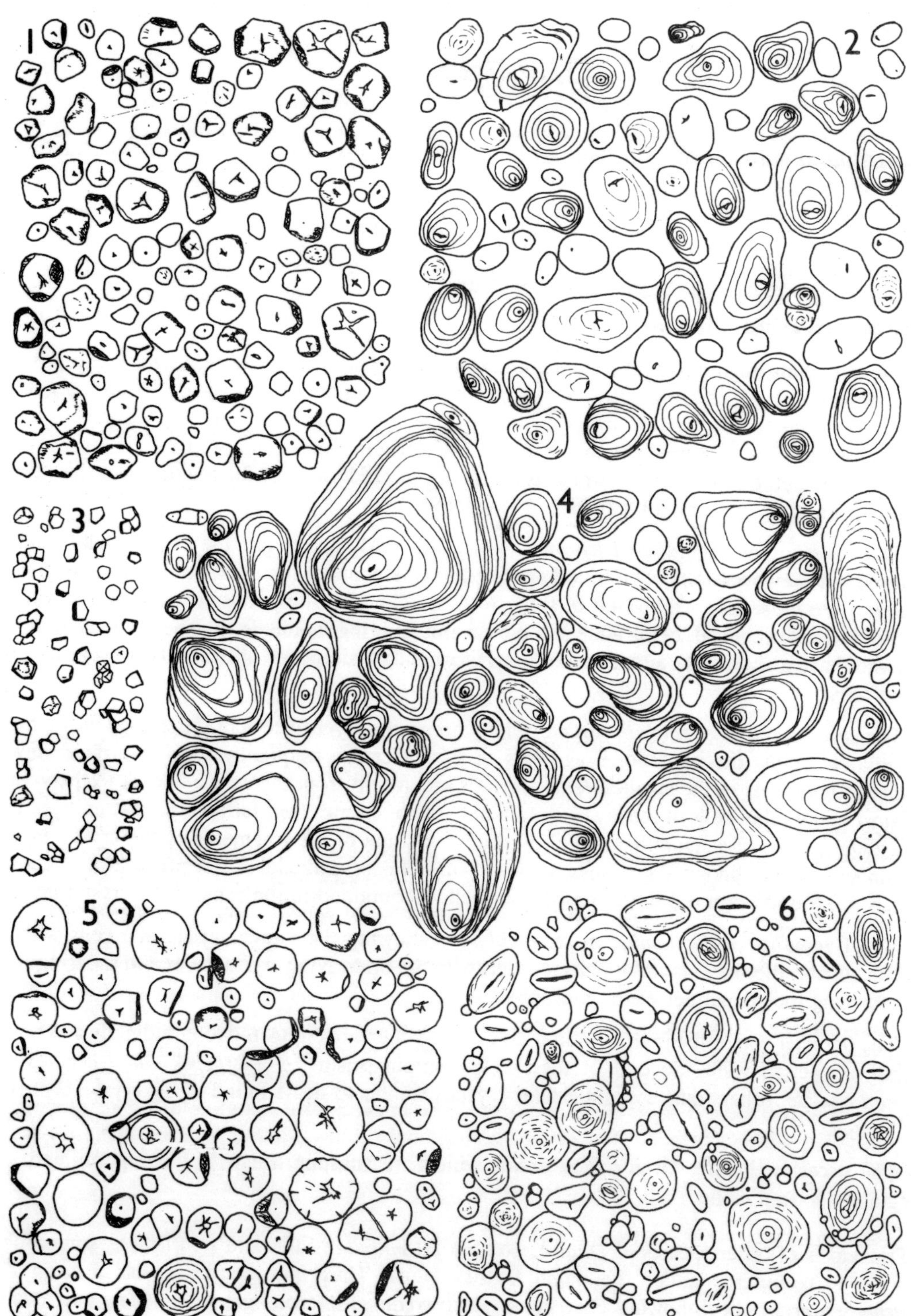

Starches

×330

1 Maize starch granules.
2 Maranta starch granules.
3 Rice starch granules.
4 Potato starch granules.
5 Tapioca starch granules.
6 Wheat starch granules.

STRAMONIUM

Datura stramonium L. and *Datura stramonium* var. *tatula* (L.) Torr. — Solanaceae

Stramonium Leaf, Thornapple Leaf

A greyish-green powder with a slight odour and a bitter taste.

The diagnostic characters are:

(*a*) The abundant fragments of the *leaf lamina in surface view*. The *upper epidermis* is composed of thin-walled cells which are slightly sinuous in outline; the underlying palisade cells are irregular in size and rather loosely packed. The cells of the *lower epidermis* have markedly wavy walls and may occasionally show very slight thickening at the corners. *Anisocytic stomata* are present on both surfaces, being rather more numerous on the lower epidermis. In the regions over the veins the epidermal cells are straight-walled and elongated.

(b) The *covering* and *glandular trichomes*, which are fairly abundant; they are usually found scattered but may occasionally be found attached to fragments of the epidermises. The covering trichomes are uniseriate, composed of three to four cells with thin, conspicuously warty walls; they are markedly conical, being wide at the base and tapering rapidly to the apex. The glandular trichomes have a short stalk and an ovoid to pyriform head composed of from four to seven thin-walled cells.

(*c*) The *cluster crystals of calcium oxalate*, which occur in a layer of cells in the spongy mesophyll immediately below the palisade. Fragments of this layer are frequently seen in surface view, attached to portions of the smaller veins; crystals are absent from the cells adjacent to the veins but most of the other cells of the layer contain one, or sometimes two, fairly large cluster crystals. Occasional *prisms* of calcium oxalate also occur and some of the fragments of the crystal layer contain somewhat abnormal crystals composed of a cluster embedded in a prism. All of these crystals are found scattered in the powder as well as contained in the cells of the crystal layer.

(*d*) The fragments of the *lamina in sectional view* showing the tabular epidermal cells with a smooth cuticle, the single layer of palisade cells with the underlying crystal layer and the irregular cells forming the remainder of the mesophyll.

(*e*) The *parenchyma* of the midrib composed of cells which are elongated longitudinally and have slightly thickened walls. Several of these cells contain prisms or *microsphenoidal crystals of calcium oxalate*; others may contain cluster crystals similar to those found in the crystal layer of the lamina.

(*f*) The occasional fairly large *pollen grains* which are subspherical with three pores and an irregularly warted exine.

The leaves of other species of *Datura*, notably *D. innoxia* Miller and *D. metel* L. sometimes occur in commerce under the name Datura Herb. They may be distinguished from *D. stramonium* by the following characters. *D. innoxia*: numerous glandular trichomes occur composed of a two- to four-celled uniseriate stalk and a unicellular, spherical head. The basal cell of the covering trichomes measures less than 50 μm in diameter; (in Stramonium the basal cell frequently measures up to 80 μm in diameter). *D. metel*: the basal cell of the covering trichomes rarely exceeds 35 μm in diameter. Irregular crystalline masses, sometimes of considerable size, occur in the mesophyll.

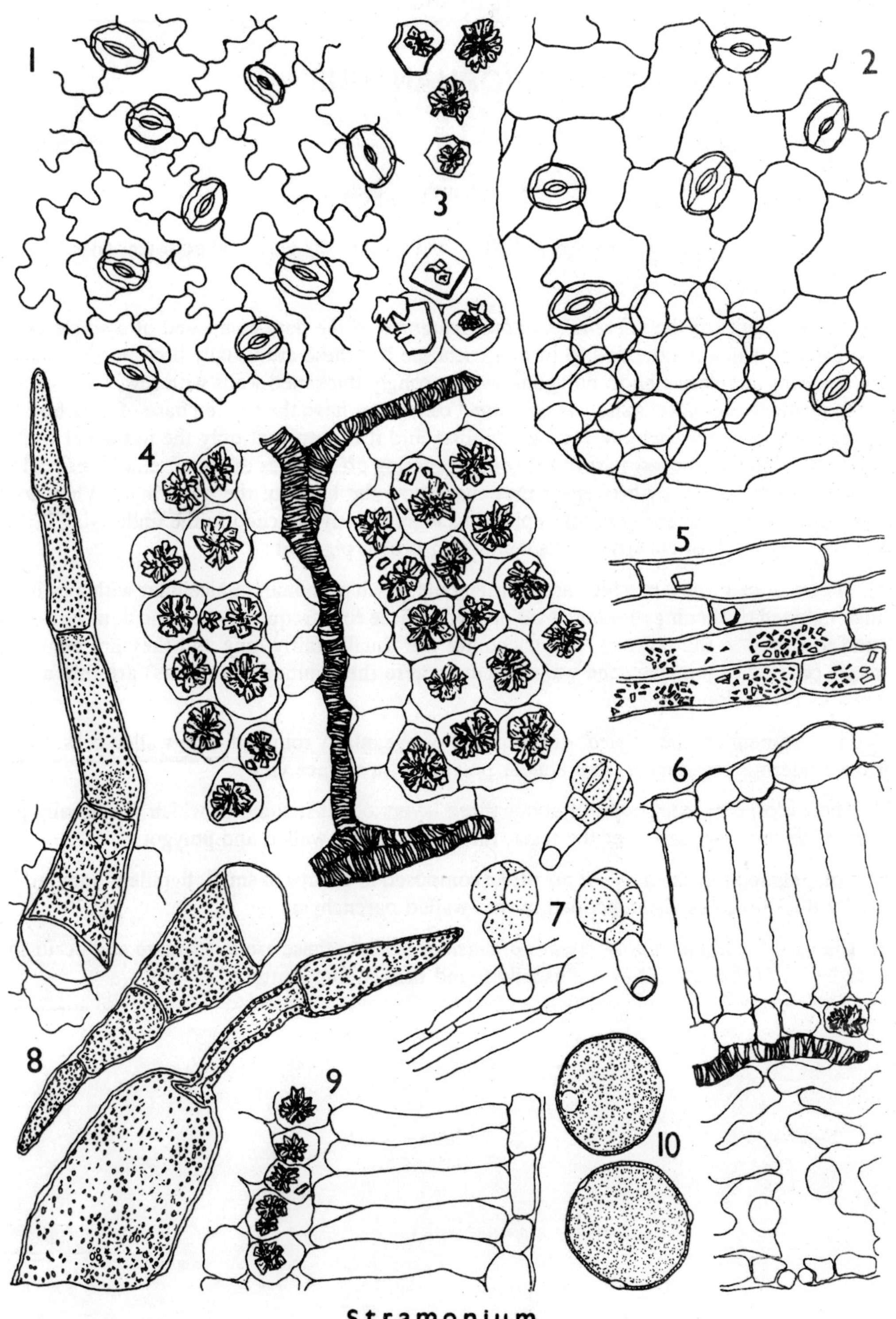

Stramonium

×330

1 Lower epidermis in surface view showing anisocytic stomata.
2 Upper epidermis in surface view showing anisocytic stomata and part of the underlying palisade.
3 Calcium oxalate crystals, some contained in the cells of the crystal layer.
4 A fragment of the crystal layer in surface view showing part of a vein and the absence of crystals from the cells adjacent to the vein.
5 Parenchyma of the midrib in longitudinal view showing prisms and microsphenoidal crystals of calcium oxalate in some of the cells.
6 Part of the lamina in sectional view, including part of a small vein, showing the upper epidermis with underlying palisade, the spongy mesophyll and the lower epidermis with a stoma.
7 Glandular trichomes, one attached to part of the epidermis over a vein.
8 Covering trichomes.
9 Part of the lamina in sectional view showing the upper epidermis, palisade and crystal layer.
10 Pollen grains.

STROPHANTHUS

Strophanthus kombé Oliver — Apocynaceae

Strophanthus Seeds

A dark, greyish-green powder with a rancid odour and an intensely bitter and persistent taste.

The diagnostic characters are:

(*a*) The fragments of the *sclerenchymatous epidermis of the testa* composed of a single layer of cells, each of which is extended to form a trichome but these are usually broken off. In surface view the cells are elongated to polygonal with strongly thickened walls with few, faint striations and no pits; occasional cells show an indistinct cicatrix or have the broken base of a trichome still attached. In sectional view the cells are tabular and it is seen that only the anticlinal walls are thickened, with the thickest part in the centre tapering off towards the outer and inner walls; the outer walls are frequently broken or they may show the bases of the trichomes. When seen in sectional view the sclerenchymatous epidermis is frequently attached to the underlying layers of the testa composed of collapsed cells containing brown pigment.

(*b*) The *trichomes*, most of which are in fragments. Each trichome is unicellular with a cylindrical rod of lignified thickening running down one side; these rods frequently become detached and are found scattered in the powder. The trichomes are usually fairly long and they are conical and sharply pointed at the apex; the walls (except where the lignified rod occurs) are thin and give only a faint reaction for lignin.

(*c*) The fragments of the *cotyledons* composed of irregularly rounded, thin-walled cells; the cells of the epidermis are smaller, and appear polygonal in surface view.

(*d*) The *endosperm*, composed of about three layers of cells, some of which are usually found attached to the inner layers of the testa; the cells are thin-walled and polygonal.

(*e*) The fragments of the *tissue of the raphe* composed of groups of small, lignified, annularly and spirally thickened vessels embedded in thin-walled parenchyma.

(*f*) The very occasional *cluster crystals of calcium oxalate*; these are fairly large and occur in the inner layers of the testa; they are usually found broken and scattered.

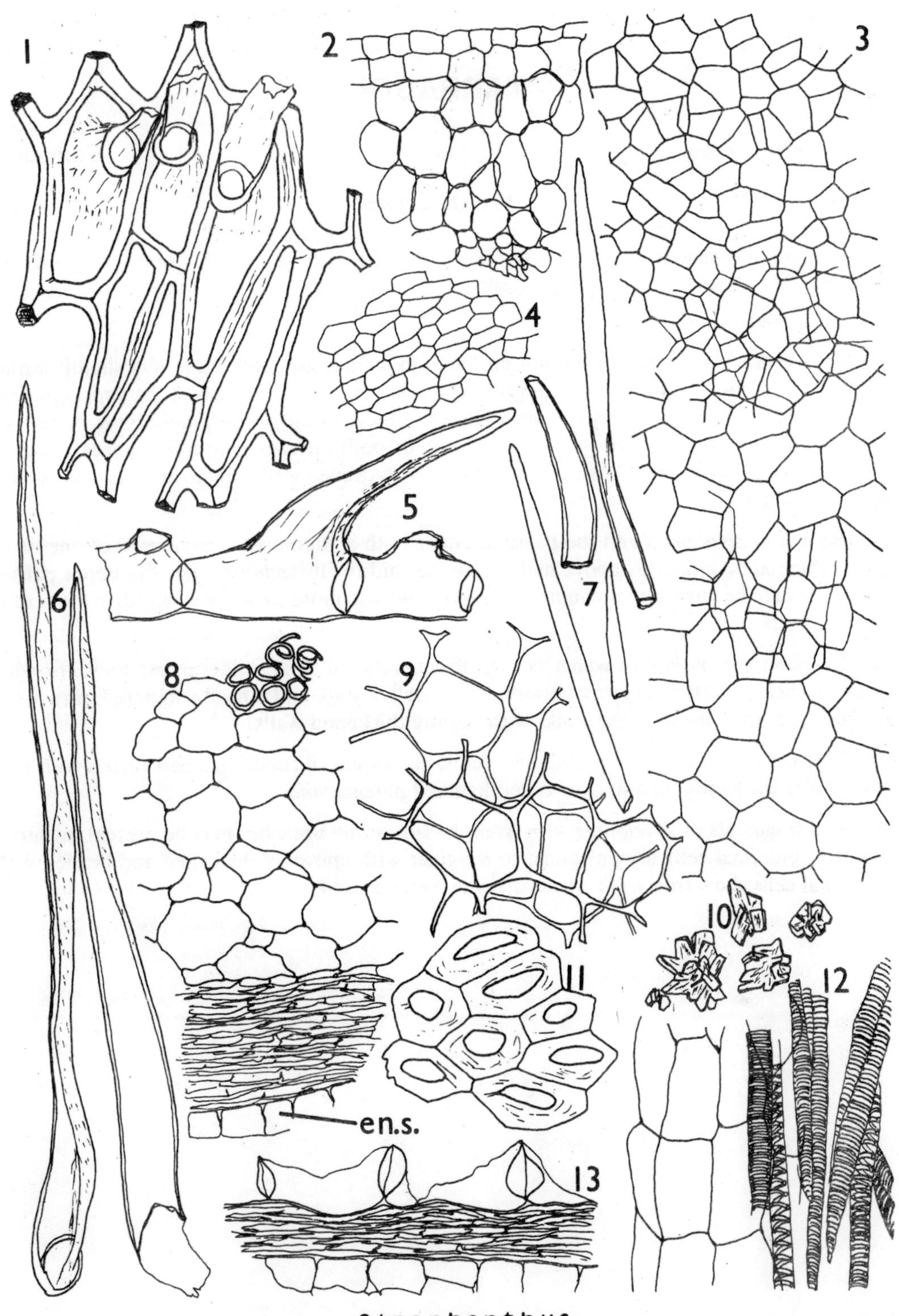

×330

1 Sclerenchymatous epidermis of the testa in surface view showing the remains of the trichomes on some of the cells.
2 Part of a cotyledon in sectional view.
3 Layers of the endosperm in surface view.
4 Epidermis of a cotyledon in surface view.
5 Sclerenchymatous layer of the testa in sectional view showing an attached trichome.
6 Trichomes.
7 Fragments of trichomes.
8 Tissues of the raphe in sectional view showing a group of vessels, parenchymatous cells, collapsed layers of the testa and the outermost layer of the endosperm (en.s.).
9 Parenchyma of the cotyledons.
10 Calcium oxalate cluster crystals.
11 Sclerenchymatous epidermis of the testa in surface view.
12 Parenchyma and vessels of the raphe.
13 Outer part of the seed in sectional view showing broken epidermal cells, collapsed pigment layers of the testa and the outer layer of the endosperm.

TARRAGON

Artemisia dracunculus L. Compositae

French Tarragon

Usually occurs in commerce as dried, broken leaf fragments, bright green with a strong, aromatic odour reminiscent of anise and a slightly pungent taste.

The diagnostic characters are:

(*a*) An exceptionally thick *cuticle* is present on both epidermises and this is very slightly striated on the upper epidermis and more strongly striated on the lower. The cells of the *upper epidermis* in surface view have thin, slighty sinuous walls while those of the *lower epidermis* are more wavy-walled; numerous large, *anomocytic stomata* occur on both surfaces. The epidermal cells over the midrib and larger veins are elongated with unevenly thickened walls which, in surface view, show distinct beading.

(*b*) The leaf is *isobilateral* and the palisade under both epidermises is composed of one or two layers which are continuous above and below the midrib. In *sectional view* the upper palisade cells are seen to be narrower and more elongated, and also more closely packed, than those of the lower palisade.

(*c*) The *glandular trichomes* which occur infrequently on both epidermises; they are small, yellowish-brown, with a very short biseriate, two-celled stalk and a head composed of two cells, slightly larger than those of the stalk, with slightly thickened walls.

(*d*) The *vascular tissue* of the midrib and veins, composed of small, lignified *vessels* with spiral and annular thickening and narrow-celled lignified *parenchyma*.

(*e*) Small fragments of *developing stem* from the tips of the branches may be present; in surface view the epidermal cells are polygonal to irregular with unevenly thickened and beaded walls; occasional cells show thin *septa* where division has occurred.

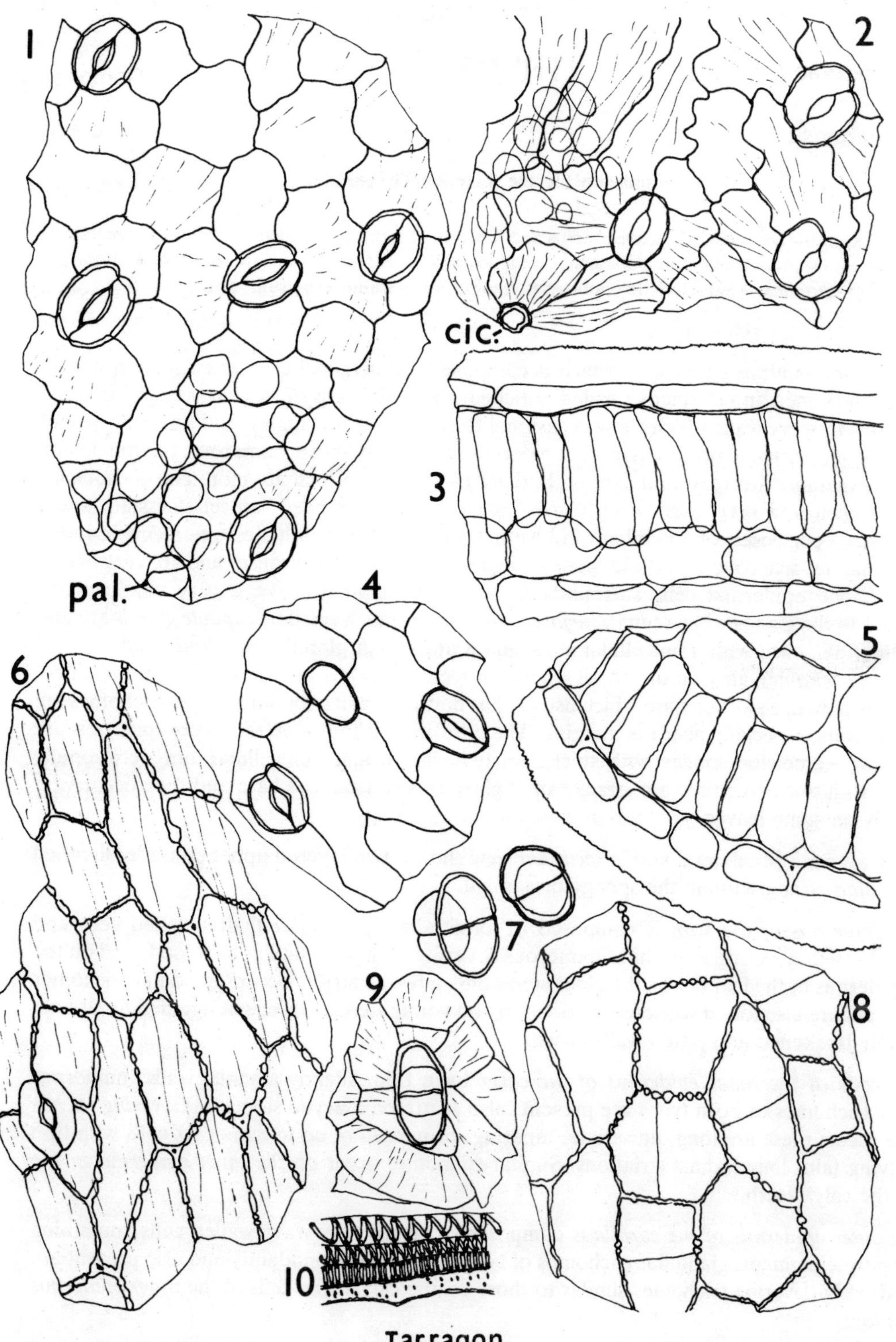

Tarragon

×330

1 Upper epidermis in surface view with stomata and part of the underlying palisade (pal.).
2 Lower epidermis in surface view with stomata, a cicatrix and part of the underlying palisade.
3 Part of the lamina in sectional view showing the thick cuticle, upper epidermis, upper palisade and spongy mesophyll.
4 Epidermis in surface view showing the stalk of a glandular trichome.
5 Part of the lamina in sectional view showing the thick cuticle, lower epidermis, lower palisade and spongy mesophyll.
6 Lower epidermis over a vein in surface view.
7 Glandular trichomes.
8 Epidermis of developing stem in surface view.
9 Lower epidermis in surface view with an attached glandular trichome.
10 Vascular tissue from the midrib.

THYME

Thymus vulgaris L. Labiatae

Common Thyme, Garden Thyme

Thyme consists of the fresh or dried leaves, stems and flowering heads. The leaves are distinctly punctate on both surfaces and sometimes densely pubescent on the lower surface; the flowers are small, pinkish-purple. It has a strong, aromatic, characteristic odour of thymol and a warming persistent taste.

The diagnostic characters are:

(*a*) The *upper epidermis of the leaf*, which is composed of polygonal cells when seen in surface view, with thickened and distinctly beaded anticlinal walls; the cells of the *lower epidermis* have thin, sinuous to wavy walls which show occasional thickening at the angles, and a faintly striated cuticle; *diacytic stomata* occur on both epidermises but are more numerous on the lower. *Glandular trichomes* are very abundant on both surfaces; those which are more conspicuous are yellowish-brown and very large, each consisting of a short, rounded, unicellular stalk and a glandular head composed of a number of indistinct, radiating cells with a common cuticle raised to form a bladder-like covering; these occur in depressions in the epidermises and are very widely distributed; the epidermal cells surrounding the stalk radiate to give a very characteristic appearance to the glands when seen in *surface view*. Other, much smaller, *capitate glands* are also fairly numerous, each with a unicellular stalk and a unicellular globular to ovoid head.

Covering trichomes also occur; those on the upper epidermis are unicellular, thin-walled, shortly conical with a swollen base which usually has dense granular contents; these trichomes are fairly numerous, especially near the margins. The covering trichomes on the lower epidermis are also conical, somewhat longer with thick, warty walls, usually unicellular but occasionally uniseriate with two cells; they are straight or slightly curved from the base and they occur very abundantly on some leaves.

(*b*) The leaves are isobilateral and in *sectional view* show a two-layered upper palisade; lignified *fibro-vascular tissue* occurs in the spongy mesophyll.

(*c*) The *epidermis of the stem* is composed of longitudinally elongated, thin-walled cells and occasional stomata; young stems have numerous covering trichomes similar to those found on the lower epidermis of the leaf but on the older stems only a few cicatrices occur; glandular trichomes of both types are also found scattered, particularly on young stems. Groups of lignified *fibres* with moderately thickened and pitted walls occur.

(*d*) The cells of the *outer epidermis of the calyx* have thin, slightly sinuous walls; numerous glandular trichomes of both types are present, also scattered diacytic stomata. *Covering trichomes* also occur; these are long, uniseriate, tapering, composed of up to five or six cells with thin walls having faint longitudinal striations. Similar trichomes occur on the *inner epidermis* at the base of the calyx teeth.

(*e*) The *outer epidermis of the corolla* is composed of small, very wavy-walled cells containing pinkish-purple pigment; glandular trichomes of both types occur abundantly and also present are scattered, long covering trichomes similar to those on the calyx. The cells of the *inner epidermis* are *papillose*.

(*f*) The *pollen grains* are spherical with six pores and rather indistinct furrows; the exine is smooth or slightly warty.

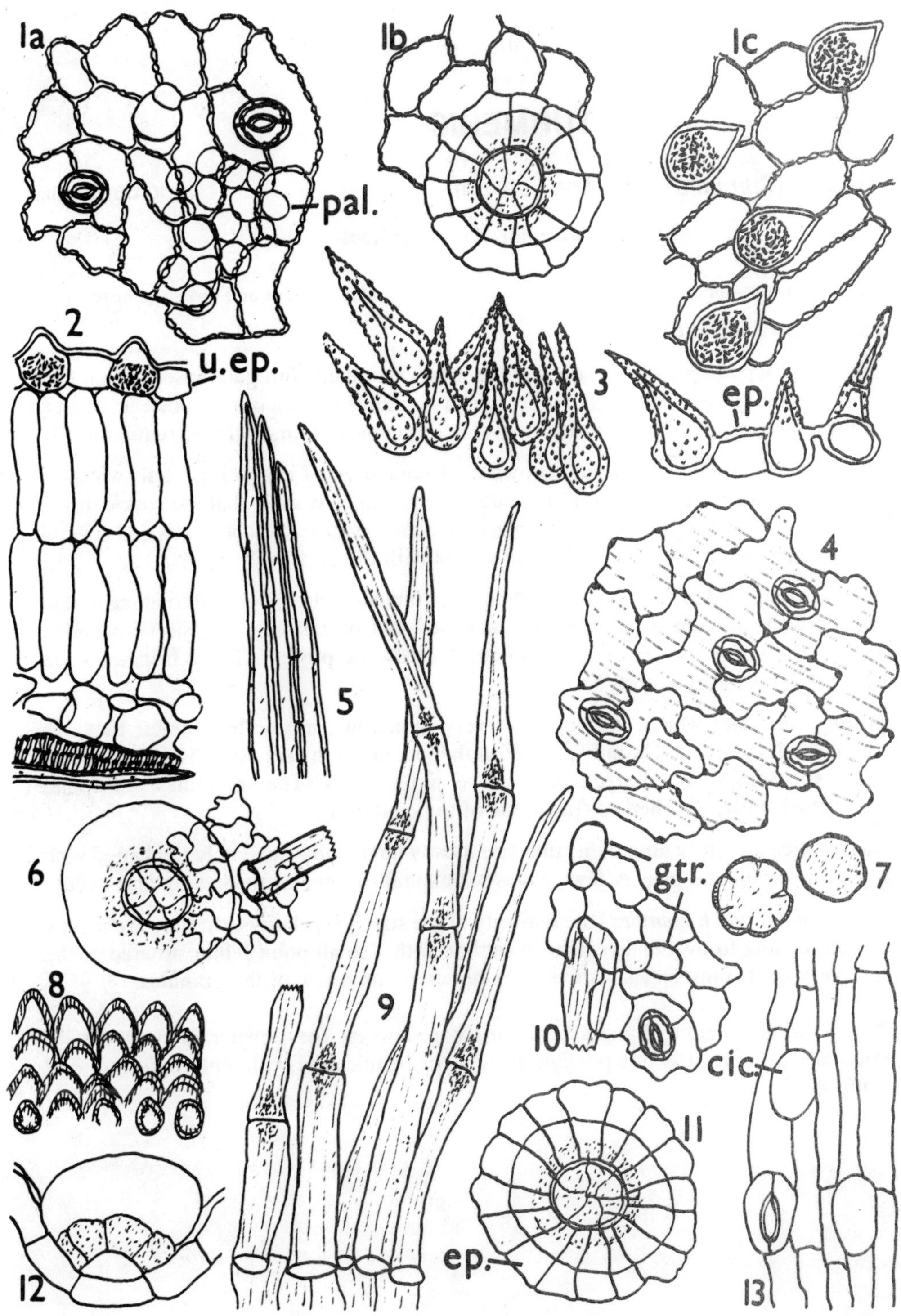

Thyme

×330

1 Upper epidermis of the leaf in surface view showing (a) diacytic stomata, a capitate glandular trichome and part of the underlying palisade (pal.); (b) a multicellular glandular trichome; (c) conical covering trichomes.

2 Part of the lamina in sectional view showing conical trichomes in the upper epidermis (u.ep.).

3 Covering trichomes on the lower epidermis (ep.) of the leaf.

4 Lower epidermis of the leaf in surface view.

5 Part of a group of fibres from the stem.

6 Outer epidermis of the corolla in surface view showing a multicellular glandular trichome and part of a covering trichome.

7 Pollen grains.

8 Inner epidermis of the corolla in oblique surface view.

9 Covering trichomes from the inner epidermis of the calyx.

10 Outer epidermis of the calyx in surface view with capitate glandular trichomes and part of a covering trichome.

11 A multicellular glandular trichome in surface view with surrounding epidermal cells (ep.).

12 A multicellular glandular trichome in sectional view.

13 Epidermis of the stem in surface view showing cicatrices (cic.).

TURMERIC

Curcuma longa L. (*Curcuma domestica* Valeton) Zingiberaceae

Turmeric Rhizome, Turmeric Root

A bright golden-yellow powder with an aromatic, pleasant odour and a pungent and aromatic taste.

The diagnostic characters are:

(*a*) The abundant groups of *parenchymatous cells*, which are filled with gelatinised starch and permeated with a *bright yellow colouring matter* which is soluble in aqueous mounts; in cleared preparations the cells are seen to be rounded to oval in outline with thin, slightly irregular walls.

(*b*) The fairly abundant fragments of pale brown *cork* composed of thin-walled cells which in surface view appear large and polygonal. Fragments in sectional view show that the cork consists of from two to five layers of cells and that it occurs inside the cortex; the epidermis and several layers of cortical cells are occasionally found associated with the cork.

(*c*) The *epidermis* composed of a layer of straight-walled tabular cells, polygonal to elongated in surface view; the walls are sometimes slightly thickened and pitted; very occasional rounded *stomata* and *cicatrices* occur and covering trichomes may also be present. These fragments are rather indistinct and not easily detected.

(*d*) The *covering trichomes* which, although not very numerous, are quite distinct; they are unicellular, elongated, conical and bluntly pointed with moderately thickened walls which may be faintly striated; the somewhat enlarged bases have pitted walls. The trichomes are found scattered and, occasionally, attached to fragments of the epidermis.

(*e*) The *vessels*, which are fairly abundant; they are mostly large and reticulately thickened with regularly arranged rectangular pits. A few vessels with spiral or annular thickening also occur.

(*f*) The very occasional *starch granules* (the majority of the starch is gelatinised); they are mostly simple, flattened, oblong to oval or irregular in outline with a small point hilum situated at the narrower end; very faint transverse striations may be visible on a few of the granules.

The yellow colouring matter changes to a bright red when the powder is treated with concentrated acids, hence it is not possible to test for lignification with *Phloroglucinol and Hydrochloric Acid*.

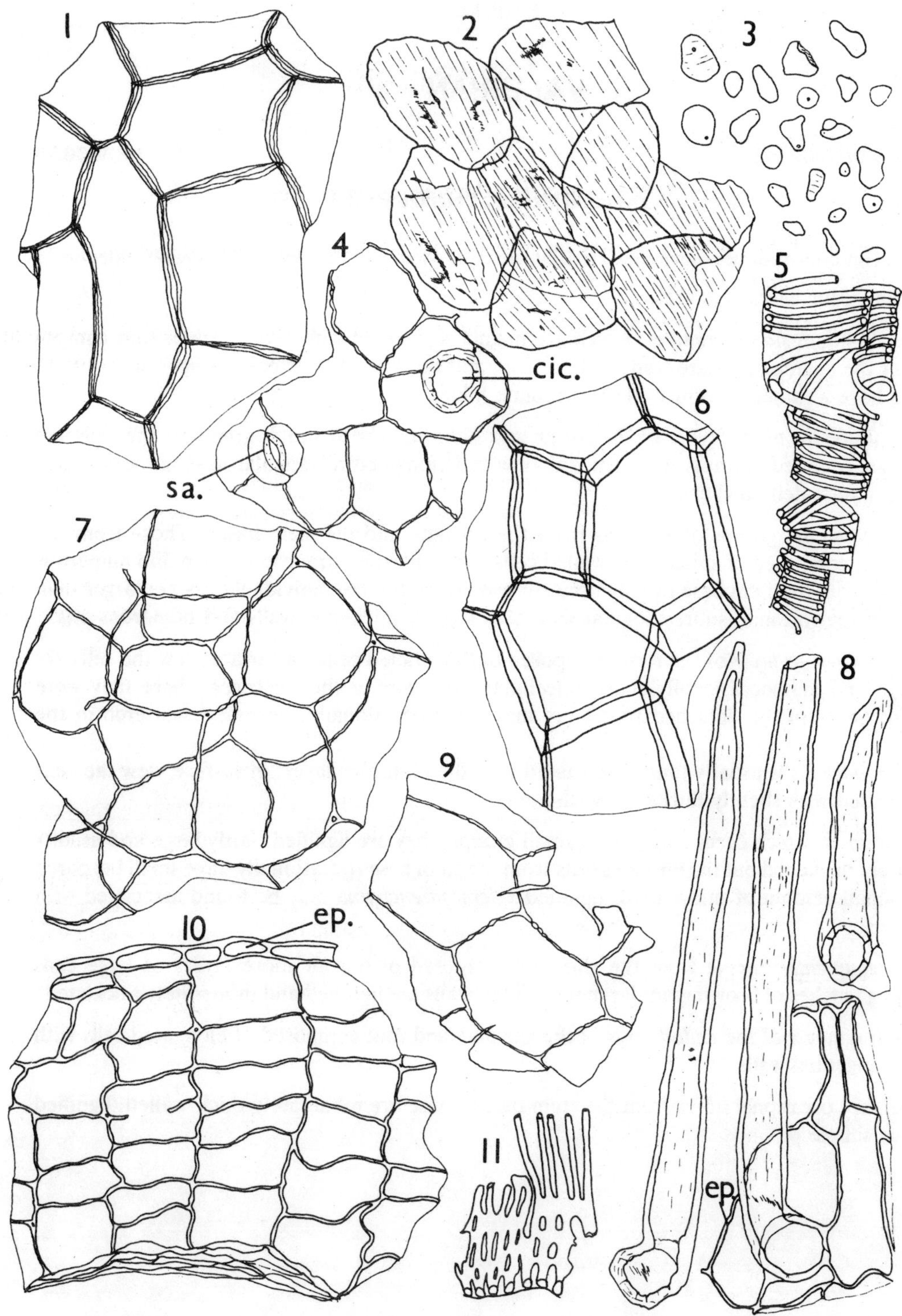

×330

1 Cork in surface view.
2 Parenchymatous cells filled with gelatinised starch and yellow colouring matter, as seen in an uncleared mount.
3 Starch granules.
4 Epidermis in surface view showing a stoma (sa.) and a cicatrix (cic.).
5 Fragmerts of spirally thickened vessels.
6 Cork in oblique surface view.
7 Parenchymatous cells as seen in a cleared mount.
8 Covering trichomes, one attached to a fragment of the epidermis (ep.).
9 Epidermis in surface view.
10 Part of the outer tissues in sectional view showing the epidermis (ep.), cortex, cork and a layer of collapsed cells.
11 Fragment of a reticulately thickened vessel.

VALERIAN

Valeriana officinalis L. s.l Valerianaceae

Valerian Rhizome, Valerian Root

A light greyish-brown powder with a characteristic, aromatic odour and an aromatic and slightly bitter taste.

The diagnostic characters are:

(*a*) The abundant *starch granules*, which are mainly compound with two, three or four components but the aggregations are frequently broken and the components occur singly; most of the granules have a rather indistinct, cleft or radiate hilum.

(*b*) The abundant *parenchyma of the cortex* and *pith*, filled with starch granules; the cells are fairly large, rounded in transverse sectional view and elongated rectangular in longitudinal view and have moderately thickened walls.

(*c*) The occasional groups of *sclereids* from the rhizome and the stem bases. Those from the rhizome are composed of small thick-walled cells with a narrow, branched lumen and numerous pits; those from the stem base usually occur in two layers and the individual cells are larger than those from the rhizome, subrectangular with only slightly thickened walls and numerous pits.

(*d*) The *piliferous layer* of the roots composed of thin-walled cells; in surface view the cells are elongated and may occasionally show unicellular *root hairs* or the cicatrices where they were attached. Some of the detached root hairs may, very occasionally, be found scattered in the powder.

The *hypodermis* is usually found associated with the piliferous layer; in surface view the cells are elongated with slightly thickened walls.

(*e*) The *vessels*, which occur singly or in small groups; they are lignified, fairly large and usually reticulately thickened but the larger vessels from the stem bases occasionally have small bordered pits. A small amount of thin-walled, lignified *xylem parenchyma* may be found associated with the vessels.

(*f*) The *tegumentary tissue* from the rhizome composed of one or more layers of large cells containing patches of brown granular material; the walls are lignified and moderately thickened.

(*g*) The fragments of the *endodermis* of the rhizome and root composed of elongated cells with sinuous tangential walls.

(*h*) The very occasional *fibres* from the stem bases; these are moderately thick-walled, lignified and have simple pits.

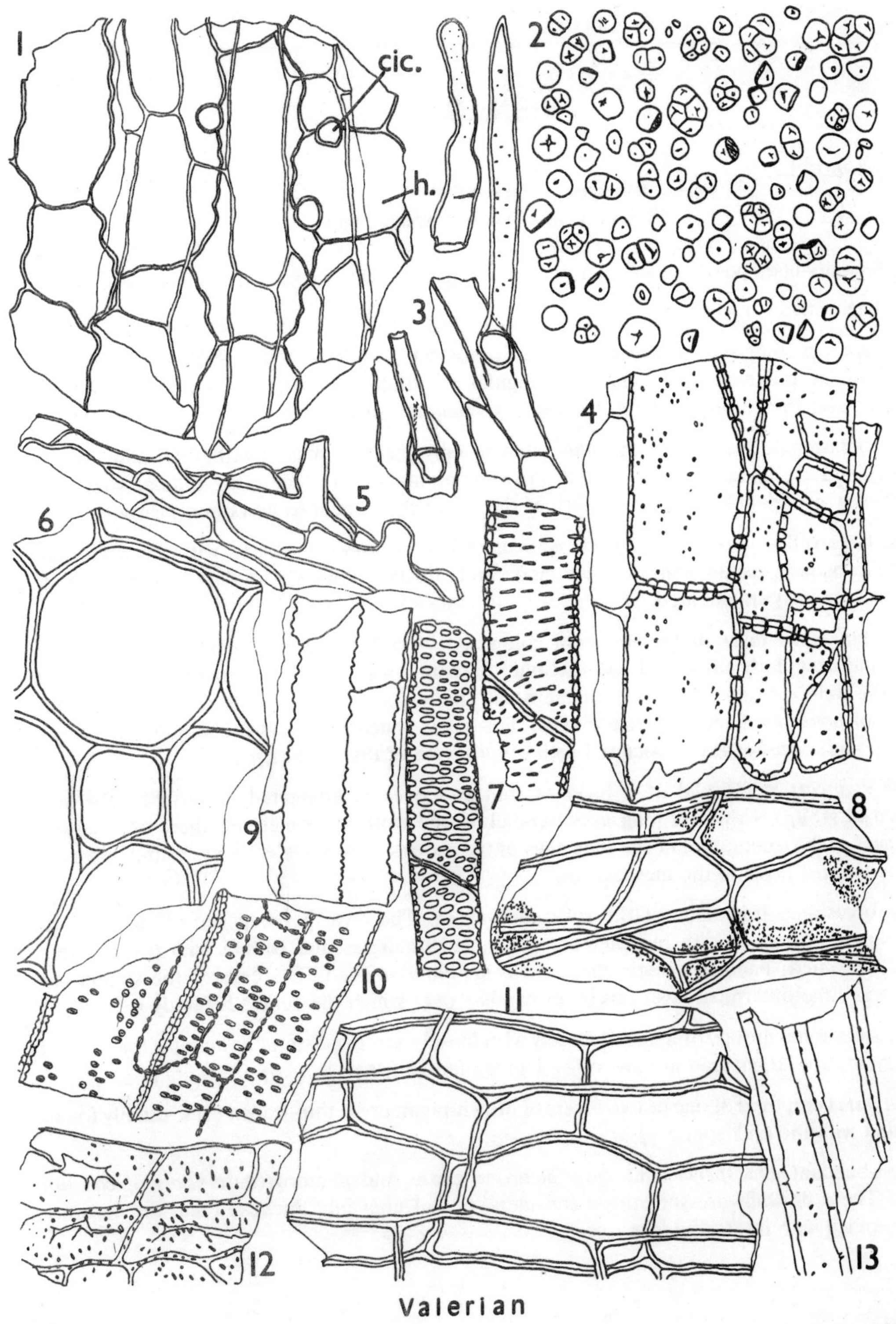

Valerian

×330

1 Piliferous layer of the root in surface view showing scars of root hairs (cic.) and underlying hypodermis (h.).
2 Starch granules.
3 Fragments of the piliferous layer with attached root hairs and a detached root hair.
4 Two layers of sclereids from the stem base.
5 Piliferous layer in oblique sectional view showing broken root hairs.
6 Parenchyma in transverse sectional view.
7 Reticulately thickened vessels.
8 Two layers of tegumentary tissue from the rhizome in surface view.
9 Endodermis in tangential longitudinal view.
10 Bordered pitted vessels with associated xylem parenchyma from the stem base.
11 Parenchyma in longitudinal view.
12 Part of a group of sclereids from the rhizome.
13 Parts of fibres from the stem base.

VISNAGA

Ammi visnaga L. Umbelliferae

Visnaga Fruits, Ammi Visnaga Fruits

A dark brownish-black powder, gritty in texture, with a faint aromatic odour and a bitter taste.

The diagnostic characters are:

(*a*) The *epicarp* composed of a layer of rather indistinct, colourless cells, which in surface view are thin-walled, polygonal and somewhat irregular in outline; the cells are slightly papillose and the *cuticle* over the papillae is faintly striated; *stomata* are infrequent.

(*b*) The occasional fragments of the *vittae*; they usually occur associated with other tissue of the mesocarp and are filled with dense, dark brown contents which obscure the cellular structure. Fragments which include the whole width of the vittae show them to be rather narrow.

(*c*) The large-celled *parenchyma of the mesocarp* which is found associated with the vittae; the cells are irregularly rectangular and have moderately thickened walls with dark brown pigment; they are frequently fragmented.

(*d*) The *innermost layer of the mesocarp* composed of cells in which the anticlinal walls are slightly and irregularly thickened and the inner periclinal walls are considerably thickened and pitted; the walls contain pale brown pigment and the pits in the inner walls are very numerous and conspicuous when seen in surface view. This layer is nearly always found adherent to the endocarp and, occasionally, associated with other layers of the mesocarp.

(*e*) The *endocarp* composed of a layer of thin-walled cells, elongated in surface view and arranged in groups with their long axes parallel to one another; sometimes there are marked differences in the orientation of the long axes of the groups. This layer is always found adherent to the innermost layer of the mesocarp.

(*f*) The occasional fragments of the *style* and *stigma*. The style is composed of thin-walled, longitudinally elongated cells in which are embedded small vascular strands with two or three spirally thickened, lignified vessels; the cuticle is faintly striated. The cells of the stigma are rounded and the outermost layer has small papillae over which the cuticle is faintly striated.

(*g*) The occasional groups of lignified *vessels* with loosely arranged spiral or annular thickening; the elements are larger than in most other Umbelliferous fruits.

(*h*) The *testa* composed of one or two layers of brown-pigmented, thin-walled cells, usually found associated with the endosperm.

(*i*) The abundant *endosperm* containing *aleurone grains* and *microrosette crystals of calcium oxalate*. The cells walls are sometimes considerably and unevenly thickened and the cells are often rounded with intercellular spaces.

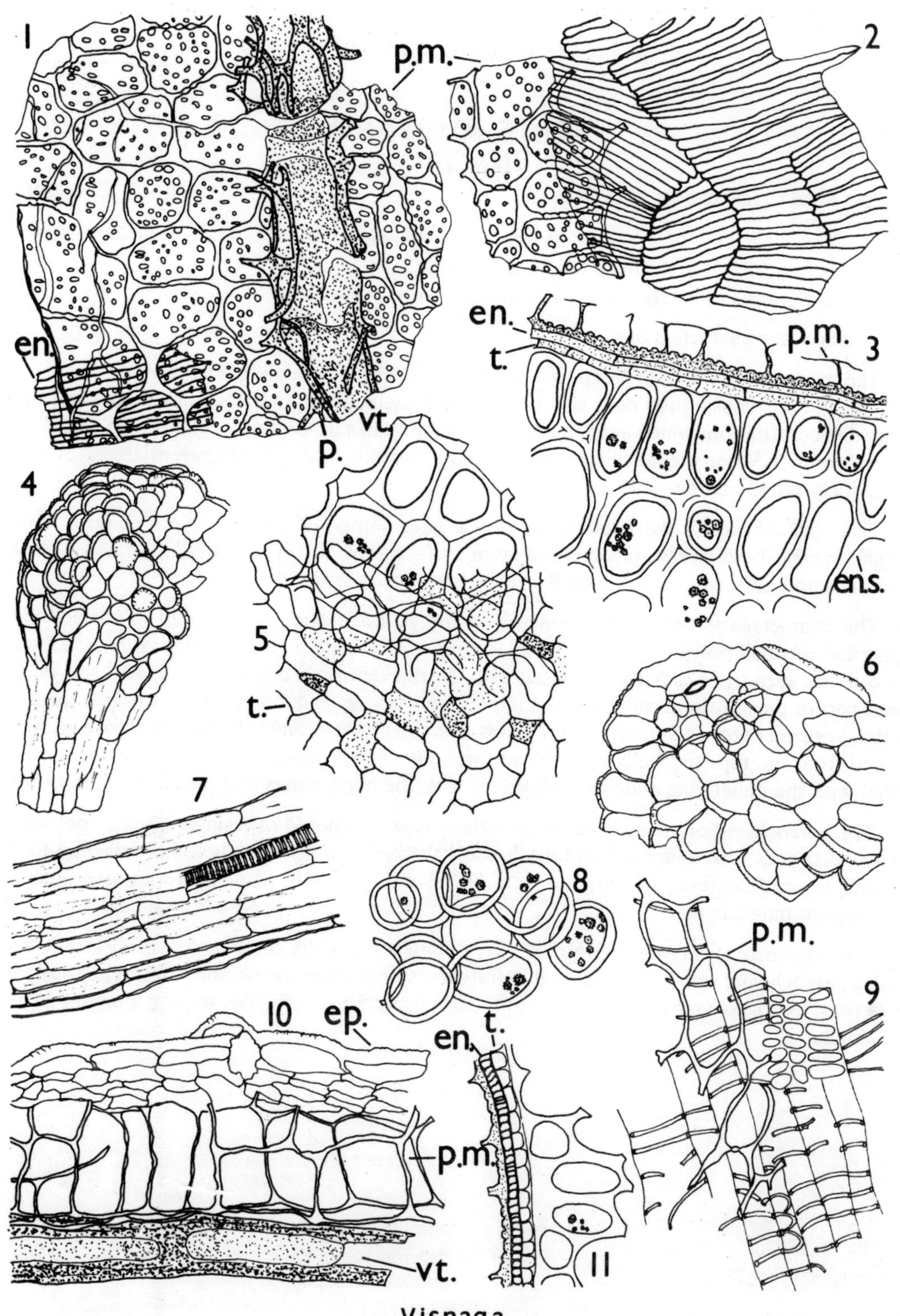

Visnaga

×330

1 Pitted cells of the innermost layer of the mesocarp (p.m.) in surface view, with part of the underlying endocarp (en.) and a vitta (vt.) with associated large-celled parenchyma (p.).

2 Endocarp in surface view with underlying pitted parenchyma of the mesocarp (p.m.).

3 Part of the pericarp and seed in longitudinal sectional view showing the innermost layer of the mesocarp (p.m.), the endocarp (en.), the testa (t.) and the endosperm (en.s.).

4 Part of the style and stigma in surface view.

5 Testa (t.) in surface view with underlying endosperm.

6 Epicarp in surface view showing stomata and underlying parenchyma.

7 Style in longitudinal view showing part of a small vein.

8 Endosperm containing microrosette crystals of calcium oxalate.

9 Group of vessels with associated parenchyma of the mesocarp (p.m.).

10 Part of the pericarp in longitudinal sectional view showing the epicarp (ep.), large-celled parenchyma of the mesocarp (p.m.) and a vitta (vt.).

11 Part of the pericarp and seed in transverse sectional view showing fragments of the innermost layer of the mesocarp, the endocarp (en.), the testa (t.) and endosperm.

WHITE MUSTARD

Sinapis alba L. (*Brassica alba* Boiss.) Cruciferae

White Mustard Seeds

A dull yellow powder with little odour and a strongly pungent taste.

The diagnostic characters are:

(*a*) The *epidermis of the testa* composed of thin-walled cells containing *mucilage* which swells in aqueous mounts causing the cells to enlarge and sometimes rupture; as it swells the mucilage forms distinct striations which appear as concentric rings in surface view; it stains with *Solution of Ruthenium Red*. When the mucilage is removed the anticlinal walls of the epidermal cells are seen to be finely pitted and beaded.

(*b*) The *collenchyma of the hypodermis of the testa* composed of two layers of fairly large, irregular cells; these layers are usually seen in surface view and are usually associated with the epidermis and also, frequently, with the underlying palisade layer.

(*c*) The characteristic yellowish fragments of the *palisade layer of the testa* in surface view composed of small polygonal cells with thickened, very slightly lignified walls. *In sectional view* the cells are seen to be radially elongated with the thickening on the basal walls and also on the lower part of the anticlinal walls, which then become thinner and more sinuous towards the apex so that *in surface view*, when seen from below, the cells have straight, thickened walls but, when viewed from the top, the walls are thin and sinuous. This layer is sometimes found associated either with the underlying endosperm layer or with the hypodermis and epidermis of the testa.

(*d*) The *parenchyma of the endosperm* in surface view composed of a single layer of polygonal to irregular cells with uniformly and moderately thickened walls, usually found attached to the palisade layer of the testa. In sectional view this layer is seen to be associated with several layers of collapsed parenchyma.

(*e*) The *fragments of the embryo* which are very abundant and are composed of fairly small, thin-walled parenchyma; some of the cotyledon fragments, in sectional view, show differentiation into epidermis, palisade and spongy mesophyll and, in surface view, developing stomata in the epidermis.

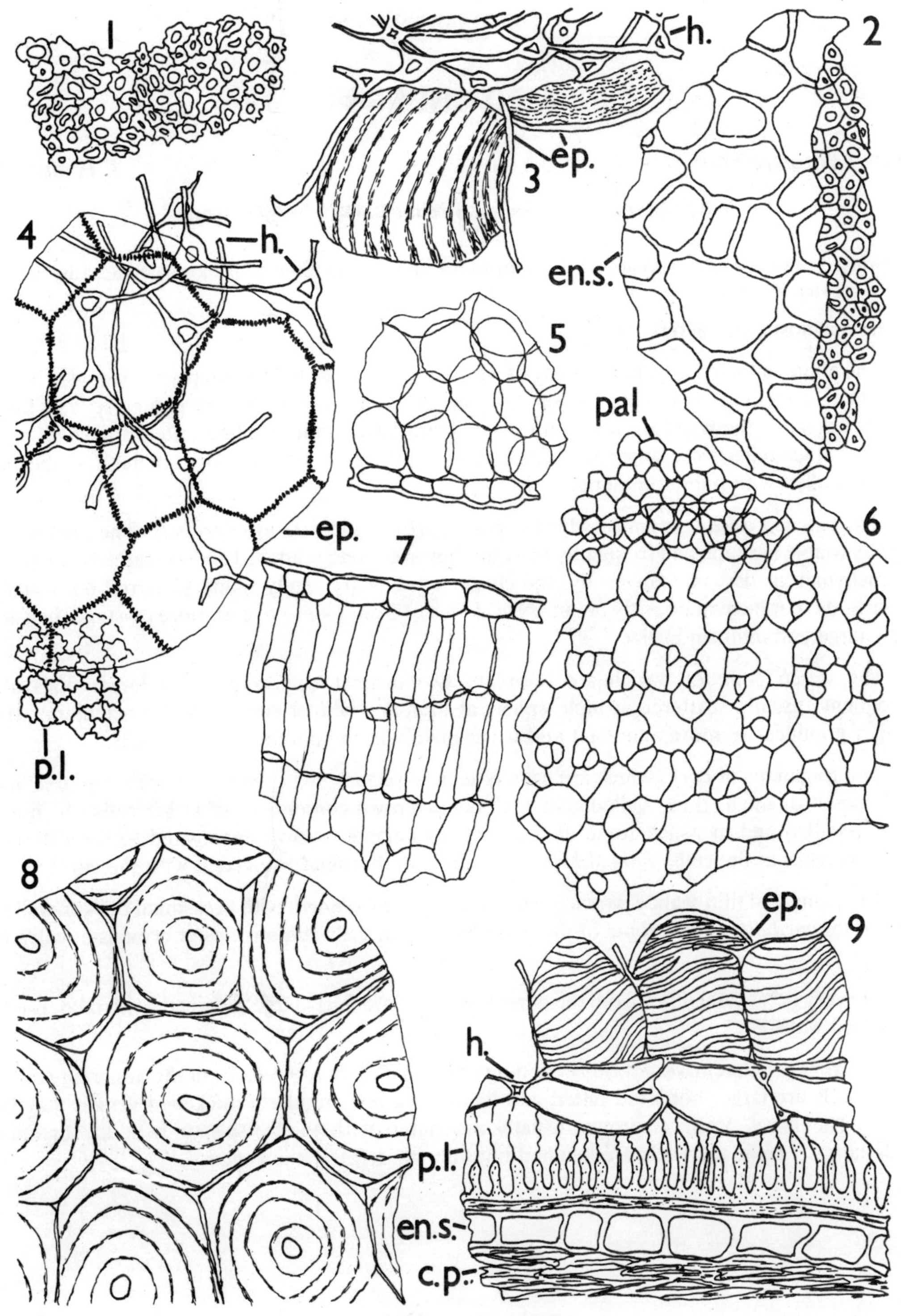

White Mustard

×330

1 Palisade layer of the testa in surface view, seen from above.
2 Endosperm layer in surface view (en.s.) with part of the adjacent palisade layer of the testa seen from below.
3 Ruptured epidermal cells of the testa (ep.) containing striated mucilage, and part of the underlying collenchyma of the hypodermis (h.).
4 Epidermis of the testa (ep.) in surface view showing pitted and beaded walls, with part of the underlying hypodermis (h.) and a fragment of some of the upper parts of cells of the palisade layer (p.l.).
5 Part of a cotyledon in sectional view showing the lower epidermis and cells of the mesophyll.
6 Epidermis of a cotyledon in surface view showing developing stomata and part of the underlying palisade (pal.).
7 Part of a cotyledon in sectional view showing the upper epidermis and underlying palisade.
8 Epidermal cells of the testa in surface view containing swollen mucilage in concentric layers.
9 Part of the seed in sectional view showing the epidermis (ep.) containing striated mucilage, collenchymatous cells of the hypodermis (h.), palisade layer (p.l.), endosperm (en.s.) and collapsed parenchymatous layers (c.p.).

WILD CHERRY

Prunus serotina Ehrh. Rosaceae

Wild Cherry Bark, Virginian Prune Bark, Virginian Prune

A fawnish-brown powder, gritty in texture, with an odour and taste resembling bitter almonds; the taste is also somewhat astringent.

The diagnostic characters are:

(*a*) The abundant *sclereids*, the majority of which occur in large dense groups; individual cells are branched, sometimes markedly so and forming *astrosclereids*; a few are elongated and form *fibrous sclereids*; the walls are thick and striated and have numerous fine, often branched, pits. Occasional sclereids occur singly or in smaller groups; these are usually more regular in shape and thinner-walled with numerous simple pits.

(*b*) The *calcium oxalate crystals*, which occur as *prisms* and as *cluster crystals*. The prisms are large, variable in shape and frequently broken; they are found scattered and are rarely seen in the parenchymatous tissues. Conversely, the cluster crystals are rarely found scattered but usually occur in the parenchymatous tissue, in vertical files of from two to five or more crystals; they are fairly large and uniform in size.

(*c*) The *starch granules*, which are found in two distinct size ranges; the larger ones are infrequent, usually scattered, simple spherical granules with a small but distinct hilum; the smaller granules are more abundant and occur mainly in the parenchymatous cells.

(*d*) The fragments of *cork*, which are usually seen in surface view. The structure is variable and may consist of small, thick-walled cells with dense brown contents or of larger cells which are thinner-walled and in which some of the contents appear to have aggregated to form darker brown patches in the cells. *Fungal hyphae* are frequently found associated with the cork.

(*e*) The elongated thin-walled *parenchymatous cells of the phloem* with occasional thicker-walled cells of the *medullary rays*; some of the parenchymatous cells contain cluster crystals of calcium oxalate.

(*f*) The very occasional *fibres* from the pericycle; these are fairly large, lignified, with moderately thickened walls.

(*g*) The very infrequent *vessels, fibres* and lignified *medullary ray cells* from the adherent wood. The vessels are large, bordered pitted and lignified; a few annularly thickened vessels may be found. The fibres occur in groups usually associated with the vessels or with the lignified medullary ray cells; the walls are lignified but only moderately thickened.

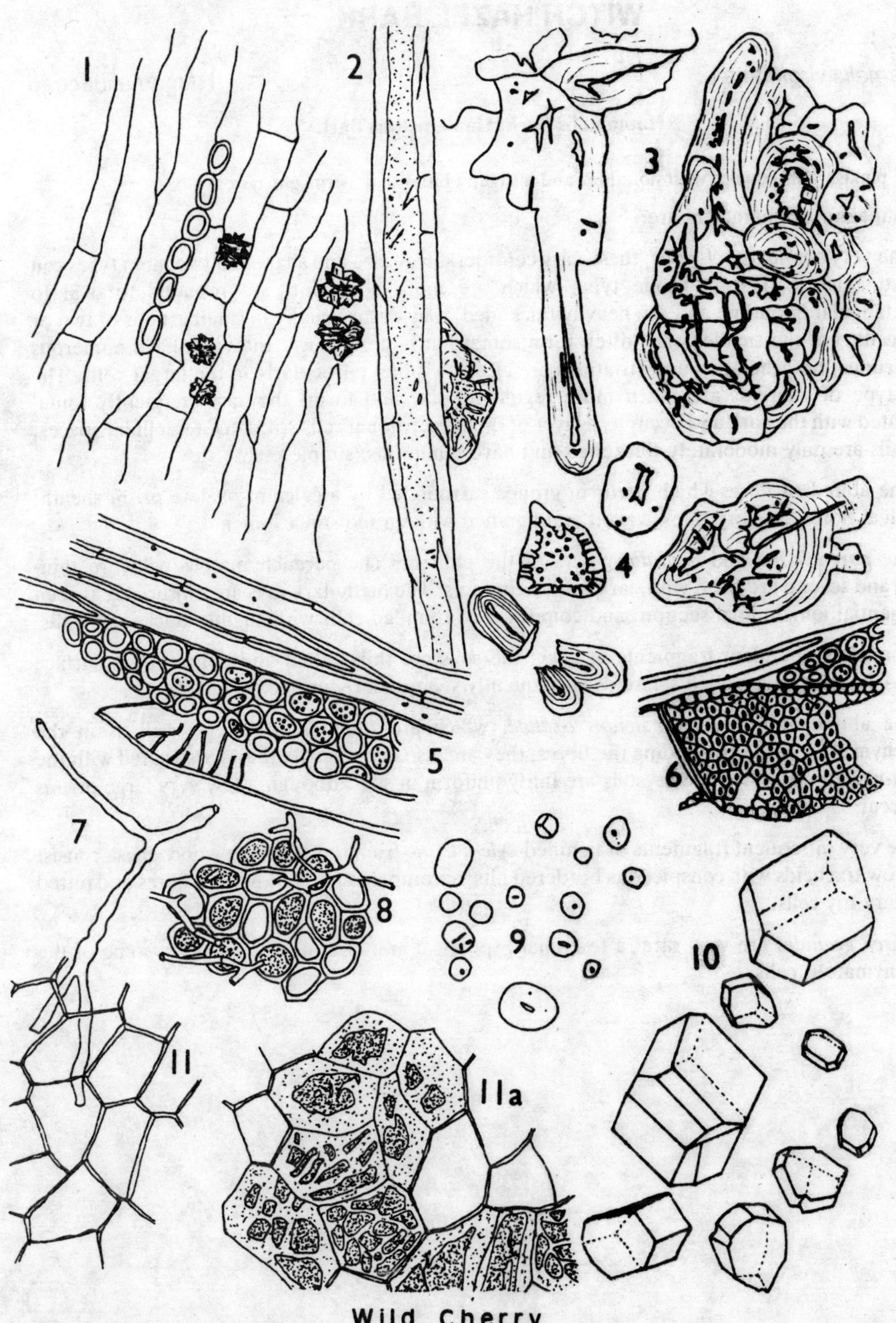

×330

1 Phloem parenchyma with cluster crystals of calcium oxalate and a medullary ray in tangential longitudinal section.
2 Part of a fibre and sclereids of the pericycle.
3 Groups of astrosclereids.
4 Single sclereids and fragments from astrosclereids.
5 Fibres, part of a medullary ray and part of a vessel from the adherent wood, in tangential longitudinal section.
6 Fragment of a bordered pitted vessel, a medullary ray and a fibre from the adherent wood.
7 Fungal hypha.
8 Cork in surface view with associated fungal hyphae.
9 Starch granules.
10 Prisms of calcium oxalate.
11 Cork in surface view.
11a Cork in surface view showing aggregated pigment in the cells.

WITCH HAZEL BARK

Hamamelis virginiana L. Hamamelidaceae

Hamamelis Bark, Hamamelidis Bark

A pale pinkish-buff powder with no odour and a slightly bitter and astringent taste.

The diagnostic characters are:

(*a*) The very abundant *sclereids*; these vary considerably in size and shape but two main types can be distinguished. Those of one type, which are more abundant, are rounded to oval to subrectangular in outline and are heavily thickened; they occur usually in small groups of two or three cells, but the smaller ones often form somewhat larger groups; the walls have numerous conspicuous, branched pits and striations are clearly visible, particularly in the larger cells. The other type of sclereids are much more regular in size and form; they are frequently found associated with the cork and occur as a layer of small, polygonal cells with no intercellular spaces; the walls are only moderately thickened and have numerous, simple pits.

(*b*) The abundant *fibres* which occur in groups surrounded by a calcium oxalate prism sheath; individual fibres are very thick-walled and lignified with an indistinct lumen.

(*c*) The *parenchyma* and *medullary rays* of the phloem. The parenchymatous cells are thin-walled and several are filled with dark brown contents. The medullary rays are uniseriate, as seen in tangential longitudinal section, and composed of rounded cells with slightly thickened walls.

(*d*) The fairly abundant fragments of *cork*; the cells are thin-walled and polygonal in surface view. A layer of thin-walled sclereids is frequently seen underlying the cork cells.

(*e*) The abundant *prisms of calcium oxalate*, which are found scattered as well as in the parenchymatous cells surrounding the fibres; they are also occasionally found associated with the thicker-walled sclereids. The crystals are fairly uniform in size although a few very large prisms may occur.

(*f*) The very infrequent fragments of lignified *xylem tissue* from the adherent wood; these consist of narrow tracheids with conspicuous bordered pits, accompanied by thin-walled fibres and pitted medullary ray cells.

(*g*) *Starch granules* are very rare; a few small, spherical granules may be found in some of the parenchymatous cells.

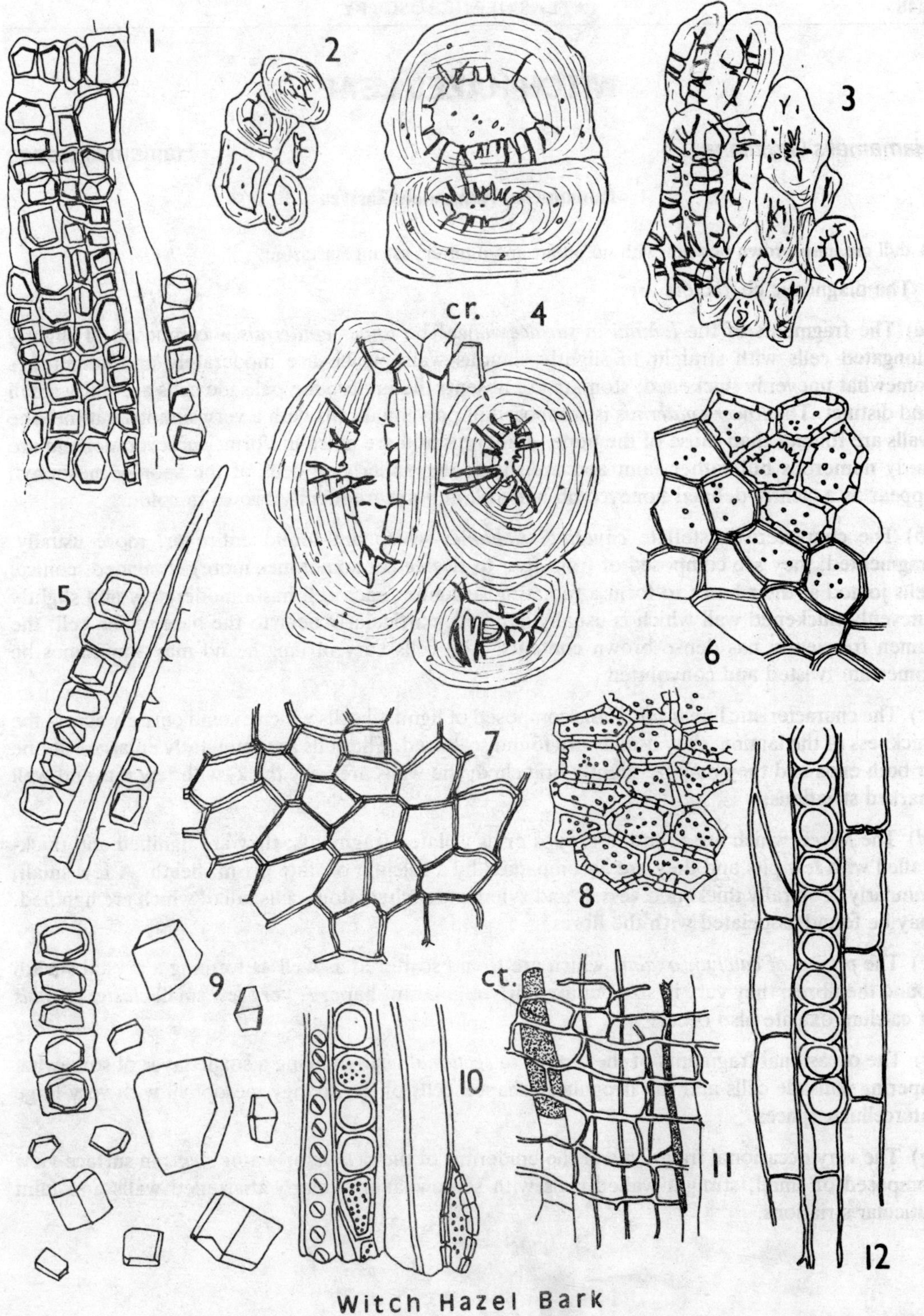

Witch Hazel Bark

×330

1 Part of a group of fibres with calcium oxalate prism sheath.
2 A group of smaller, thick-walled sclereids.
3 A group of thick-walled sclereids showing distinct pits.
4 Large, thick-walled sclereids with associated prisms of calcium oxalate (cr.).
5 Part of a single fibre with part of the crystal sheath.
6 Cork in surface view with part of the underlying layer of thin-walled sclereids.
7 Cork in surface view.
8 Part of the layer of thin-walled sclereids in surface view.
9 Calcium oxalate crystals.
10 Part of the xylem showing a tracheid with bordered pits, medullary ray cells and fibres in tangential longitudinal section.
11 Phloem parenchyma with some of the cells containing dark brown contents (ct.) and an overlying medullary ray in radial longitudinal section.
12 Phloem parenchyma and a medullary ray in tangential longitudinal section.

WITCH HAZEL LEAF

Hamamelis virginiana L. Hamamelidaceae

Hamamelis, Hamamelis Leaves

A dull greenish-brown powder with no odour and a bitter, astringent taste.

The diagnostic characters are:

(*a*) The fragments of the *lamina in surface view*. The *upper epidermis* is composed of slightly elongated cells with straight to slightly sinuous walls which are moderately and sometimes somewhat unevenly thickened; stomata are absent; the underlying palisade cells are fairly small and distinct. The *lower epidermis* is composed of polygonal cells with a very sinuous outline; the walls are thinner than those of the upper epidermis and are more uniform; *paracytic stomata* are fairly numerous but rather faint and indistinct; the underlying cells of the spongy mesophyll appear as a clearly defined honeycomb network and are frequently brown in colour.

(*b*) The characteristic stellate *covering trichomes* which are found entire or, more usually, fragmented; they are composed of from four to twelve (or sometimes more) elongated, conical cells joined at their bases to form a radiating structure; each cell has a moderately and slightly unevenly thickened wall which is usually lignified, particularly near to the base of the cell; the lumen frequently has dense brown contents. The cells vary in length and may sometimes be somewhat twisted and convoluted.

(*c*) The characteristic linear *idioblasts* composed of lignified cells which extend entirely across the thickness of the lamina; they usually are found scattered. The cells are frequently enlarged at one or both ends and they may be slightly branched; the walls are very thick, with few pits and well marked striations.

(*d*) The *fibres*, which are found in groups or as isolated fragments; they are lignified and thick-walled with few pits and they are accompanied by a calcium oxalate prism sheath. A few small, annularly or spirally thickened vessels and xylem parenchymatous cells, all of which are lignified, may be found associated with the fibres.

(*e*) The *prisms of calcium oxalate* which are found scattered as well as forming a crystal sheath round the fibres; they vary in size but are fairly regular in shape. A very few small *cluster crystals* of calcium oxalate also occur.

(*f*) The occasional fragments of the *lamina in sectional view* showing a single layer of somewhat tapering palisade cells and the irregularly shaped cells of the spongy mesophyll with very large intercellular spaces.

(*g*) The very occasional fragments of the epidermis of the *petiole* or *young stems* in surface view composed of small, straight-walled cells with somewhat irregularly thickened walls and faint cuticular striations.

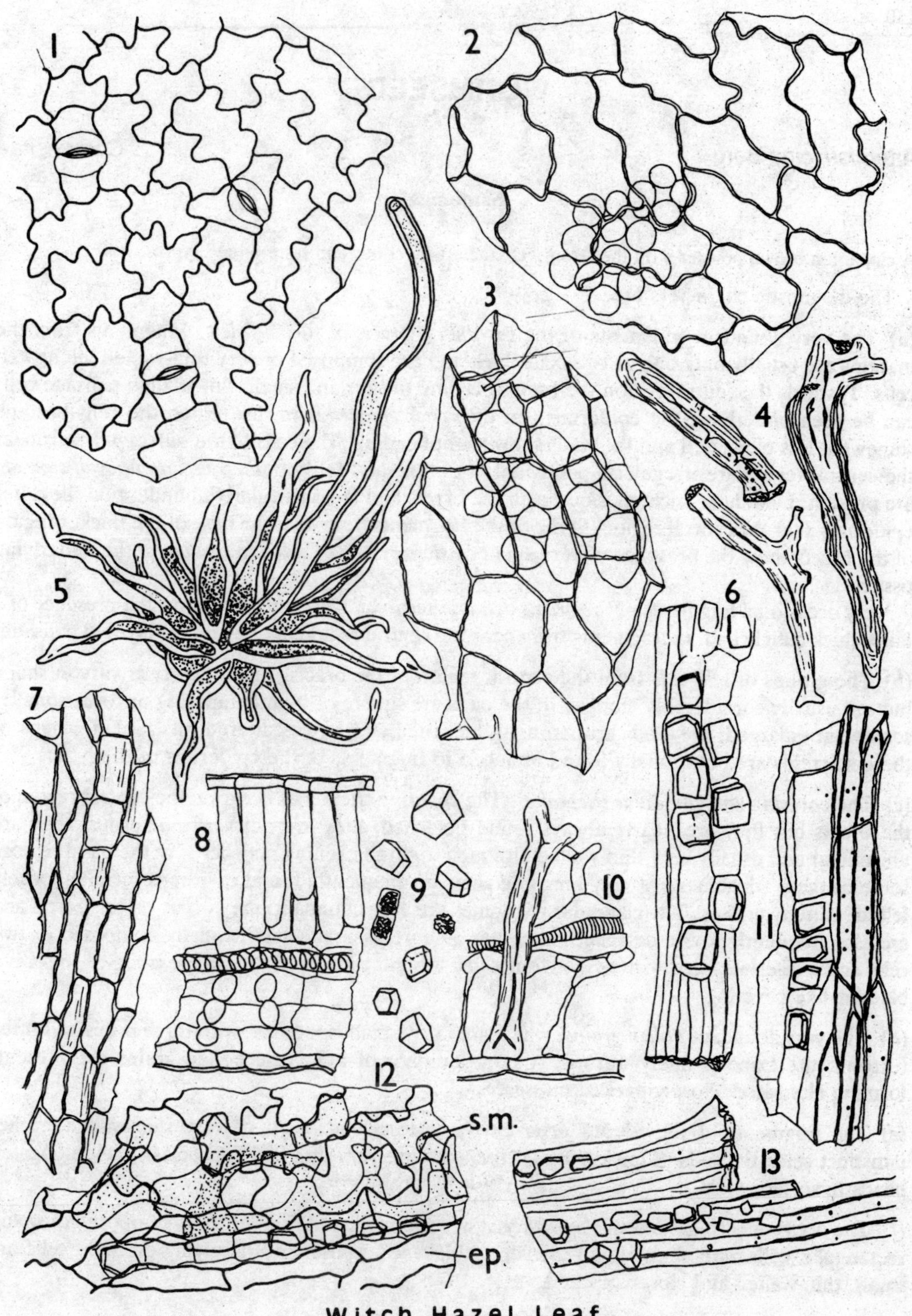

Witch Hazel Leaf

×330

1 Lower epidermis in surface view, with paracytic stomata.
2 Upper epidermis in surface view, with part of the underlying palisade.
3 Upper epidermis in surface view showing straight-walled celis with uneven thickening and part of the underlying palisade.
4 Isolated idioblasts.
5 Stellate trichome.
6 Part of a group of fibres with calcium oxalate prism sheath.
7 Epidermis of the petiole in surface view.
8 Part of the lamina in sectional view.
9 Calcium oxalate crystals.
10 Fragment of the lamina in sectional view showing an idioblast.
11 Fibres and xylem elements with part of a calcium oxalate prism sheath.
12 Lower epidermis (ep.) over a vein in surface view with underlying spongy mesophyll (s.m.) and part of a calcium oxalate prism sheath.
13 Part of a group of fibres with an incomplete sheath of small prisms of calcium oxalate.

WORMSEED

Artemisia cina Berg Compositae

Santonica

A cinnamon brown powder with the strong, characteristic odour and taste of eucalyptus.

The diagnostic characters are:

(*a*) The very abundant fragments of the *involucral bracts in surface view*. Fragments from the margins are usually only one or two cells thick and are composed of very thin-walled, elongated cells. Towards the central region the bracts become thicker and small, thin-walled palisade cells can be seen underlying the epidermis; on the *inner epidermis* in this region the cells become somewhat less elongated and the walls show slight beading. The cells of the *outer epidermis* near the central region are irregularly polygonal in outline and fairly numerous *anomocytic stomata* are present. Glandular trichomes occur on the bracts and are particularly abundant on the outer epidermis near the central region. Some of the fragments from near the base of the thicker region of the bracts show the presence of very small *cluster crystals of calcium oxalate* in the underlying tissues.

Very occasional fragments of the *bracts* occur *in sectional view* and these show the presence of a fairly thick cuticle and, in fragments from near the central region, a one- or two-layered palisade.

(*b*) The groups of *sclereids* from the central region of the bracts. Individual cells vary in shape but are usually considerably elongated; the ends are square or bluntly tapering or, occasionally, somewhat enlarged; the walls are strongly thickened and have scattered pits. Small groups of these sclereids are occasionally found attached to fragments of the epidermis of the bracts.

(*c*) The *covering* and *glandular trichomes*. The covering trichomes occur on the central region of the bracts but they are nearly always found detached; they are not very numerous; they are unicellular and usually very thin-walled although slight thickening may occur in the basal region; some of these trichomes are very long and they are frequently found in groups forming loosely felted, cottony masses. The glandular trichomes are very abundant; they occur on the bracts and are also frequently found detached; each has a short, biseriate stalk, usually composed of two cells and a biseriate head with two or four cells; around each head the cuticle is raised to form a bladder-like covering.

(*d*) The very abundant *pollen grains*, which are fairly small, spherical, with three pores and three furrows; the exine is finely warted. A large number of immature pollen grains are present, forming elongated, closely packed masses.

(*e*) The fragments of the *fibrous layer of the anthers* composed of very thin-walled, rather indistinct cells; the rods of thickening on the walls are very thin and appear as small, elongated beads in surface view.

(*f*) The occasional fragments of the *pedicels*; in surface view the epidermis is composed of small, rectangular cells with slightly and unevenly thickened walls; the underlying palisade cells are small, thin-walled and closely packed.

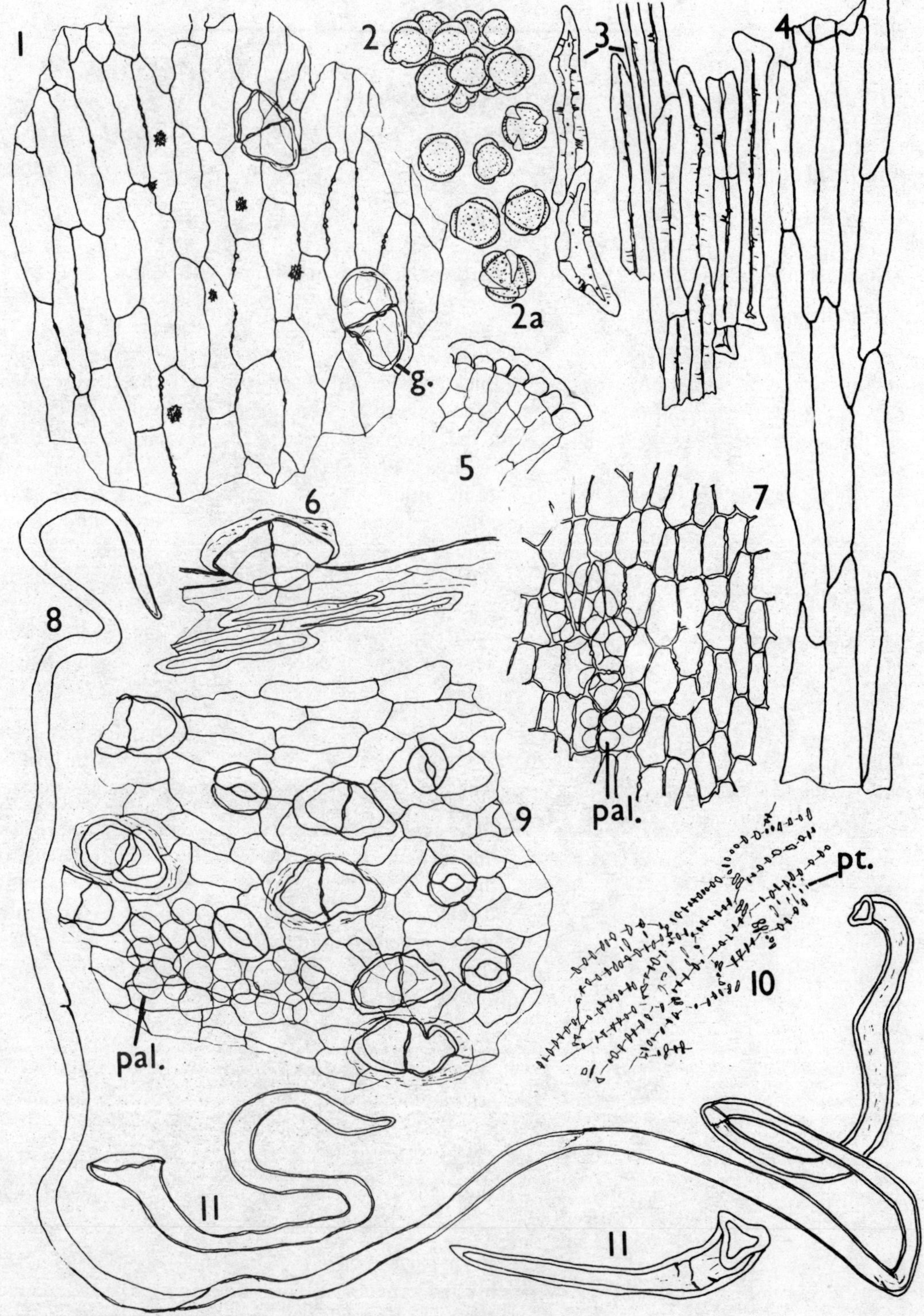

Wormseed

×330

1 Inner epidermis from near the central region of a bract in surface view showing glandular trichomes (g.).
2 Part of a group of immature pollen grains.
2a Mature pollen grains.
3 Groups of sclereids from the central region of a bract.
4 Epidermis near the margin of a bract in surface view.
5 Part of a bract in sectional view.
6 Part of the central region of a bract in sectional view showing the epidermis with an attached glandular trichome and part of a group of sclereids.
7 Epidermis of the pedicel in surface view with part of the underlying palisade (pal.).
8 A large covering trichome.
9 Outer epidermis from near the central region of a bract showing stomata, glandular trichomes and part of the underlying palisade (pal.).
10 Fibrous layer of the anther in surface view showing pits (pt.).
11 Small covering trichomes.

INDEX OF ENGLISH NAMES AND SYNONYMS

INDEX OF BOTANICAL SOURCES